APR 98

PHARMACOLOGY

PHARMACOLOGY
DRUGS AFFECTING BEHAVIOR

CONAN KORNETSKY
Boston University
School of Medicine
Boston

A Wiley-Interscience Publication
JOHN WILEY & SONS
New York / London / Sydney / Toronto

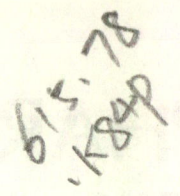

Copyright © 1976 by John Wiley & Sons, Inc.

All rights reserved. Published simultaneously in Canada.

No part of this book may be reproduced by any means, nor transmitted, nor translated into a machine language without the written permission of the publisher.

Library of Congress Cataloging in Publication Data:

Kornetsky, Conan.
   Pharmacology.

   "A Wiley-Interscience publication."
   Includes bibliographical references and index.
   1. Neuropsychopharmacology. I. Title.
[DNLM: 1. Behavior—Drug effects. 2. Psychotropic drugs—Pharmacodynamics. QV77 K84p]
RM315.K67   615'.78   76-6062
ISBN 0-471-50410-6

Printed in the United States of America

10 9 8 7 6 5 4 3 2

To Marcia, David, and Lisa

PREFACE

The purpose of this book is to provide the clinical psychologist and others in the mental health professions who do not have a medical background the necessary knowledge of pharmacology needed to adequately function in any clinical setting. It is also hoped that counselors and educators may find this text a useful source of information concerning the major classes of drugs that many of their clients or students may be using, either licitly or illicitly. Although psychiatrists have taken a course in pharmacology as part of their medical education, they may find this to be a useful book for the review of drugs that affect behavior.

Drugs are used extensively in our society, both for legitimate medical purposes as well as for nonmedical reasons. Whether drugs are taken for specific medical reasons, simply to produce a feeling of well-being, or as intoxicants, their actions follow certain well-defined principles. Knowledge of these basic principles of pharmacology will help the therapist, counselor, or educator be more effective in serving those for whom they have responsibility. Furthermore, since most of the drugs discussed in this book have marked effects on behavior, they have proved to be useful tools for many experimental and physiological psychologists in their study of behavior.

With some exceptions, much of the information contained in this book can be found in any standard text of pharmacology. However, those trained in the behavioral sciences usually find that such a text is much too detailed and assumes a comprehensive background in chemistry and physiology on the part of the reader. In writing this book I have made the assumption that the readers may have had little or no background in chemistry and that their knowledge of physiology is, at most, rudimentary.

Chapters 1 to 4 are designed to give the reader the basic vocabulary of pharmacology, plus some basic concepts concerning the autonomic and central nervous system that will make subsequent chapters more understandable. However, many of the chapters do stand alone in that someone wishing to learn about a particular class of drugs may do so without reading the entire text. Although I have attempted to define most of the medical terms when they are first used in the text, I suggest that all those in the mental health field have a standard medical dictionary at their disposal.

In Chapter 12, which deals with the nonmedical use of drugs, and Chapter 13, which reviews the pharmacological treatment of the hyperkinetic child, the discussion encompasses much more than the pharmacology of the drugs involved. Chapter 12 not only briefly describes the pharmacology of drugs of abuse not previously discussed in the text, but also examines the social and psychological aspects of illicit drug use. In Chapter 13 I have presented the various aspects of the hyperkinetic syndrome as well as a consideration of the drugs used in treatment.

This text is not a treatise on psychopharmacology. The purpose in writing this text was not to review the extensive literature on the effects of drugs on behavior in man and animals, but as I originally stated, my intent was to provide the nonmedical reader with an understanding of the general pharmacology of drugs that affect behavior.

C. KORNETSKY

Boston, Massachusetts
April, 1976.

ACKNOWLEDGMENTS

I would like to thank all those members of the Laboratory of Behavioral Pharmacology at Boston University School of Medicine who were most giving of their time in critically reviewing and suggesting changes in the text. These include George Bain, Robert Markowitz, Richard Marcus, Maressa Hecht Orzack, and Janet Tarika. The role of Marjorie O'Connell must be acknowledged for her patience in typing the manuscript. Special thanks must be given to Robert Markowitz who contributed extensively during the many revisions of the text. It is unlikely that this book would have been finished without his help. I would also like to thank Gladys Friedler and Allan F. Mirsky of the Division of Psychiatry who critically reviewed specific chapters and made many useful suggestions.

The photographs of old drug advertisements in Chapter 2 were obtained with the generous help of Richard Wolfe, rare books librarian, Countway Library, Harvard Medical School. Most of the original drawings were done by William O'Leary, medical artist at Boston University School of Medicine.

Finally, I would like to acknowledge the Career Scientist Program of the National Institute of Mental Health for its continued support (NIMH Career Scientist, MH 1759) and NIHM grant NH 12568 and NIDA grant DA 00377 that supported much of my research referred to in the text.

The following publishers and authors are thanked for their permission to reproduce figures and quotations from indicated works:

Chapter 1:
Kornetsky, C. An overview of drug action. In A. DiMascio and R. I. Shader (Eds.) *Clinical Handbook of Psychopharmacology.* New York, Science House, 1970, pp. 105-119 (Figures 1-7).

Chapter 4:
Bradley, P. B. The central action of certain drugs in relation to the reticular formation of the brain. In H. H. Jasper, L. D. Proctor, R. S. Knighton, W. C. Noshay, and R. T. Costello (Eds.) *Reticular Formation of the Brain.* Boston, Little, Brown, 1958 (Figure 3; also Chapter 5, Figure 7).

Cooper, J. R., Bloom, F. E. and Roth, R. H. *The Biochemical Basis of Neuropharmacology.* New York, Oxford University Press, 1970 (Figure 8).

Penfield, W. and Jasper, H. *Epilepsy and the Functional Anatomy of the Human Brain.* Boston, Little, Brown, 1954 (Figures 4 and 5).

Chapter 5:

Eliasson, M. and Kornetsky, C. Interaction effects of chlorpromazine and reticular stimulation on visual attention behavior in rats. *Psychonomic Science,* **26,** 1972.

Kornetsky, C. and Bain, G. Effects of chlorpromazine and pentobarbital on sustained attention in the rat. *Psychopharmacologia (Berlin)* **8,** 1965, 277-284 (Figure 5).

Kornetsky, C. and Eliasson, M. Reticular stimulation and chlorpromazine: An animal model for schizophrenic over-arousal. *Science,* **165,** 1969, 1273-1274 (Figure 8).

Chapter 7:

Hill, H., Kornetsky, C., Flanary, H., and Wikler, A. Effects of anxiety and morphine on discrimination of intensities of painful stimuli. *The Journal of Clinical Investigation,* **31,** 1952, 473-480 (Figure 3).

Kornetsky, C. and Bain, G. Morphine: Single-dose tolerance. *Science,* **162,** 1968, 1011-1012 (Figure 4).

Marcus, R. and Kornetsky, C. Negative and positive intracranial reinforcement thresholds: Effects of morphine. *Psychopharmacologia (Berlin),* **38,** 1974, 1-13 (Figure 6).

Chapter 8:

Dews, P. Studies on behavior, I. Differential sensitivity to pentobarbital of pecking performance in pigeons depending on the schedule of reward. *Journal of Pharmacology and Experimental Therapeutics,* **113,** 1955, 393-401 (Figure 2).

Chapter 9:

Mello, N. K. and Mendelson, J. H. Drinking patterns during work-contingent and noncontingent alcohol acquisition. *Psychosomatic Medicine,* **34,** 1972, 139-164 (Figure 2).

Chapter 12:

Chayet, N. L. Legal aspects of drug abuse. *Suffolk University Law Review,* **3,** 1968, 1-22, (quotation, p. 190).

Hofmann, A. Psychotomimetic drugs chemical and pharmacological aspects. *Acta Physiologica, et Pharmacologica Neerlandica,* **8,** 1959, 240-258 (quotation, pp. 205-206).

Klüver, H. *Mescal and Mechanisms of Hallucinations.* Chicago, The University of Chicago Press, 1966. Originally published as *Mescal, the 'Devine' Plant and Its Psychological Effects.* London, Kegan Paul, Trench, Trubner and Co. Ltd., 1928 (quotation, pp. 204-205).

Lasagna, L. Addicting drugs and medical practice; Toward the elaboration of realistic goals and the eradication of myths, mirages and half-truths. In D. M. Wilner and G. K. Kassenbaum (Eds.) *Narcotics.* New York, McGraw-Hill, 1965, pp. 53-66. (quotation, p. 210).

Chapter 13:-reprinted in part from:

Kornetsky, C. Minimal brain dysfunction and drugs. In W. M. Cruickshank and D. P. Hallahan (Eds.) *Perceptual and Learning Disabilities in Children.* Syracuse University Press, 1975, 447-481.

C. K.

CONTENTS

1	Introduction and Basic Principles	1
2	The Placebo and Nonspecific Factors as Determinants of Responses to Drugs	22
3	The Autonomic Nervous System and Autonomic Drugs	45
4	Neurophysiology and Biochemistry of the Central Nervous System	63
5	Antipsychotic Drugs	81
6	Drugs Used in the Treatment of Depression and Anxiety	103
7	Narcotic Analgesics	117
8	Hypnotics and Sedatives	137
9	Alcohol	149
10	The Amphetamines	164
11	Antiepileptic Drugs	175
12	The Nonmedical Use of Drugs	185
13	Minimal Brain Dysfunction (The Hyperkinetic Syndrome) and Drugs	223

Appendix Glossary of "Street Terms"	253
Author Index	259
Subject Index	265

1 INTRODUCTION AND BASIC PRINCIPLES

The aim of this book is to provide for psychologists and those in allied fields a basic understanding of the principles and methods of the science of pharmacology as well as to present the essential pharmacology of those drugs that may have relevance to both clinical and experimental psychologists.

Pharmacology, broadly defined, is the study of the action of any chemical agent on living systems. It involves the chemical and physical properties of substances, their absorption, distribution, and excretion as well as their biochemical, physiological, and psychological effects, and finally their mechanism of action. Pharmacology is concerned with therapeutic as well as toxic effects of these chemicals. Since not all chemicals are used in the treatment and diagnosis of disease or are endogenous substances that play a role in the functional organization of living protoplasm, only those chemicals that are so used are called drugs.

As one might imagine, pharmacology is a very broad field. The methodology of the field relies heavily on both physiology and biochemistry, and in more recent years the procedures, techniques, and attitudes of the psychologist have found their way into the discipline of pharmacology. The need for psychologists to become more familiar with the discipline of pharmacology is particularly important for those who work in medical or paramedical settings. It is important that clinical psychologists be aware of and knowledgeable about the actions of drugs used in the treatment of mental illness if they are to interpret intelligently the results of various diagnostic tests, use psychotherapy and counseling of patients or clients who are also being treated with these drugs, and counsel people who may be abusing drugs. The experimental psychologist who is using drugs as tools in the study of behavior as well as the psychologist who is simply interested in the very important empirical problems of the types of behaviors that drugs affect not only should have some knowledge of the specific drugs that are being used in their experiments but also should be familiar with the principles of the discipline of pharmacology. And finally, it is important in our medicated society that the layman be informed so that he can more intelligently evaluate the claims and counterclaims that continually appear in the lay press.

ABSORPTION

Absorption is that process by which drugs are made available to the body fluids that distribute the drugs to organ systems. This process depends not only on the method of administration and physical properties of the drug but also on their interaction. Most of us think that drug administration is primarily by the oral route (absorption from the gastrointestinal tract) and by means of injection (parenteral administration). However, other methods are frequently used: absorption through the oral mucosa (sublingual administration), absorption via the lungs (inhalation), absorption through the skin (cutaneous administration), and administration of rectal and vaginal suppositories. Each of these methods has advantages as well as disadvantages. For example, oral administration is much safer than parenteral administration; however, there are many drugs that are not readily absorbed from the gastrointestinal tract. Furthermore, when speed of action is essential, parenteral administration is preferred.

Absorption from the Gastrointestinal Tract

Absorption can occur all along the gastrointestinal tract; however, maximum absorption for most agents is from the small intestine because of the enormous surface area available. For a drug to pass from the lumen of the gastrointestinal tract to the blood stream, it must pass through the epithelial lining and the blood capillary wall. The blood capillary wall is readily permeable to all crystalloids (most drugs are crystalloids, and crystalloids in solution readily pass through animal membranes). Thus the epithelial lining of the lumen probably is the main barrier to drug absorption from the gastrointestinal tract. Since drugs that are more lipid soluble (a lipid is a fatlike substance relatively insoluble in water but soluble in organic solvents, e.g., ether, chloroform, or some alcohols) are absorbed more rapidly, it is believed that the epithelial lining acts like a lipid sieve between the contents of the lumen and the blood plasma.

An important variable is the pH of the drug as well as that of the gastrointestinal tract. The pH (negative logarithm of the concentration of hydrogen ions) is the relative acidity or alkalinity of a solution. The pH scale goes from 1 to 14, with 1 being most acid, 14 most base (alkaline), and 7 being neutral. Most drugs are weak acids or bases. The pH of the media determines the extent to which a drug will remain ionized or nonionized. Ionization is the process of dissociation of substances in solution into constituent ions (charged particles). The nonionized form of a drug passes more readily through membranes. At low pHs, weakly acidic drugs are, for the most part, nonionized and are absorbed relatively rapidly in proportion to their lipid solubility. However, many drugs are basic (high pH) and hence ionized at the gastric pH. Thus despite the lipid solubility of those molecules that are

ABSORPTION

nonionized, they are so few in number that overall drug absorption is extremely slow.

Absorption from the stomach, small intestine, and colon all follow the same principle; however, the stomach is highly acid (pH near 1), whereas the small intestine and the colon are more neutral (pH approximately 5-7). Because basic drugs are less likely to undergo ionization in a more neutral or basic environment, with the reverse for acidic drugs, basic drugs are more readily absorbed in the small intestine or colon than acidic drugs, and the latter are more readily absorbed in the stomach.

Other factors besides the diffusion across a membrane influence the rate of absorption of a drug. The rate will vary depending on the contents of the stomach or the presence of enzymes that affect the stability of the drug. Rate of gastric emptying may be quite important. Thus if gastric emptying is retarded or speeded up it will have different effects on bases and acids. The rate of absorption of some drugs from the gastrointestinal tract is far greater than one would expect from simple diffusion. Thus it is believed that there may be an active process requiring metabolic energy. This type of absorption is called *active transport*.

Generally, drugs are administered via the enteric route (oral) unless specifically contraindicated. Some drugs cause emesis or may be especially irritating to the gastrointestinal tract; others may not be readily absorbed from the gastrointestinal tract; still others are destroyed by compounds present in the gastrointestinal tract. This route of administration is not used if immediate effects are desired or if the patient is unconscious or delirious. Not only is this route the simplest method of getting drugs into the body since no special equipment is needed, but it is probably the safest route and least likely to produce allergic responses.

Although most research laboratories do not use this mode of drug administration with animals, it can easily be done, and many drug-manufacturing laboratories use this method if the drug is to be used orally in man. In animals oral administration calls for either a plastic tube on the end of a syringe or a curved metal tube with a bulb on the end. The animal is firmly held, with pressure on the side of the jaw causing its mouth to open. The cannula is then gently pushed over the tongue and into the esophagus where the material is placed by the depression of the plunger on the syringe.

Absorption from Parenteral Administration

Parenteral administration has both disadvantages and advantages over oral administration. Absorption is usually more rapid and more predictable, giving one greater control over the effective dose. It is the method most frequently used in animal experimentation because of the factor of dosage control. The disadvantages include the necessity of sterile technique in man, local irritation, and the greater possibility of a systemic reaction, especially when potent drugs are given intravenously. It can be painful, and when chronic administration is needed, it demands either continual trips to the physician's office or self-administration, which may be difficult, if not impossible, for some people.

Intravenous. The intravenous route of drug administration provides not only for the most rapid rate of introduction of the material into the blood stream, but also for the most accurate control of dosage. Usually, only drugs in an aqueous solution may be given intravenously. Effects are usually immediate. Often the dose is slowly infused so that the exact dosage is determined by the response of the patient.

In Pentothal (thiopental sodium) interviews, this was the method of drug administration. Despite the advantages of this method, it is probably the most dangerous, because once the drug is injected there is no way to inhibit absorption and thus obtund or reverse an adverse reaction. Also, the occurrence of serious systemic reactions is more likely with intravenous injections.

Intramuscular. This method requires the injection of the drug deep into muscle tissue. Drugs in aqueous solution are rapidly absorbed; however, this route is often used when slow absorption is desired. This is done by either dissolving or suspending the drug in an oil vehicle. Penicillin is often given in this fashion.

Subcutaneous. This method calls for the placing of the drug just under the skin and can only be used for those compounds that are not irritating to tissue. Lipid-insoluble drugs are absorbed by their penetration of the relatively large aqueous pores in the endothelial membrane. The method provides for a fairly even and slow rate of absorption, and the rate may be manipulated by the use of different vehicles. Massaging the site of injection will increase absorption; placing a tourniquet proximal to the site of injection will impede the distribution of the drug, as is true also for the intramuscular route. Since this method depends on adequate peripheral circulation, the drug does not enter the circulation when a patient is in shock (a massive physiological reaction to body trauma or disease characterized by marked depression of vital signs, i.e., blood pressure, pulse, and respiration).

Intraperitoneal. Because of the large absorptive surface of the peritoneal cavity, this method provides a rapid means of getting drugs into circulation. However, it is a procedure rarely used in man and finds its main use in the animal laboratory.

Intracerebral. By the use of cannulae appropriately placed by means of a stereotaxic instrument, drugs either in solution or as crystals themselves are delivered directly to specific sites in the brain. This method is being more frequently used in the behavior-drug-brain interaction studies. (For a review of the use of intracerebral drug administration, see Routtenberg, 1972.)

Inhalation

Inhalation provides a very rapid way for a drug to gain access to the circulation. Inhalation may be used when the material is atomized and the fine droplets then inhaled. The difficulty with the inhalation technique is the inability to accurately regulate dose. However, despite the shortcomings of the method, it is used extensively in the administration of gaseous anesthetics and by means of an aerosol, drugs used in the treatment of bronchial asthma. An example of self-administration of a drug by inhalation is the use of tobacco or marihuana where there is rapid onset of action. This is related to the exposure of the material to the large surface area of the lungs with their rich supply of capillaries. Although people who do not inhale obtain an effect from nicotine, the onset of action is much slower and is the result of passage of the material through the mucosa of the oral cavity.

DISTRIBUTION OF DRUGS IN THE BODY

The main body fluid of distribution for a drug is the plasma. However, once it reaches the plasma it must cross various barriers before it can reach its final site of action. Most drugs rapidly cross the capillary wall by means of diffusion and filtration. Drugs do not uniformly distribute to all body sites. Some compounds may bind with the plasma proteins. The protein-bound fraction is usually inactive; however, the drug is then slowly released thereby giving long action to these drugs. Also, drugs may bind to a cell for which they have a particular chemical affinity.

In addition, for drugs to have effects in the CNS, they must be able to cross the *blood-brain barrier*. Thus a drug may enter into the cerebral circulation, yet may not enter into the cells of the brain. The blood-brain barrier was originally postulated from experiments in which dyes were injected into the systemic circulation but were found not to reach the cells of the brain. Subsequent work has indicated that although there is such a barrier (some have referred to it as the blood-brain sieve), it is not an all-or-none phenomenon, and the actual manner by which blocking takes place is not known. However, it is an empirical fact that many drugs that easily penetrate other body organs do not appreciably enter the brain.

Excretion and Metabolism

Once a drug finds its way into the body, it must also find a way out. The single most important route of excretion taken by most drugs is through the kidneys.

Some drugs are excreted into the bile, but this usually results in recycling through the intestine. The lactating mother may excrete drugs in the milk, but this has more importance for the child than the mother. Some drugs are blown off by the lungs, and there is some excretion via perspiration.

Most drugs are not excreted unchanged by the body but undergo a biotransformation. The purpose, teleologically, for this biotransformation is to metabolize a drug to a compound that can be more readily excreted by the kidneys. Thus a highly nonionized drug is more likely to be reabsorbed or bound by the plasma rather than be excreted. Biotransformation that converts a relatively more lipid soluble compound into a less lipid soluble form will increase the likelihood of its excretion. This biotransformation, for the most part, is the result of enzymatic action in the liver. Usually, drugs are excreted as metabolites as well as in the unchanged form. Although biotransformation for most drugs involves metabolism of an active compound to an inactive one, metabolism may result in an active drug being changed to an even more active compound. Also, there are relatively inactive drugs that may be changed to active compounds.

The presence of liver disease may often interfere with the metabolism of a drug so that repeated dosing may result in the build-up of toxically high levels of the drug in the body. Often the administration of two drugs together may result in one of the drugs inhibiting the enzymatic metabolism of the other drug, resulting in severe toxic reactions.

MECHANISMS OF DRUG ACTION

The study of the mechanisms of drug action is really the heart of pharmacology. Most explanations of the mechanisms are superficial or incomplete because of the lack of knowledge of what actually occurs in the cell. Although the terms drug action and drug effect are considered synonymous by most people, there is a distinction made by some pharmacologists. It is believed that most drugs produce their effects either by combining with enzymes, with cell membranes, or with some other part of the cell. Thus, the drug interacts with some component of the cell that initiates a sequence of biochemical and physiological events that characterizes the pharmacological effects of the drug. Only the initial result of the drug-cell interaction is defined as the action of the drug. Although the ultimate goal of understanding the pharmacology of drugs is to have intimate knowledge of the drug-cell interaction, for the most part, only the physiological effects of a drug can be described. Despite a lack of knowledge of the molecular biology that is necessary for any real understanding of the mechanism of drug action, a number of general concepts have been proposed and these hypothetical constructs have had value in generating a framework for further work.

Structure-activity Relationships

The chemical structure of a drug is closely related to the action of that drug. Sometimes the relationship between chemical structure and pharmacological action is so close that only a slight change in the structure results in an entirely different profile of action. With other compounds a slight change in the molecular makeup of the drug results in only a slight alteration in the pharmacological effects, except for a change in potency. Often certain types of unwanted side effects can be attenuated by a slight change in the molecular configuration. What is sometimes quite disturbing is that drugs of entirely different structure may have quite similar pharmacological effects. Despite a lack of perfect correlation between chemical structure and activity, many potent drugs have been developed by systematic manipulation of chemical structure.

The Receptor

The cell or, more strictly speaking, the cell component that is intimately involved in the drug-cell interaction is called the *receptor*. Such receptor sites with which drugs are postulated to combine to produce their effects are hypothetical constructs, and they may be within the cell or on the cell surface. The initial action of a drug is postulated to be at the receptor. Examples of drug-cell interactions that do not result in drug action are such things as the binding of drugs to plasma and cell proteins and to enzymes, whose main function is the transport or biotransformation of drugs. The assumption is that there are specific receptors for specific chemical structures, that this drug-receptor interaction is chemical in nature, and that this chemical reaction is usually reversible.

Included in the receptor theory are the following principles: A drug that interacts with the receptor and also initiates drug action is called an *agonist*. A drug that combines with the receptor but fails to show any action is called an *antagonist*. The tendency to combine with a receptor with or without a response is called *affinity*. Both antagonist and agonist have affinity for a receptor. However, the ability to combine with a receptor and initiate drug action is called *intrinsic activity* or *efficacy*, and only the agonist has intrinsic activity. The belief that most drug effects are due to the occupation of receptors by drugs is generally accepted. However, the receptor-occupation theory has difficulty in explaining certain types of drug effects in which initial receptor stimulation is followed by tachyphylaxis (rapidly developing tolerance). A more recent receptor theory explains the drug action in terms of the rate of the drug-receptor combination. Many drugs will affect the nerve cell by causing it either to release or to inhibit release of a specific endogenous substance (neurotransmitter). (This is discussed in Chapter 3).

DRUG EFFECTS

Drugs are often characterized by their primary effect and use, for example, analgesics, psychotomimetics, and hypnotics. If drugs are to be evaluated and compared, their effects must be related to dose (amount administered), time course (time to onset and duration of effect), and half-life (time it takes for half of the active drug to be removed from body tissues). The time course includes such things as the latency of onset, time to maximum effect, and duration of effect. Most of these characteristics are related to dose.

Dose Effect

If one wishes to compare the effects of two different drugs on some measure of effect, it is not enough simply to take a single dose of the first drug and compare it to a single dose of the second drug. If, for example, one were interested in the relative effects of morphine and secobarbital on simple reaction time and it was found that 5 mg of morphine impaired reaction time significantly more than 50 mg of secobarbital, one could not conclude that morphine has a greater effect on reaction time than secobarbital; further study might indicate that 250 mg of secobarbital has a greater effect on reaction time than 5 mg of morphine. Thus it is obvious that one cannot generalize from the effects of a single dose of a drug.

If, in the foregoing example, one were to study a variety of doses and plot dose on the abscissa against reaction time on the ordinate, the curve would be called a dose-response curve or a dose-effect curve. In this text the terms will be used interchangeably. However, some pharmacologists refer to the dose-response curve as a plot of the mean effect of some continuous variant (e.g., reaction time, blood pressure, or heart rate) against dose. They refer to the dose-effect curve as the percentage of subjects exhibiting some defined effect plotted against dose. An example of this would be the percentage of animals unable to exhibit a righting reflex after various doses of pentobarbital.

Implicit in the above definitions is the concept of biological variability. If variability between members of a single species did not exist, no subject would have the specifically defined effect until some threshold dose was reached, and at this dose, all subjects would exhibit the effect. Any variability in response could then be attributed to errors in the observation method.

The dose-effect curve is a *sine qua non* of pharmacology. One can easily conceptualize it in terms of psychophysics. Increasing the level of stimulation, in this case the dose of a drug, gives greater effect. As in psychophysics, the slope of the curve approaches a straight line if the units of stimulation are transformed to log units. To determine the lethal dose of a drug gradually increasing doses could be administered, each to a different group of animals. Plotting the percentage of animals that were killed at any particular dose would yield a frequency polygon that is skewed to the right as in Figure 1.

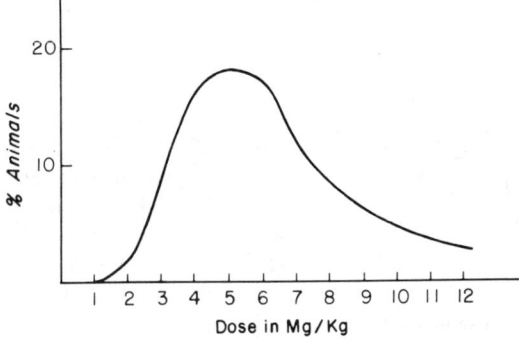

FIGURE 1. A hypothetical arithmetic plot of percent animals killed as a function of dose (from Kornetsky, C. An overview of drug action. In A. DiMascio and R. I. Shader (Eds.). *Clinical Handbook of Psychopharmacology*. New York, Science House, 1970, pp. 105–119).

If the dose levels were converted to log units, the frequency polygon would lose its skewed form and it would appear as in Figure 2.

From such a frequency polygon the median lethal dose (LD50) can be obtained and if the distribution were normal, this would be equal to the mean lethal dose. This method of determining the LD50 is not particularly parsimonious with respect to its use of animals nor the time involved; it is also difficult to make direct comparisons between drugs or types of effects with the frequency polygon.

The same curve shown in Figure 1 can be rectified by plotting cumulative frequency of percent against dose. This would give a skewed sigmoid curve as in Figure 3. Changing the dose units to log units reduces the skewness as in Figure 4. Here the LD50 dose could be easily obtained and comparisons of the dose-effect curve and LD50 of other drugs could be made. However, if this cumulative plot was made of z-scores against log dose a straight line would be obtained (Figure 5) which would then be described in terms of slope. The use of a *z* score results in negative values, and to avoid this the *z* scores are usually transformed to probit scores. Probit scores have a mean of 5 and a standard deviation of 1. Thus with a probit plot the LD 50 can be easily obtained as well as any other LD percentage (e.g., the LD 84, that dose of the drug that would be expected to kill 84 percent of the animals). The LD 84 is plus-1 standard deviation above the mean and thus has a probit value of 6.

The slope of the dose-effect curve is quite important. The steeper the slope of the line, the greater will be the effect of small increments in the dose of the drug. Thus a drug with a steep dose-effect curve is potentially more dangerous than one with a shallow dose-effect curve.

The term *potency* is often used to describe a drug, but it is only meaningful in terms of a comparison, in other words, *relative potency*. Relative potency

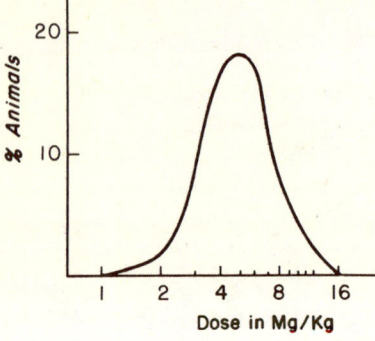

FIGURE 2. The same curve as in Figure 1, plotted with dose in log units (from Kornetsky, C. An overview of drug action. In A. DiMascio and R. I. Shader (Eds.). *Clinical Handbook of Psychopharmacology.* New York, Science House, 1970, pp. 105–119).

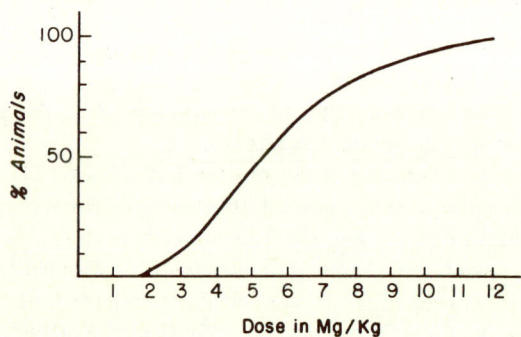

FIGURE 3. The cumulative plot of data in Figure 1 (from Kornetsky, C̄. An overview of drug action. In A. DiMascio and R. I. Shader (Eds.). *Clinical Handbook of Psychopharmacology.* New York, Science House, 1970, pp. 105–119).

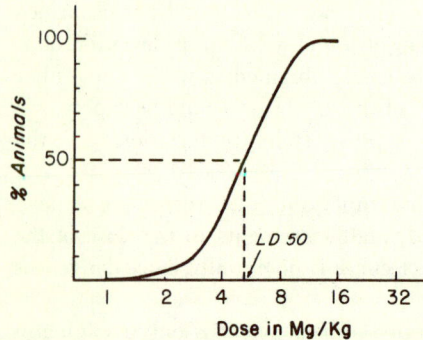

FIGURE 4. The cumulative plot of data in Figure 3 with dose in log units. Also indicated is the LD 50 (from Kornetsky, C. An overview of drug action. In A. DiMascio and R. I. Shader (Eds.). *Clinical Handbook of Psychopharmacology.* New York, Science House, 1970, pp. 105–119).

DRUG EFFECTS

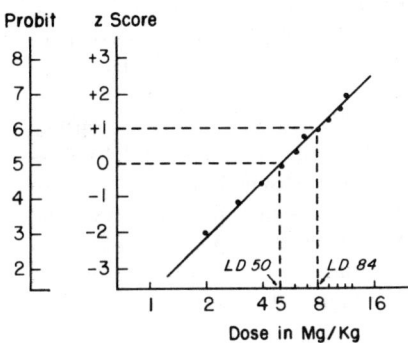

FIGURE 5. The dose-response curve of the previous data. The ordinate is in standard score units and equivalent probit scores. Note that this allows an accurate determination of not only that LD 50, but also any other LD desired. Indicated is the LD 84 (from Kornetsky, C. An overview of drug action. In A. DiMascio and R. I. Shader (Eds.). *Clinical Handbook of Psychopharmacology*. New York, Science House, 1970, pp. 105–119).

can easily be determined by the comparison of the dose-effect curves of two drugs. The drug whose curve lies to the left of the other is the more potent of the two. By plotting the dose-effect curves for two drugs it is quite simple to ascertain which are equipotent doses. In Figure 6 the dose of drug *B* which is equipotent to 5 mg/kg of drug *A* is illustrated.

Potency of a drug is not by itself a very important consideration as long as equal effects can be obtained with two drugs and the side effects are about the same.

Thus far we have been discussing the dose-effect curve for lethality. The same type of analysis may be made for the effective dose (ED). The ED 50 is that dose which produces a specifically described effect in 50 percent of the subjects. If the LD 50 is divided by the ED 50, the result is called the *therapeutic index*. Obviously, the larger the therapeutic index, the safer the drug. The therapeutic index can be misleading if the slope of the dose-effect curve for therapeutic effect is different than the slope of the dose-effect curve for the lethal effect, as shown in Figure 7.

It should be noted that all drugs, including such common agents as aspirin,

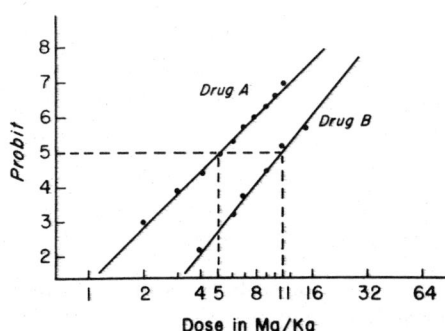

FIGURE 6. The log probit dose-response plot of two hypothetical drugs. With such a plot equipotent doses of the two drugs can be obtained. The example shows that 5 mg/kg of drug A is equivalent in effect to 11 mg/kg of drug B (from Kornetsky, C. An overview of drug action. In A. DiMascio and R. I. Shader (Eds.). *Clinical Handbook of Psychopharmacology*. New York, Science House, 1970, pp. 105–119).

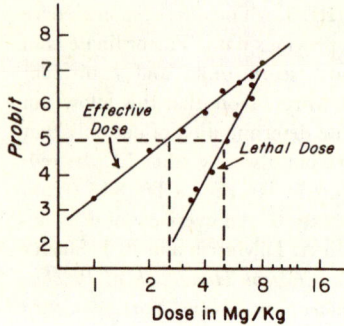

FIGURE 7. A plot of the effective dose and lethal dose when the slopes are different. In this example animals requiring a large dose for effect will be receiving a dose that is close to a lethal dose. In this case the therapeutic index (LD 50/ED 50) is not a valid indication of safety (from Kornetsky, C. An overview of drug action. In A. DiMascio and R. I. Shader (Eds.). *Clinical Handbook of Psychopharmacology.* New York, Science House, 1970, pp. 105–119).

have some risk when given to man. The probability of an untoward response to aspirin is so slight that we consider it relatively harmless. The risk of giving a drug must always be balanced against the consequences of not giving the drug. Obviously, in cases of carcinoma in which the prognosis is very poor, one might use a drug in which the ED50 and the LD50 are very close. However, one does not kill a fly with a sledge hammer; morphine is not used for the treatment of the common headache. Many of the drugs used in the treatment of the mentally ill are highly toxic and may even cause irreversible blood dyscrasias (pathological changes in the cellular components of the blood), yet they are used because it is believed that as a result of the severity of the illness and the poor prognosis in the absence of drug treatment, the risk is worth taking.

It is clear from the previous discussion that not all biological organisms respond to the same degree to a fixed dose of a drug. A dose of d-amphetamine, a CNS stimulant, that will produce only mild alerting in one individual may keep another awake all night. Most adults and even some children have observed the variability in responses to alcohol ingestion. The cocktail party is a beautiful example of this. Some of the variability here could be attributed to differences in the amount of alcohol consumed and some to differences in the number of hors d'oeuvres eaten; however, a great deal of the variance is simply due to intrinsic differences in the psychobiology of people. Not only do people differ in their responses to alcohol, but the same individual may respond quite differently to the drug in different situations. The college student who has three drinks at a fraternity party, for example, may respond quite differently to the same amount of alcohol ingested at a Christmas party when mother, father, and grandparents are present.

Hyper- and Hyposensitivity

Hypo- or hypersensitivity simply refers to the characteristics of those individuals who fall at either end of the normal distribution curve for drug effects. The hyposensitive person, although a challenge, is not too great a problem for

DRUG EFFECTS

the clinician. Dose of a drug can simply be increased until an effective dose is reached. The hypersensitive individual is, on the other hand, a marked therapeutic problem. If a drug has a very steep dose-effect curve, a markedly hypersensitive person may experience severe toxic effects at a dose that would be therapeutic for the average individual. Sensitivity is related simply to quantitative differences in response. Depression caused by a CNS stimulant would not be hypersensitivity, rather, it would be a qualitatively different response that is called an *idiosyncratic response.*

Predicting where a person will fall on the dose-effect curve without prior knowledge of a previous experience with the drug is almost impossible. There is some slight experimental evidence suggesting that there are certain individuals who are drug sensitive and others who are drug resistant. It does not seem to matter what CNS drug they receive; if they are hyposensitive to one, they are likely to be hyposensitive to several others. In studies with human subjects there has been some evidence suggesting that personality plays a role.

Predicting clinical success with a drug is most important. Understanding why some patients improve with chlorpromazine, for example, and others do not is of both clinical and experimental value. Many attempts have been made to determine what variables can be used to predict outcome. These are described in Chapter 2.

Idiosyncratic Responses

There are responses to a drug that are qualitatively different from those that are normally seen. They are not allergic responses. They are usually not predictable except for the fact that it is known that a small percentage of subjects will probably exhibit such idiosyncracies. It is possible that they may be determined genetically or that they may be related to some particular personality type. It is possible that with some drugs the idiosyncratic response may be the result of the multiple action of the drug. For example, the usual effect of morphine is one of depression; however, it is known that morphine acts simultaneously as a depressant and a stimulant. The stimulating effects of the drug are usually completely overridden by the depressant effects, and thus the resultant gross effect is one of depression. If an individual's biochemistry and physiology are such that the stimulating effects are greater than the depressant effects, the resultant effect will be stimulation. In rodents and cats the stimulating effects of morphine are much more apparent than in other species. In man some idiosyncratic responses may, in fact, be due to just such a selective sensitivity to some aspects of the drug effect.

Allergic Responses

An antigen-antibody reaction to a drug can be one of the most acute situations that a physician may encounter. These dangerous anaphylactic reactions occur within minutes after the patient receives the drug and are characterized by marked hypotension (fall in blood pressure) and bronchial constriction. In many instances this type of allergic response has been fatal. The reaction rarely occurs after oral administration. It is usually assumed that a previous small dose of the drug was administered which then sensitized the allergic individual. Less dangerous but still serious are such skin manifestations as hives and/or angioneurotic edema (temporary swelling of areas of skin, mucous membranes, and occasionally the viscera). Also commonly seen is a contact dermatitis.

Other Toxic Drug Effects

All drugs have toxic effects. These may be exaggerated manifestations of the normally expected response to the drug (hypersensitivity), or they may be idiosyncratic or allergic manifestations. It is important to determine if the toxic effects are simply a manifestation of too large a dose for the individual or are of the idiosyncratic or allergic types. If the toxic manifestations are simply dose related, then a reduction in the dose level will reduce the number and severity of the toxic reactions. The presence of idiosyncratic or allergic responses may call for an immediate cessation of the medication. The difficulty that faces the physician is that he often cannot make the distinction between hypersensitivity and an idiosyncratic response to a drug.

Side Effects

Since all drugs have multiple actions, some of these actions may be undesired. These undesirable effects are called side effects.

These effects are often toxic in nature and may run the gamut from slightly annoying to life threatening. A drug given for its antihistaminic effects may cause drowsiness; however, the same drug may be used by some physicians specifically because of its soporific action. In the latter case the main action is hypnosis, and the side effect is the antihistaminic action. Often, side effects are severe enough to preclude the use of a particular medication. Unless the side effect is an allergic or an idiosyncratic response, a reduction in the dosage will often be sufficient to reduce the side effect to a clinically acceptable level. At times other medications are given to counteract the side effects of a particular drug. Many of the drugs used in chemotherapy of schizophrenic patients will cause Parkinson-like symptoms, and antiparkinsonian agents are administered in conjunction with the antipsychotic medication. Parkinsonism is a disease characterized by muscular rigidity, immobile facies, tremor that tends to disappear on volitional movement, and loss of fine motor control.

Presence of Disease

A drug will vary in its effect as a result of the presence or absence of disease. Many hypotensive agents do not lower blood pressure in normo-tensive (normal blood pressure) individuals. Antipyretics such as aspirin do not lower body temperature unless there is an abnormal elevation of temperature present. The presence of abnormally functioning kidneys and liver will have marked manifestations when drugs are excreted and detoxified by these organs. Hyperactive children often are sedated by amphetamines. As a result of the lack of knowledge concerning the role of pathological conditions, the physician often has few guidelines in determining the proper chemotherapeutic dose.

Age and Weight

Although weight of an individual may be important when administering drugs, for the most part, drugs are not given according to the weight of the adult human. Weight may not be as critical as the ratio of lean body mass to fat since many drugs are stored in fat and then slowly released over time. However, in animal experiments drugs are usually administered in doses calculated as milligram/kilogram of body weight. Children usually receive lower doses of medication than adults. However, children are not simply small adults, and although the rough rule of thumb is for smaller dosages, the dosage should depend on the drug and the physical development of the youngster. Pediatricians have been surprised to find that even when they reduce a dose of phenobarbital for a child, proportional to his weight, the effect is excitement rather than sedation. Older people sometimes respond differently to drugs than younger people. Some of the differences seen in the response of older people to drugs can be attributed to the presence of disease or changes in the distribution of fat and muscle. For a review of drugs in the aged, the reader is refered to Jarvik, Gritz, and Schneider, (1972).

Set and Expectation

Until recent years very little attention was paid to this aspect of variability in the response of subjects to drugs. The term *nonspecific drug factors* has been used to encompass all those factors that are not directly related to the chemistry of the drug and physiology of the organism. However, it is reasonable to assume that such things as set and expectation may so alter the physiological system that what we consider a nonspecific factor is really an alteration in the functional physiology, so that the drug now has a different effect because it is acting on an altered system (see Chapter 2).

Drug Interactions

Drugs are often given in combinations, both by design and (occasionally) inadvertently. When drugs are combined, the result may be an additive or antagonistic effect, or the effects may be completely independent. At times combinations of drugs may result in marked toxic effects. As an example, highly toxic effects are often seen when antidepressants of different chemical structures are combined or when one is substituted for the other without a relatively long interval in between. Various terms have been used to describe the types of combined effects that are seen. There is not complete agreement concerning the definitions of such terms as *synergism, additive,* and *potentiation.* Thus the following definitions may be at variance with those found in some textbooks:

Synergism. When selected doses of each of two drugs have a measurable effect and when combined, their effect is greater than the algebraic sum of the individual actions of the two drugs, this is called synergism.

Additive Effect. When the combined effect of two drugs is the simple algebraic sum of their individual actions, this is called an additive effect.

Potentiation. When the selected dose of one drug is ineffective alone but when combined with another drug produces an effect that is greater than the algebraic sum of their individual effects, this is called potentiation.

Additive effects are often seen when both drugs have similar actions. Synergism or potentiation may occur when one of the drugs inhibits the detoxification or excretion of the other.

Antagonism. When one drug blocks the effect of another, this is called antagonism. The antagonism of one drug by another can be achieved by chemical, physiological, or pharmacological mechanisms.

Chemical antagonism is the least frequent type of antagonism. It is simply the combining of one chemical with another in the body to make an inactive complex.

Physiological antagonism is the resultant effect of two drugs that have opposite physiological effects but whose actions are on different receptors. The supposed action of caffeine in the inebriated individual is an example of this type of antagonism.

Pharmacological antagonism is the result of two drugs competing for the same receptor. It is believed that one of the compounds prevents the access of the second compound to the receptor. The antagonism of endogenous histamine by an antihistaminic agent is believed to be this type of antagonism.

Tolerance and Physical Dependence

Tolerance to a drug may be defined either as the need to increase the amount of drug taken to obtain a given initial effect or, conversely, as the decrease in the effect of a drug as a result of repeated administration of a given dose. Tolerance does not develop to all drugs, but an argument could be made for the development of a behavioral tolerance to almost all drugs that affect the central nervous system.

Behavioral tolerance may be defined as the development of alternative func-

DRUG EFFECTS

tions that compensate for the pharmacological effects of a drug. Although it may often be difficult to differentiate between pharmacological tolerance and behavioral tolerance, both types are probably present when central nervous system drugs are given chronically. Tolerance is not a unitary mechanism; often, some response systems in an organism show evidence of tolerance, whereas other systems respond to the same or near same degree as they did initially. This can lead to some difficulty, because the dose may be continually raised to overcome the development of tolerance in one system, but in some other system, where tolerance has not developed to the same degree, the increased dosage may approach toxic levels.

Very rapid development of tolerance is called *tachyphylaxis*. It is not generally seen with drugs; however, when observed, it appears when the second dose of the drug is given while the effects of the first dose are still present. It is believed to be the result of the first dose occupying the receptor surfaces, so that additional drug is blocked from the receptor. Another type of tachyphylaxis is seen when the effect of a drug is dependent on the depletion or release of some endogenous substance in the body. Once depletion is already complete from previous doses, no additional effect can occur. This type of tachyphylaxis has been called *desensitization*.

Physical dependence is defined as that condition in which cessation of drug administration or reduction of the dose results in a syndrome characterized by an altered physiological state, the *withdrawal syndrome*. The syndrome may take many forms, but it is often manifested as a rebound effect so that during withdrawal from a drug that causes a rise in blood pressure, there may be a fall in blood pressure. The syndrome may be quite mild with some drugs with the subject exhibiting only mild discomfort. With other drugs, however, the syndrome may be characterized by grand mal seizures and delirium. In such cases the withdrawal syndrome may be life threatening. In recent years the term *psychological dependence* has appeared. Psychological dependence may occur in the absence of physiological dependence. It has been defined as a continual craving for a drug; this craving may be accompanied by irritability, anxiety, and inability to concentrate, and so on. It is characterized by drug-seeking behavior not necessarily motivated by a need to alleviate a physical withdrawal syndrome. Although it is not clear that there is physical dependence on cigarettes, abrupt termination does seem to cause psychological discomfort in people. Tolerance to and dependence on drugs will be discussed in more detail in Chapters 7, 8, and 12.

Cumulative Effects

If a second dose of drug is given before the first dose has been detoxified or excreted from the body, there will be an accumulation of the drug resulting in an increased effect (unless it is a rare instance of tachyphylaxis). If the drug is repeatedly administered, increased effects will occur until an equilibrium occurs between the amount ingested and the amount excreted unless rate of intake exceeds elimination capacity. The number of doses that are necessary before this equilibrium occurs will be dependent on the half-life of the drug (the time it takes for the concentration of drug in the body to be reduced by one half) and the interval between doses. Figure 8 shows how the equilibrium is achieved when repeated doses are used.

Genetic Factors

In recent years a field of pharmacology has evolved called *pharmacogenetics*. It is believed that much of the normal variance seen after drug administration may be due to genetic differences in subjects. The occurrence of certain types of side effects seen with some drugs may very well be related to some genetic predisposition. It is a well-known fact that in studies done with animals in the laboratory, different strains of rats and mice have different sensitivities to certain drugs. McLaren and Michie (1956) (in Kalow p. 62) demonstrated that an inbred strain of mice had greater variability in response to pentobarbital (this was measured by sleep time) than did either random-bred or hybrid mice. This is the opposite of what would be expected, for inbreeding would be expected to produce animals with a more homogenous response to the drug. It was therefore concluded that drug effects result from a combination of both genetic and environmental factors. The finding of McLaren and Michie cannot be generalized, however; for if one measures less global response systems than sleep-wakefulness the opposite results occur: less variance is seen with the more homogenous strains. Geneticists have been interested in pharmacology longer than pharmacologists have been interested in genetics. Geneticists have employed drugs as tools to demonstrate the presence of specific genes.

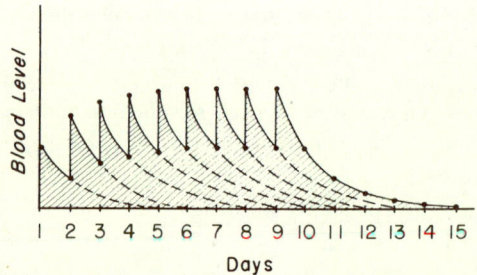

FIGURE 8. Hypothetical curve of blood levels of a drug given once a day with a half-life of 24 hours. The last dose is given on day 9. Note that by day 7 blood levels have reached equilibrium. The time that it takes blood levels to reach such an equilibrium will depend on the half-life of the drug and the frequency of drug administration.

GENERAL INFORMATION

Many students of psychology are completely unfamiliar with certain practical aspects of administering drugs, such as dosage form, and calculation of concentration and dosage in animal experiments.

Concentration, Dosage, and Dilution

In man drugs are often given in the form of pills or capsules. These are ways of giving drugs in solid form. When drugs are given in this manner, expression of dose in weight is sufficient. In recent years almost all drug weights have been in the metric system, but occasionally, the older apothecary form is used. The apothecary system uses a more colorful terminology such as grain, scruple, dram, and ounce for measures of weight and minim, fluid dram, and fluid ounce for measures of volume. The following table shows the various weights and measures for both the metric and apothecary systems and their equivalents.

TABLE OF WEIGHTS AND MEASURES

Weight

METRIC

1000.0 grams (gm)	=	1 kilogram (kg)
0.001 gram	=	1 milligram (mg)
.000001 gram	=	1 microgram (μg)

Approximate metric to English (avoirdupois) conversions

1 kilogram	=	2.2 pounds (lb)
454 grams	=	1 pound

APOTHECARY

20 grains (gr)	=	1 scruple
60 grains	=	1 dram
480 grains	=	1 ounce
1 grain	=	60 milligrams

Fluid Volume

METRIC

1 liter (l)	=	1000 milliliters (ml)
1 milliliter	=	1 cubic centimeter (cc)

Approximate metric to English conversions

1 liter	=	1.06 quarts (qt)
1 liter	=	33.8 fluid ounces (fl oz)

APOTHECARY

1 minim	=	0.06 milliliter
1 fluid dram	=	3.7 milliliters
1 fluid ounce	=	29.57 milliliters

When drugs are given in solution, it is necessary not only to prescribe the concentration of drug but the vehicle in which the drug is dissolved. Concentration is either expressed as mg/ml or in terms of percent. With respect to weight, percent always means grams per 100 ml of solution. Thus a 10-percent solution means that there are 10 gm per 100 ml of solution.

Drug Preparations

Most drugs currently being marketed have two names. The first is the nonproprietary name that is the official name of the drug, and the second is the proprietary name that is the trade name of the drug. The term generic name has been incorrectly used to refer to the nonproprietary name. The generic name refers to a class of compounds. Thus phenothiazine is the generic name, chlorpromazine is the nonproprietary name, and Thorazine is the trade name.

Many drugs are prepared and marketed in the form of salts, for example, morphine sulfate, caffeine citrate, and sodium amobarbital. This is done because these salts will more readily dissolve in water than will the uncombined drug, and aqueous solubility facilitates most forms of drug administration. A drug may be prepared in different salt forms, for example, dextroamphetamine sulfate and dextroamphetamine phosphate. These salts dissociate in solution, thereby freeing the drug, amphetamine in this case, to act at the appropriate receptors. The amount of phosphate or sulfate introduced into the system exerts a negligible pharmacologic effect. In general, it may be said that the use of different salt forms does not alter the basic pharmacology of a drug. Different salts may, however, dissociate at different rates or to different degrees and thereby affect absorption. Usually, the pharmaceutical houses use this to their advantage, compounding the salt form whose solubility characteristics provide for the most reliable and predictable absorption pattern.

SUMMARY

This review of some of the basic concepts in pharmacology is, by its nature, a gross oversimplification of many of the areas. Each of the areas mentioned is, in itself, a highly elaborated field, and only the relevant points have been discussed in this chapter. The basic concepts that have been reviewed are common to all drugs whether the drug is a major tranquilizer, aspirin, or marihuana.

Action of drugs on living organisms cannot be intelligently discussed or understood without familiarity with the presented concepts. Something as obvious as the dose-response relationship is often ignored both in clinical practice and in research. In the former it may often result in the appropriate drug given at an inappropriate dose, and in the latter it often precludes meaningful interpretation of an otherwise sound experiment.

REFERENCES

Fingl, E., and **Woodbury, D. M.** General principles. In L. S. Goodman and A. Gilman (Eds.) *Pharmacological Basis of Therapeutics.* (4th ed.). New York, Macmillan, 1970, pp. 1-35.

Goldstein, A., Aronow, L., and **Kalman, S. M.** *Principles of Drug Action: Basis of Pharmacology.* (2nd ed.). New York, Wiley, 1974.

Goth, A. Principles and concepts. In *Medical Pharmacology.* (6th ed.). Saint Louis, Mosby, 1972, pp. 1-50.

Jarvik, M. E., Gritz, E. R., and **Schneider, N. G.** Drugs and memory disorders in human aging. *Behavioral Biology,* 7, 1972, 643-668.

Kalow, W. Heredity and the response to drugs. In *Pharmacogenetics.* Philadelphia, Sanders, 1962.

Kornetsky, C. An overview of drug action. In A. DiMascio and R. I. Shader (Eds.) *Clinical Handbook of Psychopharmacology.* New York, Science House, 1970, pp. 105-119.

Levine, R. R. *Drug Actions and Reactions.* Boston, Little, Brown, 1973.

Routtenberg, A. Intracranial chemical injection and behavior: A critical review. *Behavioral Biology,* 7, 1972, 601-641.

2 THE PLACEBO AND NONSPECIFIC FACTORS AS DETERMINANTS OF RESPONSES TO DRUGS

INTRODUCTION

The *placebo effect* may be defined as any effect of medical intervention that cannot be attributed to the specific action of a drug or the treatment given. This definition implies that the placebo effect is unique to medicine; however, an argument could be made that all of us are responding in some way and to some degree to placebos in our daily lives. Many of the testimonials that we give to a particular brand of cigarette, coffee, soap, and so on, could be considered to be the result of a type of placebo effect. Often the major difference between many consumer products is the advertising that is used to entice us. Despite this presence of a placebo effect in our daily lives, the formal use of the term placebo has been limited to medical and clinical pharmacological use. Although the importance of the placebo in clinical research and medicine was not emphasized until the beginning of the last decade, the term did appear in Hooper's 1811 *Medical Dictionary*. The definition given there gave a negative connotation to the term—"an epithet given to any medication adopted more to please than to benefit the patient."

History

Despite the early lack of formal attention to the placebo, the history of medical treatment up to the last 70 to 80 years could be considered to be the history of the placebo effect. Even today the physician finds that dissimilar drugs, or even different therapeutic measures, will act with equal effectiveness on certain symptoms or disease states. This may in part be attributed to placebo responding. There is a remark attributed to Voltaire, "A doctor is a person who administers drugs he does not know, to an organism he knows even less." However, the physician of today gives more or less adequate relief to those he treats. In some cases this relief is due to a direct pharmacological action; in others it is due to the combination of pharmacological actions and placebo effects; and in still other instances, relief is a direct effect of the placebo. Modell (1955, p.55) has stated that the placebo effect "is the only action which all drugs have in common, and in some cases it is the only useful one that a medication can exert."

The term placebo is derived from the Latin infinitive *placere* which means "to please." Early reference to the use of the placebo can be found in the ninth verse of the 116th psalm of the *Vulgata*, a verse that was sung at the start of the vespers for the dead during the middle ages: "Placebo domino in regione vivorum." Geoffrey Chaucer used the word placebo to define a mocker and a hypocrite. The word also crept into the writing of Sir Walter Scott: "With this placebo she concluded her note," meaning that she concluded her note with a soothing sentiment. Even prior to the 1811 *Hooper Medical Dictionary,* the word was found in medical dictionaries without the negative connotations of the Hooper definition. The 1787 edition of Quincy's *Lexicon* and John Redman Coxe's *Philadelphia Medical Dictionary* of 1808 defined placebo as a "commonplace method of medicine." In the 1965 edition of the *Dorland Medical Dictionary* there is still the negative element in the definition of placebo, although there is a mention of its use in controlled clinical studies: "An inactive substance or preparation, formerly given to please or gratify a patient, now also used in controlled studies to determine the efficacy of medicinal substances."

Much of the effectiveness of many of the early treatment methods could be attributed to the placebo effect. According to Shapiro (1959), the *Papyrus Eber,* circa 1500 B.C., gives a long list of treatments for a variety of diseases. These included such things as "Lizards' blood, crocodile dung, the teeth of swine, the hoof of an ass, putrid meat with fly specks." Later in medical history more sophistication appeared. In the 7th century A.D. therapy had evolved to the point where certain types of blood were used for specific conditions. Pigeon and turtle blood were used for ocular hematomas, owl blood for dyspnoea, bat blood for preserving the breasts of virgins.

Some medications had to be given or obtained at a specific time of day, month, or year. During the middle ages Pope Boniface VIII was cured of kidney colic by his physician who hung a gold seal bearing an image of a lion around the thigh of the Pope. The seal was fashioned while the sun was at its zenith. The effect was excellent.

One treatment that was very popular in the sixteenth and seventeenth centuries was prepared from powdered mummy (Egyptian variety). This preparation was reported to taste like ground raisins. Since the demand was so great it was often counterfeited, and when the therapy did not work its failure was attributed to the use of the counterfeit product.

The nineteenth century was one of great expansion of the patent medicine field. Patent medicine manufacturers anticipated many of the more modern advertising techniques. In the first half of the nineteenth century patent medicine manufacturers had a number of firsts in merchandising. They sought a national market for their products and helped promote their sale by going directly to the consumer with messages extolling the virtues of the medications. These promotions were vivid, if not lurid, whereas most advertising of the period was drab (see Figure 1). The proprietary medicine industry spent more for advertising than any other industry in the United States throughout the 19th century.

Very popular during this period and even up to the present time were various purges. There were many remedies on the market then and still today "... whose chief mission appeared to be to open men's purses by opening their bowels." This quotation was first written in 1838. The obvious advantage of a laxative in a patent medicine over a completely inert medicine is that it provides irrefutable evidence that the "drug" is doing something.

Placebo effects have not been confined to medicinals. Many gadgets have been used through the years. Often symptoms would disappear after the use of these gadgets simply because many diseases are self-limiting or because of the strong suggestion accompanying the treatment, although this latter effect may only be temporary. In many cases, however, patients have died because of the substitution of quackery for adequate medical care. Early in this century a New York "clinic" treated, by a form of shock therapy, young men who believed they were suffering from syphillis or from weakness due to self-abuse (masturbation) (Young, 1967, p. 244). Although this therapy did not produce convulsions, the treatment was probably as traumatic as if it had. The patient would sit on a type of toilet bowl with his bare back resting against a metal plate and his scrotum emersed in a whirling pool of water. The pool and plate would then be connected to an electric battery. Although this method would not cure syphillis, it probably did have some effect on the malaise (ill-defined feelings of lethargy and illness) attributed to self-abuse. Despite such an array of painful or distasteful therapies of questionable value, the healer in all cultures has been respected and, for obvious reasons, feared.

Current Therapies

Although a review of these early practitioners and gullible consumers seems somewhat humorous, we find in current therapies many things reminiscent of these early therapies. An editorial in the *British Medical Journal* in 1961 stated that "At the present time, many of the medicines commonly administered are placebos." It was estimated that 20 to 40 percent of prescription medicines are really placebos. An argument could be made that the placebo is probably the most therapeutic armament of the physician, and for many patients, it may be the only useful tool that the physician has at his dis-

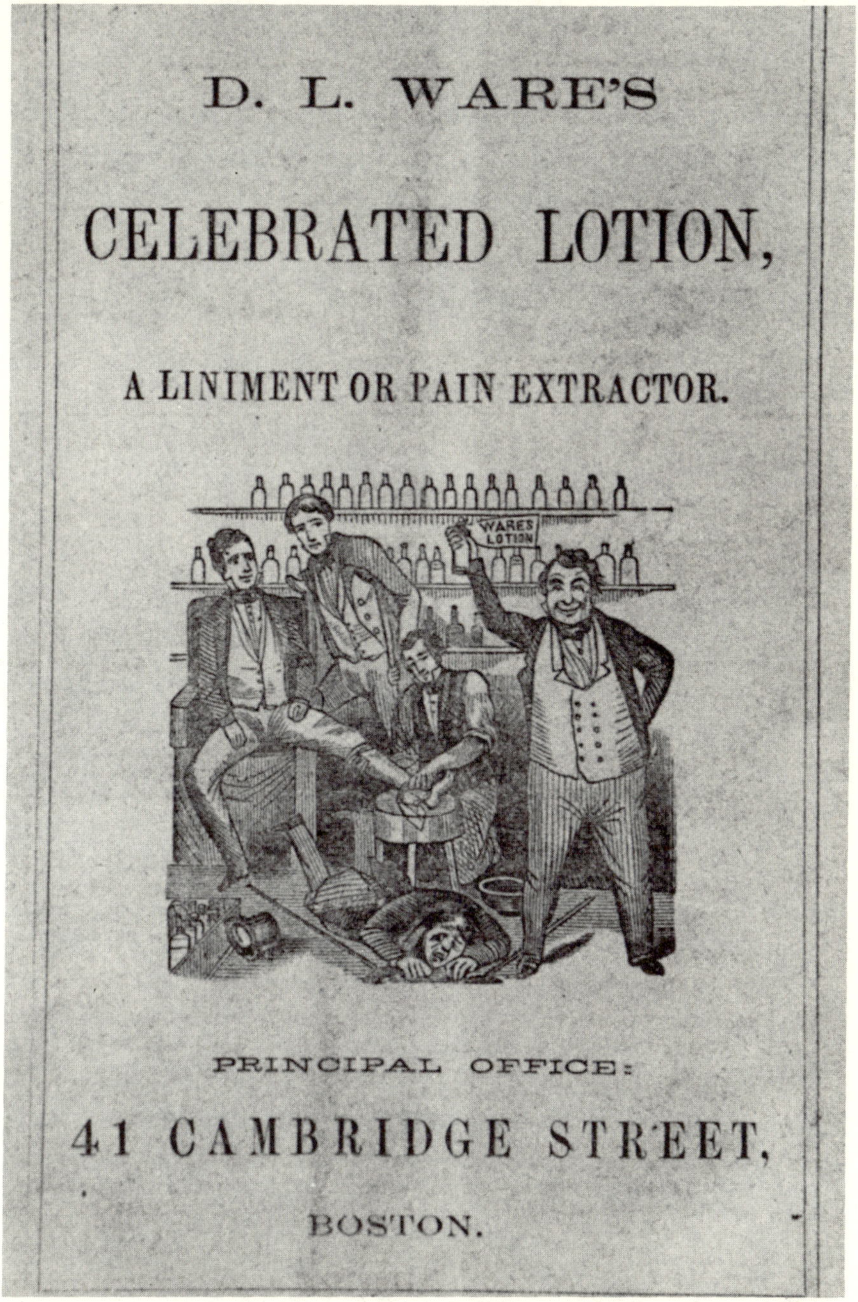

FIGURE 1a. Example of drug advertising during the latter part of the nineteenth century.

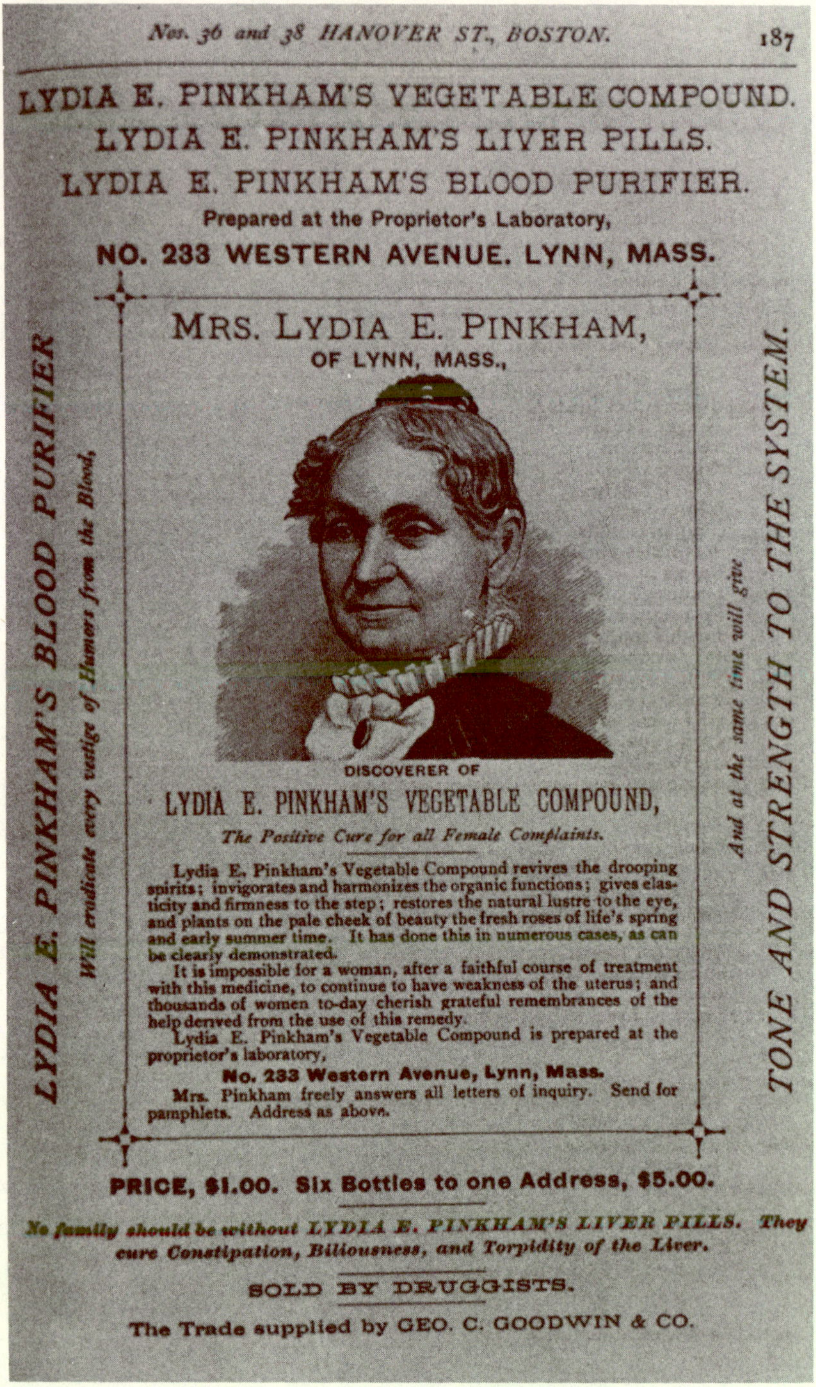

FIGURE 1b. Nineteenth-century drug advertising.

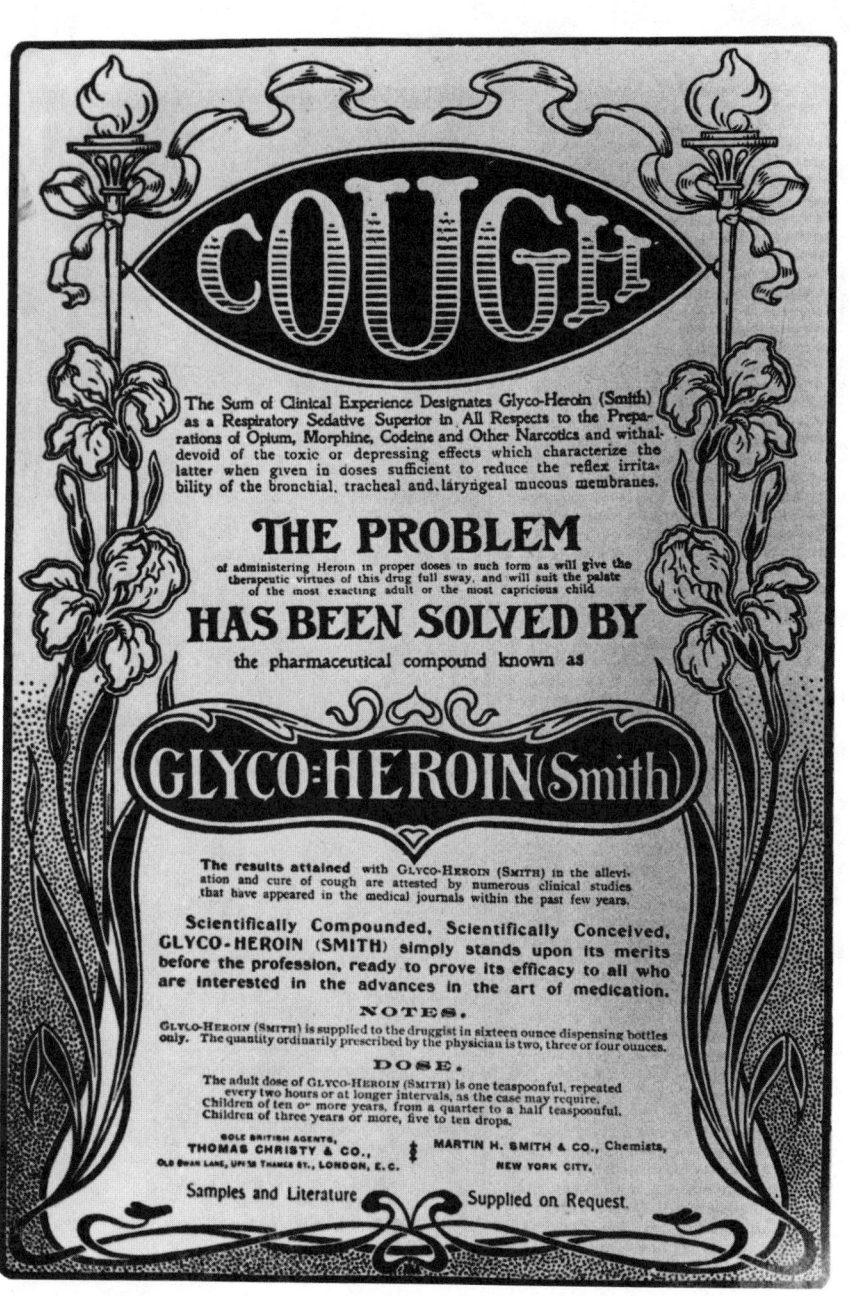

FIGURE 1c. Nineteenth-century drug advertising.

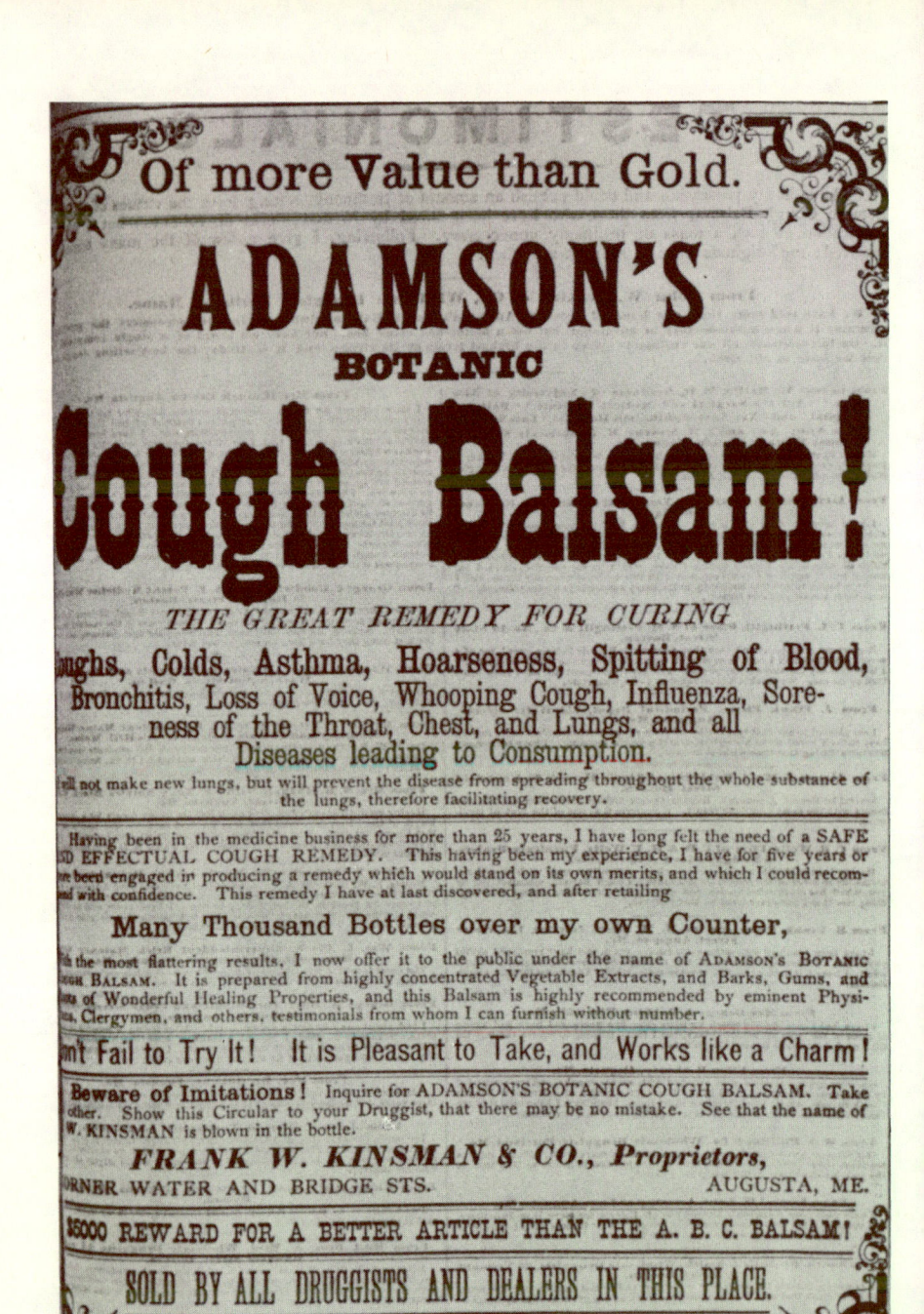

FIGURE 1d. Nineteenth-century drug advertising.

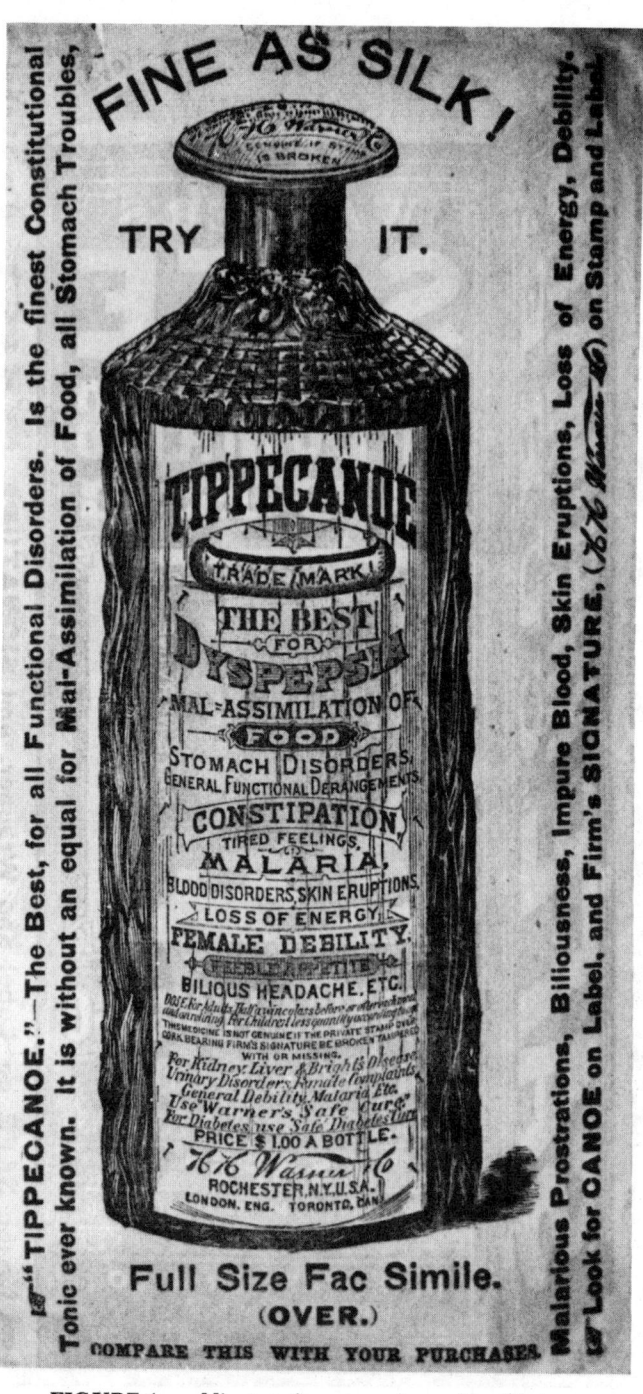

FIGURE 1e. Nineteenth-century drug advertising.

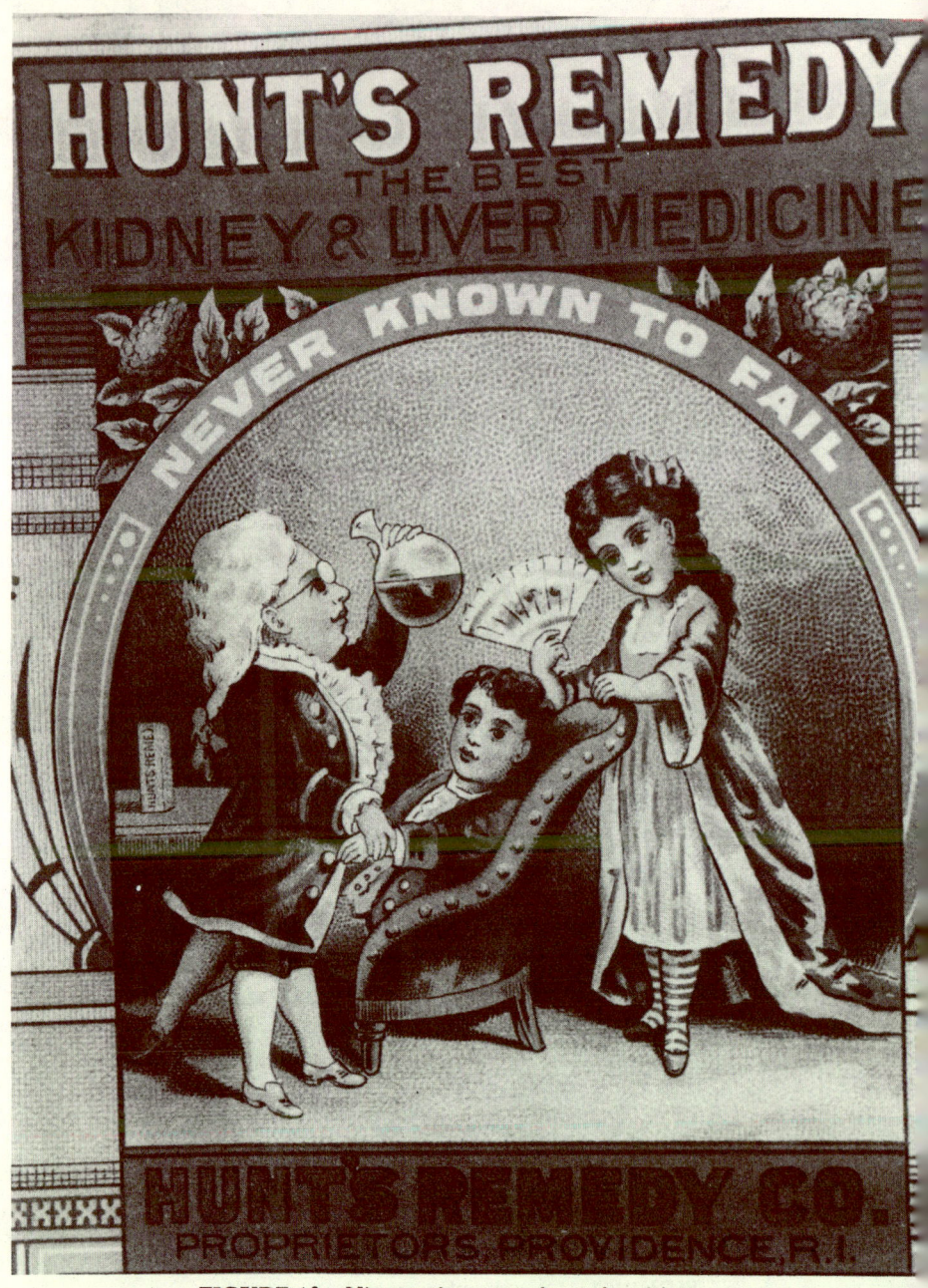

FIGURE 1f. Nineteenth-century drug advertising.

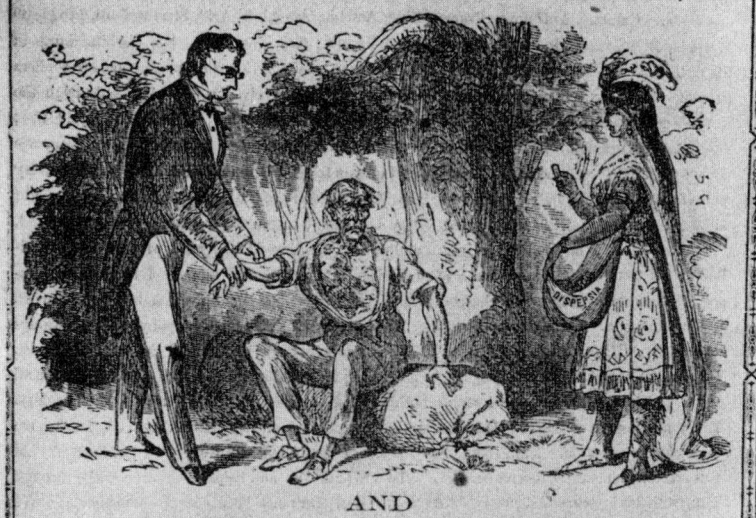

FIGURE 1g. Nineteenth-century drug advertising.

posal. The efficacy of many of the lotions, vitamins, laxatives, suppositories, and so on, found on the patent medicine shelf of the pharmacy or written into the prescription of the physician could be attributed to the placebo effect. There is a great deal of evidence from published reports on the efficacy of new treatments that they should be used soon after their introduction to the market while they still have the power to heal.

Schindel (1962) has defined two types of placebo in medical use, the *pure* placebo and the *impure* placebo. The pure placebo is given with full knowledge by the physician that what is given is a placebo. It is used extensively in the evaluation of pharmacologically active compounds for their clinical efficacy. The impure placebo is a drug which both the patient and the doctor believe to be therapeutically effective, although no pharmacological basis for the drug's effectiveness in the disease under treatment exists. Another type of impure placebo is used for clinical evaluation of new compounds. In this case, the clinical pharmacologist knows that it is not an effective drug. It is called an *active* control.

Lasagna (1955) has referred to the use of placebos, both pure and impure, as a pharmaceutical charade. To insure the success of this charade, certain measures, often punitive, are necessary. For example, the patient must be kept unaware of the deceit. Although this is generally the case, there have been studies in which the subjects were told that they were receiving a placebo, and a placebo effect was still observed. This probably could be attributed to the tremendous faith that is given to the physician in our society so that even when told that they were being given a placebo, patients were unable to accept such a possibility. (Illegible prescriptions add to the mystique of the physician's power.) The efficacy of a placebo may be influenced by the color of the capsule or pill. It has been reported that subjects respond better to treatment with capsules that are of their preferred color. Colorless capsules may not instill in the patient a feeling of confidence in the physician. Bitter or highly flavored placebos are more effective than tasteless ones. An extraordinarily large pill may impress the patient by its size while the exceptionally small one impresses the patient by its potency. Injections are often more effective than oral medication. The presence of the physician or nurse when an injection is given probably enhances the placebo effect because of the reverence that most people have for members of the healing profession. Although all of the above statements may be broad generalizations, each is supported by experimental evidence.

Similarity to Active Drugs

Although a pure placebo is an inert substance and any effect that it manifests has to be attributed to such things as suggestion, expectation, and the setting in which the drug is given, it does have many of the same characteristics as an active drug (Lasagna, Laties, and Dohan, 1958; Wolf, 1959). These include such things as a time-effect curve, cumulative effects, tolerance, side effects, and even the possibility of a dose-effect curve.

Time-effect Curve. One of the primary attributes indicating pharmacological activity of a drug is the time-effect curve. This curve represents the buildup of effect after a drug administration and includes the time of onset of the effect and the time to peak or maximum effect. These factors normally vary with drug, dose, and mode of administration. There is then a gradual decline in effect with the subject returning to basal levels of response. Reported experiments in which a placebo has been used clearly demonstrates a time-effect relationship. With an active drug the time to onset of effect and peak effect will appear earlier than with a placebo. Also the active drug will usually have a longer duration of action than the placebo.

Cumulative Effects. Although it is well known that an active drug will cause increased effects after repeated doses and that this is usually a reflection of increasing concentration of the drug in the blood or body, it is not generally appreciated that a placebo may mimic this type of effect. In a study reported by Lasagna, Laties, and Dohan (1958), in which a group of geriatric patients who complained of lack of "pep" and loss of appetite were given a daily tonic that was completely inert, there was an increase in both appetite and "pep" commencing on about the tenth day and continuing after the placebo was discontinued on the seventeenth day. The role of expectation was clear in this study for when the patients were asked why they thought the tonic took so long to have an effect, the responses contained such statements as, "You know, it takes a while for these drugs to take hold, Doc." Thus the patients show an expectation of how a drug should work. There is also the desire not to disappoint a physician who is presumably eager for the patient to show improvement. Also, especially in chronic care patients, the patient may feel that a "correct" response will result in the doctor taking a greater interest in him. Since physicians are human, it is very likely that they will take a greater interest in those patients who respond to therapy in a manner that concurs with the physician's own expectation.

Tolerance. Repeated use of a placebo in patients who initially respond to the inert substance may result in a progressive decrease in its effectiveness. For example, such "tolerance" was clearly demonstrated by Huckabee (personal communication) in studies in which hypertensive patients received "chronic administration" of a placebo.

Dose-effect Curve. Obviously, one cannot change the dose level of an inert substance, but what can be done is to increase the number of capsules that are given. Although I know of no study where this has been done, I would expect that in a carefully controlled placebo study where the number of inert capsules was systematically varied, a dose-effect curve would be generated.

Side Effects. It is the rare drug that does not have some unwanted side effects. Even aspirin may produce side effects in some people. Such things as nausea and vomiting have been reported to occur after ingestion of a normal dose of aspirin. These side effects often interfere with therapy, for in order to obtain an effective dose of the drug, it is almost impossible not to have concomitant side effects. Sometimes these side effects can be controlled by giving some other medication that is relatively specific for the treatment of the side effects. Many of the drugs used in the treatment of various forms of cancer cause nausea and vomiting, and these are often reversed by the use of low doses of chlorpromazine. Side effects are always dose related so that doses may be titrated to reduce the severity of these effects. Often the reduction in dose need be only temporary, for with some drugs, tolerance to the side effects may develop with no concomitant development of tolerance to the therapeutic effect. This seems to be true with chlorpromazine treatment of schizophrenic patients, in which a postural hypotension (also called orthostatic hypotension, drop in blood pressure upon standing) is a quite common side effect. However, with repeated administration, tolerance develops to this action of chlorpromazine while the antipsychotic actions of the drug persist.

Side effects are also somewhat arbitrarily defined. Reserpine, which formerly was used quite extensively for the treatment of schizophrenia, also had a hypotensive effect; however, the drug is also used in the treatment of hypertension, and in this case the hypotensive effect is considered a main effect.

The side effect due to the placebo was most dramatically reported by Wolf and Pinsky (1954) in a study of patients suffering from such disorders and complaints as peptic ulcers, migraine, muscle tension, headache, and backache. In all patients, anxiety and tension were prominent among the complaints, and in most of the patients, there were such objective manifestations as tremulousness, sweating, and tachycardia (increase in heart rate). In this particular study the active drug was mephenesin, a muscle relaxant. All subjects received both placebo and active medication on different occasions during the course of the study. Many of the patients had minor or equivocal complaints such as lightheadedness, drowsiness, and anorexia while they were taking either the placebo or mephenesin. The appearance of such symptoms occurred with equal frequency with either the placebo or with the active medication. Three of the patients in the study had what could be considered severe side effects. One patient had sudden overwhelming weakness, tachycardia, and nausea within 15 minutes after taking the placebo. A second had epigastric (commonly called heartburn) pain within 10 minutes of taking the pills, followed by watery diarrhea, urticaria (generalized itching in response to vascular changes in the skin), and angioneurotic edema of the lips. Subsequent administration of the placebo at 48 and again at 96 hours after the first ingestion produced the same effects. In these two cases the effects were observed after the active medication as well as after the placebo. A third patient had a diffuse itchy rash which developed after 10 days of taking the placebos. After the treatment was stopped, the eruption quickly cleared. These effects reported by Wolf and Pinsky are quite severe in contrast to the more usual reactions a placebo produces. More commonly seen are milder responses such as anxiety, tension, or sleepiness.

The Placebo Reactor

The response to a placebo raises two important questions: what percent of a given population will respond to a placebo, and can these placebo responders be identified? Beecher (1959, p. 65) reviewed 15 experiments in which a placebo was employed in clinical studies of pain. These studies involved more than 1000 subjects. He found that placebos satisfactorily relieved pain of various sorts in 35 percent of the subjects with a standard error of 2.2 percent. The power of the placebo becomes more impressive when one realizes that a large dose of morphine relieved pain in only 75 percent of the subjects. It would appear that once it has been established that a significant number of subjects will respond to a placebo, the characteristics of the placebo responder can be systematically studied. One of the difficulties is that the placebo responder in one situation may not be a placebo responder in a somewhat different situation or may not even respond in the same fashion when the first conditions are repeated. It was found (Lasagna, Mosteller, von Felsinger, and Beecher, 1954) that fewer than 50 percent of the patients who received more than a single treatment with a placebo responded consistently.

Fisher (1967) in his review of the problem of identifying the placebo reactor gives two cogent reasons for the failure to find consistency across placebo situations. The first reason he gives is the practice of use of a single placebo experience to determine the placebo reactor. Fisher, justifiably, states that the use of a placebo-reactivity score that relies on a single placebo situation is the equivalent of using only one item from a personality inventory to categorize a person's personality. The second reason is that researchers often fail to differentiate between what Fisher calls "placebo uniformity" and "placebo constancy." The former refers to the potency of the environment in causing a placebo effect, whereas the latter refers to personality traits. Thus if one is interested in the "placebo constancy," the subjects must be tested under relatively equal conditions of "placebo uniformity."

Not only is the conduciveness of the environment necessary for producing the placebo effect but the subject must be motivated to have such an effect. In clinical studies most patients are strongly motivated for the treatment to be therapeutic. There probably is more motivation for a patient in physical pain to have the symptom relieved than there is for the neurotic patient to give up his pathological defenses.

The attitude and role of the physician is also important in determining the potency of a placebo. Schindel (1962) reports an observation of Wolf that might be called an anti-placebo effect: negative attitudes of the physician toward the therapy resulted in patients who benefited least, while patients being treated by physicians who were most enthusiastic about the new drug were helped the most.

In attempts to delineate the characteristics of the placebo reactor, it was found that age, sex, and intelligence levels of the patients were not predictors. The studies by von Felsinger, Lasagna, and Beecher (1955) suggested that the placebo reactors tended to be more anxious and hostile than the nonreactors, as determined by the Rorschach test. The reactors tended to be happier with their hospital experience than nonreactors. The reactors were more cooperative in the hospital, made less of their post-operative discomfort, and had a greater tendency to develop somatic complaints such as diarrhea, headache, and nervous stomach than did the nonreactors. The main criticisms that can be made concerning most of the studies designed to determine the characteristics of the placebo reactor are that small samples of subjects were used and the failure, as Fisher pointed out, to obtain more than one index of placebo reactivity.

Nonspecific Factors

The term "nonspecific factors" has been used to define nonpharmacological variables that influence a patient's reaction to a drug. These include age, sex, personality of the subject, environment, attitude of subject as well as that of physician and staff, and so on. The following discussion regarding these factors follows closely the paper by Fisher (Nonspecific Factors as Determinants of Behavioral Response to Drugs, 1970). Fisher points out that the term "nonspecific factors" is often nothing more than a wastebasket category. If we can find no obvious pharmacologic or physiologic explanation for an observed difference in the responses of patients to a drug, we attribute the difference to nondrug factors. It is very possible that many nondrug factors are, in fact, conventional pharmacologic variables that are overlooked either because of lack of knowledge concerning the interaction of drugs and the CNS, or because of incomplete understanding of how drugs are excreted and detoxified. We, therefore, invoke personality or milieu as an explanation. This is not to say that environment and personality cannot alter drug effects but that the behavioral scientist is often too eager to make a judgement concerning the importance of these nonspecific factors.

INTRODUCTION

Conceptual Models. Fisher has proposed two models for assessing the separate and combined contributions of drug and nondrug factors in mediating response to a psychotherapeutic drug. The main method of determining nondrug factors has been to perform experiments that use placebo controls. Thus if a placebo results in five arbitrary units of improvement in a patient and a drug yields eight units of improvements, it is often assumed that only three of the units are the result of the drug. This type of *additive model* may be correct in some cases, but there is another model called the *interaction model*. Figure 2 (A & B) shows identical hypothetical effects for patients treated with a placebo as a function of the treating physician's set (positive or negative). Thus if the set is extremely negative, the placebo may result in worsening the patient's condition. At 0 units of set the assumption is made that the placebo will have 0 units of positive effect and the drug will have two units of positive effect over that seen with the placebo at all levels of the physician's set. Unfortunately, this simple model may not describe what is happening clinically as accurately as the interaction model shown in the figure. In the interaction model, a hypothetical two units of improvement are shown with drug treatment. However, depending on the set of

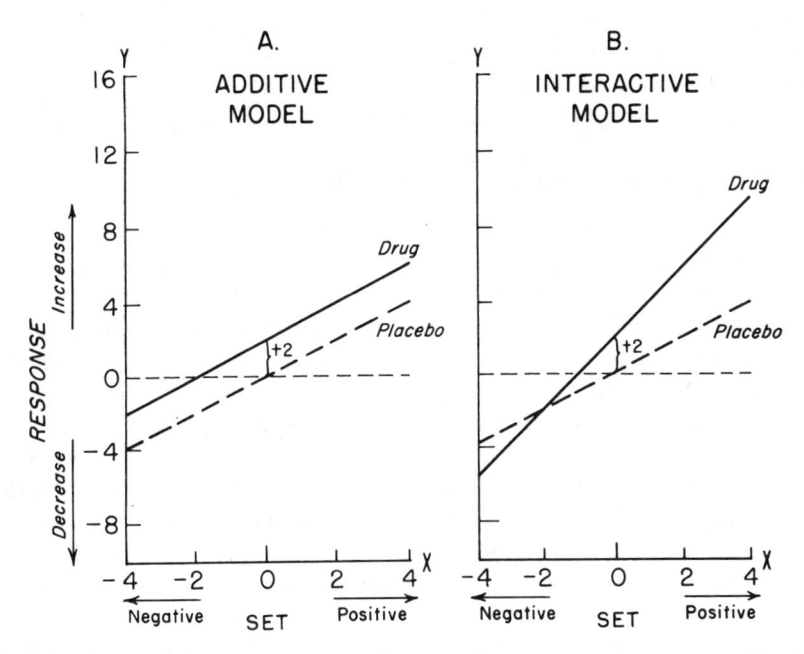

FIGURE 2. Models of drug-set combination. A. Nonspecific effect (set) and drug effect are additive. B. Postive nonspecific effect potentiates drug effect in the interaction model (after Fisher, 1970).

the subject, the clinical state will vary to a greater or lesser degree as compared to placebo conditions. In fact, there can be a situation where the patient may even do worse with a drug. These figures suggest that there is a linear relationship between set and drug or placebo effect. The probability is that these curves in reality are not linear and that the scaling of such things as set and clinical improvement is not a simple ratio scale. If we add to this the problems of dose and duration of treatment, one can easily see the complexity of clinical studies and difficulty in determining nonspecific factors. Results of clinical trials suggest that the additive model holds for studies with antipsychotic drugs, but that with the drugs used in the treatment of neuroses, the data more closely fit an interaction model.

General Principles

Fisher (1970) has postulated four general principles regarding nonspecific effects: (1) "The more the response system being measured involves cortical processes such as awareness, consciousness, and subjective feelings, the greater will be the role of nonspecific factors influencing drug response." (2) "Many apparent nonspecific influences may be reducible to (i.e., explained by) simple physiologic and pharmacologic factors." (3) "The more 'potent' a drug is, the less sensitive it will be to nonspecific factors." (4) "Most available clinical data suggest that maximum drug response can be obtained by administering the drug in the presence of the most favorable 'placebogenic' factors."

The Placebo Reactors in Nonclinical Studies

In most of the conditions referred to above, the studies were carried out in a clinical setting; that is, the subjects were people with clinical complaints that were treated with a placebo. The treatment with the placebo was usually one of many treatments, some purportedly active medications that were used to alleviate the condition or complaint. In drug studies with normal volunteers, the placebo is also used as a control. In this type of experimental study, placebo effects are rarely seen unless the experiment is expressly designed to produce potent placebo effects, or the subjects are knowledgeable about the active medications that will be used. The lack of measurable placebo effects in this type of study is probably not due to the fact that there are no placebo effects present but that the subjects do not have a consistent set of expectations for responding. The variety of ways that the human subject can respond are many, and the variety of placebo responses across subjects may result in a net zero effect. For example, one subject may respond with an increase in pulse rate, whereas another subject who is responding equally to the placebo may do so with a decrease in pulse rate. Thus if the experimental design and the information given to the subjects do not give them a uniform set, no uniformity will be seen in the placebo effects.

MECHANISM OF ACTION

Thus far we have described various phenomenological aspects of the placebo as well as some of the factors that will enhance the effects of the placebo, but the question concerning how an inert substance can have pharmacological properties has not been completely answered. The modes of action of placebo are probably of three general types, and probably all three may be acting at any single time. The first of these I would like to call animism. This is a type of magical thinking in which the inert material is endowed with a "soul" or power of its own that is capable of causing change. The second and third are suggestion and conditioning.

Animism

The effectiveness of many of the medicinals used in earlier societies were of this animistic nature. The juxtaposition of ingestion of some herb or putrid, fly-specked meat and the fortuitous remission of some symptoms led to an incorrect conclusion of cause and effect. A power was attributed to the herb or meat. Once this conclusion was accepted by the authority in the community, be it the primitive medicine man or the modern physician, the lay individual was prone to accept the efficacy of the medication. This type of magical thinking has much in common with science (Frazer, 1959, p. 649). The primary difference between magic and science is that in the former there is a lack of well-documented observations. (Unfortunately, one can still find in science observations that are not well documented.) Magic is the mistaken application of two fundamental laws of thought, the association of ideas by similarity and contiguity. Frazer in his original treatise says of these laws, "Legitimately applied they yield science, illegitimately applied they yield magic, the bastard sister of science." Thus if magical thinking utilizes the same structure as science, then continual magical thinking, in regard to medications whose actions are those of an inert placebo, is understandable.

Suggestion

Much of the placebo effect relies on straight suggestion. As mentioned earlier, if the suggestion of a specific response to a drug is made by someone in whom the patient has faith, he will respond appropriately. Many medications that owe their initial therapeutic effect to the fortuitous juxtaposition of medication and spontaneous change, continue to be therapeutic to some individuals by means of continued suggestion. If suggestion alone were the primary cause of placebo response, then it might be expected that those individuals who can be easily hypnotized would be more likely to be placebo responders than subjects who are difficult to hypnotize. Unfortunately, this is not the case. The phenomenon of hypnosis is not well understood, and purported tests of suggestability do not correlate with susceptability to hypnotic suggestion.

The role of the physician as an authority figure is most interesting. As mentioned previously, in a clinical study in which subjects (patients) were told they were being given placebos, there still was a placebo response. This was most surprising to the investigators. The subjects, when questioned, indicated that they knew what placebos were, but they did not believe that their "doctor" would really give them an inert substance.

Conditioning

Another model for explaining the placebo effect is the conditioning model. Probably both classical and instrumental conditioning play a role in the placebo response. Something akin to a placebo response has been seen in animals, and this response can only be attributed to conditioning, for it is unlikely that animals respond to suggestion. Although a type of behavior described as "superstitious" has been observed in subhuman species, it is unlikely that a placebo effect in animals could be attributed to this "superstitious" behavior. The type of placebo response that can be seen in animals is usually observed when a drug is repeatedly given by injection. The injection itself may be considered the conditional stimulus. The response to the drug itself is the unconditioned response. The administration of saline under these conditions often results in a response to saline that was not present before repeated administrations of the active drug were started. The argument for instrumental conditioning of the placebo response is probably applicable to the case of human subjects. Taking an active medication by means of the oral route can be considered the operant or instrumental response which leads to some reinforcement (e.g., the relief of a headache by aspirin). If a placebo were given instead of the aspirin, relief of the headache would be the conditioned response, and instrumental conditioning of the placebo effect would be demonstrated.

At our present stage of knowledge theories regarding the mechanism of action of placebos are, for the most part, conjectures, and, in fact, a specific placebo effect cannot be accurately predicted in an individual. However, many of the things that have been discussed do affect the potency of placebos. Thus in any large group of patients or subjects, variables can be manipulated that will increase the percent of subjects who will respond to a placebo. But, to accurately predict which subjects will and which will not respond is, at present, beyond our ability.

THE PLACEBO IN RESEARCH

At the present time it would be very difficult to have a clinical drug study published that did not use a placebo or some other equivalent control. In the absence of a placebo there are two types of control medications that might be acceptable: either an active control or a standard drug.

An *active control*, ideally, is a drug that has all of the pharmacological effects of the drug under study with the exception of the clinical activity desired. In practice, it is difficult to have the ideal active control; however, drugs that have at least some of the pharmacological activity of the compound under test have been used. Barbiturates have often been used as active control medications for clinical studies of the phenothiazines.

A *standard drug* is used for a control condition instead of a placebo in those clinical studies where there is already an effective drug and the investigator is trying to determine if a new drug is as good as, or better than, the standard. In these cases a placebo control cannot be used because it certainly could not be considered an ethical practice to withhold effective medication from a patient to test whether some new compound is clinically useful. The use of morphine as a standard for the comparison of new analgesics removes the investigator from the difficult position of not treating the often severe pain of the postoperative patient. Clinical researchers do have a problem, however, because at the present time the Food and Drug Administration of the U.S. Department of Health, Education, and Welfare requires that before a drug is approved for clinical use, it must be shown to be superior to a placebo. Simply showing that the drug is equal to or better than a standard is not sufficient. The argument for the necessity of a placebo control is that the sample selected for study may not respond to the standard, therefore, finding that the standard and the drug under study do not differ in efficacy could be misleading.

Implicit in the use of a placebo is the concept of the *single blind* experiment. In an experiment employing a single blind design, only the subject or patient is unaware that a placebo is being used. A more rigorous design is one that employs what is called the *double blind* procedure. In this type of design neither the experimenter nor the subject is aware when or if a placebo will be used. There are many variations of the degree of "blindness" involved in an experiment or clinical study.

The least blind of the double blind type of design is one in which the experimenters who made the various clinical measurements are not only aware that a placebo is being used in the experiment, but they know the number of times that the placebo will be used, they are aware of the "active" drugs that are being used, and they know that the placebos and "active" drugs are packaged in different forms. A double blind experiment of this type is almost as bad as having no controls in the experiment. It leads the nurses and physicians who make various types of clinical judgements to start guessing which medication is the placebo. Thus it is obvious that if at all possible, all medications should be packaged exactly alike, and all doses should have the same number of pills or capsules. If one knows the maximum dose that will be used this is fairly easy to do. Let us assume that the maximum number of capsules needed to provide the maximum dose of drug will be four. However, early in the experiment only one capsule of active drug will be needed; thus to provide four capsules at the start of the experiment, three capsules will be placebo and one capsule the active drug.

Often, in clinical studies, the physicians in charge of the patients do not wish to abdicate their control of the dosage level in treating a patient. For example, if the patient does not seem to respond to a dose of a drug and side effects are not present, the physician will often wish to increase the dose level. If considerable planning is done beforehand, a double blind experiment can be carried out giving the physician this type of control. The dose-effect curves of the drugs under study must be known to give the physician the flexibility he desires. For example, the physician in the study is instructed to start with two capsules every six hours, and at any time he deems it necessary, he may increase or decrease the dosage one capsule at a time. Thus not only may he increase or decrease the dosage of the active drug, but he will also be manipulating the "dose" of the placebo. In this type of design it is often necessary to set an upper limit on the total daily capsules that the physician may use with any patient. Although this design is a nightmare for the statistically inclined to analyze, its advantage is that it involves the physician much more than does a design where he has no control over the medication. In addition, this design more closely approximates the manner in which drugs are normally given in the clinical situation.

The need for properly designed double blind experiments is considerably greater when subjective ratings for clinical improvement or drug effects are being used. One is never sure what an objective measure is, but certainly the auscultation (by means of a blood pressure cuff) method of recording blood pressure cannot be considered an objective method. The need for a double blind procedure is most clearly shown in the almost apocryphal report of Stuart Wolf (1959):

"A patient who had chronic asthma for twenty-seven years had suffered almost continuous asthma for the past seventeen years. He had thus become a favorite subject on which to test new drugs. He had even become resistant to epinephrine. Finally the product of one pharmaceutical company seemed effective in his case. When he was given the agent, he was free of asthma; when it was then stopped, the asthma returned. Accordingly, the physician substituted a placebo without the patient's knowledge. Asthma was not relieved. Shifts from agent to placebo and back again were carried out several times with consistent results in favor of the agent. When the company was approached for additional supply of the material, their representative acknowledged that because they had had so much trouble with positive enthusiastic reports, they had, in this instance, sent the placebo first."

One of the problems confronting the clinical investigator who uses a placebo in a double-blind study is the possibility that the code will be revealed because of the relative lack of side effects with the placebo. Lasagna (1971) noted that only in the "perfect experiment," in which there were no drug effects other than the therapeutic effect of the experimental drug, would the double blind be "broken." He states that it is rare for a drug to cause side effects in all subjects and for the placebo not to cause side effects in some subjects. The presence of side effects is not necessarily correlated with a desired therapeutic effect.

One type of experimental approach that might circumvent the problem of easy identification of the placebo group in a clinical trial would be to start the intended placebo group on the putatively active drug, and after a number of days reduce the dose of the drug and substitute the placebo. Thus the control group always receives the same number of capsules as the experimental group, and at the beginning of the study, when the presence of side effects usually makes the identification of the experimental group relatively easy, both groups are treated identically. As far as I know this type of design has never been tried. It would be particularly useful for those drugs in which tolerance develops to many of the side effects. The disadvantage of this experimental design is that if the drug under study causes a significant clinical improvement within the first week of therapy, there would be no difference between the placebo group and the drug group. This lack of difference would make it impossible to make any statement concerning the placebo-drug treatment difference.

The question often arises when starting a clinical pharmacological study whether to use a dependent group (cross-over design) or an independent group design. In a cross-over design all subjects receive all treatments, whereas in an independent group design each group receives a different treatment. The difficulty with the dependent group design is that the assumption is made that subjects will return to their previous baseline levels when the first treatment ceases, so that the second treatment will be started on subjects who are clinically the same as when they were first treated. In most cases this assumption cannot be made. It is generally preferred that in clinical trials an independent group design be used. Further discussion of the problems of clinical trials can be found in *Principles and Problems in Establishing the Efficacy of Psychoactive Drugs,* edited by Levine, Schiele, and Bouthilet (1971).

REFERENCES

Beecher, H. K. *Measurement of Subjective Responses Quantative Effects of Drugs.* New York, Oxford University Press, 1969.

Beecher, H. K. Surgery as a placebo. *Journal of the American Medical Association,* **176,** 1961, 1102–1107.

British Medical Journal, Editorial, **66,** 1961, 44.

Fisher, S. The placebo reactor: Thesis, antithesis, synthesis, and hypothesis. *Diseases of the Nervous System,* **28,** 1967, 510–515.

Fisher, S. Nonspecific factors as determinants of behavioral response to drugs. In A. DiMascio, and R. I. Shader (Eds.) *Clinical Handbook of Psychopharmacology.* New York, Science House, 1970, pp. 17–39.

Frazer, J. G. *The New Golden Bough.* (Edited edition by T. H. Guster) New York, Criterion 1959.

Lasagna, L. Placebos. *Scientific American,* **193,** 1955, 68–71.

Lasagna, L., Laties, V. G., and Dohan, J. L. Further studies on the "pharmacology" of placebo administration. *Journal of Clinical Investigation,* **37,** 1958, 533–537.

Lasagna, L., Mosteller, F., von Felsinger, J. M., and Beecher, H. K. A study of the placebo response. *The American Journal of Medicine,* **16,** 1954, 770–779.

Levine, J., Schiele, B. C., and Bouthilet, L. *Principles and Problems in Establishing the Efficacy of Psychotropic Drugs.* U.S. Government Printing Office. Public Health Service Publication, No. 2138, Washington, D.C., 1971.

Modell, W. *The Relief of Symptoms.* Philadelphia, Sanders, 1955.

Shapiro, A. K. The placebo effect in the history of medical treatment: Implication for psychiatry. *The American Journal of Psychiatry,* **116,** 1959, 298–304.

Schindel, L. E. Placebo in theory and practice. *Antibiotica et Chemotherapia, Advances,* **10,** 1962, 398–430.

von Felsinger, J. M., Lasagna, L., and Beecher, H. K. Drug induced mood changes in man. II. Personality and reaction to drugs. *Journal of the American Medical Association,* **157,** 1955, 113–119.

Wolf, S. The pharmacology of placebos. *Pharmacological Reviews,* **11,** 1959, 689–704.

Wolf, S. and Pinsky, R. H. Effects of placebo administration and occurrence of toxic reactions. *Journal of the American Medical Association,* **155,** 1954, 339–341.

Young, J. H. *The Medical Messiahs.* Princeton, Princeton University Press, 1967.

3 THE AUTONOMIC NERVOUS SYSTEM AND AUTONOMIC DRUGS

In this chapter we review some of the anatomy and physiology of the autonomic nervous system as well as the pharmacology of those drugs whose action is primarily on this system. Although most clinical psychologists will have little contact with this class of compounds, an understanding of the autonomic nervous system and the drugs that act on it is important, since most of the agents used in the treatment of the mentally ill have actions involving the autonomic nervous system. These actions are usually considered side effects, and it is important to be able to recognize these.

The use of a term such as "autonomic drugs" incorrectly implies an isolation of the autonomic nervous system from the central nervous system and suggests that the drugs that affect the autonomic nervous system (ANS) do not have actions in the central nervous system (CNS) and vice versa. There are drugs that, as far as we know, only have action on the ANS, but it is unlikely that there is any CNS drug that does not affect the ANS. Although most of our knowledge concerning the transmission of nerve impulses has been obtained by the study of the ANS, it is reasonable to assume that within the CNS transmission is mediated in the same manner.

In this chapter we mainly discuss the autonomic nervous system; however, the autonomic nervous system cannot be discussed without some mention of the somatic nervous system or motor system (neuromuscular), which is the system concerned with voluntary control of skeletal muscles. The transmission of impulses in the somatic system is not fundamentally different from what is seen in the ANS. Those parts of the autonomic and somatic nervous system lying outside of the spinal cord are often referred to as the *peripheral nervous system*.

The Nerve Cell (Neuron)

The nerve cells are essentially different from other cells of the body because of two distinct characteristics. Nerve cells are capable of conducting bioelectric impulses over long distances without any loss in the strength of the impulse. They also have both specific input and output connections with other nerve cells and with effector organs, such as muscles and glands.

All nerve cells are made up of a nerve cell body in which there is a cell nucleus. Information from other nerve cells is transmitted to the cell body via dendrites. Information from the cell to dendrites of other neurons is by means of an axon which, in the case of a spinal motor neuron, can be as long as three feet, (See Figure 1).

The connection between the axon of one neuron and the dendrites of another is called the *synapse*. Thus impulses to the terminus of an axon are called *presynaptic*. There is actually a space between these two synapsing neurons that is called the *synaptic cleft*. A mass of synapsing neurons is called a *ganglion*. Impulses to a ganglion are called *preganglionic*, and those emanating from a ganglion are called *postganglionic*.

There are additional types of synapses, for example, axo-axonal, axo-somatic, dendro-dendritic; however, for the purpose of this text, the above definition will be sufficient for the understanding of the material that will be covered.

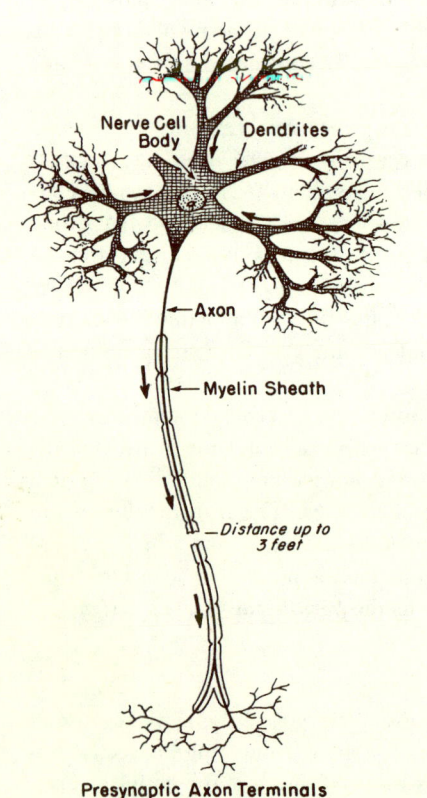

FIGURE 1. A representation of motor neuron with various parts indicated.

Synaptic Transmission

It is generally accepted that when a nerve cell is stimulated, endogenous chemical mediators are released into the synaptic cleft, and these activate the postsynaptic neuron. The theory of the transmission of nerve impulses mediated by the release of some chemical was not demonstrated experimentally until the classic experiments of Otto Loewi, published in 1921. Loewi, in his beautiful and simple experiment, found that if he stimulated the vagus nerve of a perfused frog heart, a substance was given off that slowed the heart rate of a second perfused heart that had no neural connection with the first (see Figure 2). This experiment clearly demonstrated the presence of a chemical transmitter of neural impulses. Loewi called this material "Vagusstoff." Subsequently, Loewi's "Vagusstoff" was identified as *acetylcholine*. He also observed opposite effects when a sympathetic nerve was stimulated.

About the same time that Loewi was doing his classic experiments, Cannon and Uridil, in 1921, observed that if a sympathetic nerve to the liver was stimulated, a substance was released that was similar to epinephrine. This substance was called *sympathin*. Subsequently, it was believed that this substance of Cannon and Uridil was *norepinephrine*.

These discoveries opened entirely new areas and avenues of approach to pharmacological problems and, for the most part, put to rest the idea that transmission of nerve impulses was electrical in nature. However, there is evidence for electrical synapses in some lower forms of animals, but it is clear that in mammals transmission of neural impulses is chemically mediated.

Many of the side effects seen with drugs are a function of their action on the ANS. Also, some discussion is in order concerning neural transmission and the role of chemical transmitters, since the nature of drug effects can only be understood with the transmitter concept in mind.

THE AUTONOMIC NERVOUS SYSTEM

The ANS has been called the "vegetative nervous system," "general visceral efferent system," and the "involuntary nervous system." These names reflect the functional role of the ANS, for it participates in the regulation of such vital functions as digestion, blood pressure, body temperature, sexual activity, and emotional behavior. Many of these functions are carried on continually without any conscious awareness, except when the system malfunctions.

The ANS is divided into two parts, the *sympathetic* and the *parasympathetic* nervous system. The sympathetic system is most manifest during stress situations or periods where additional energy is needed, although it functions continually in nonstress, day-to-day activities.

The main function of the sympathetic nervous system is to allow the

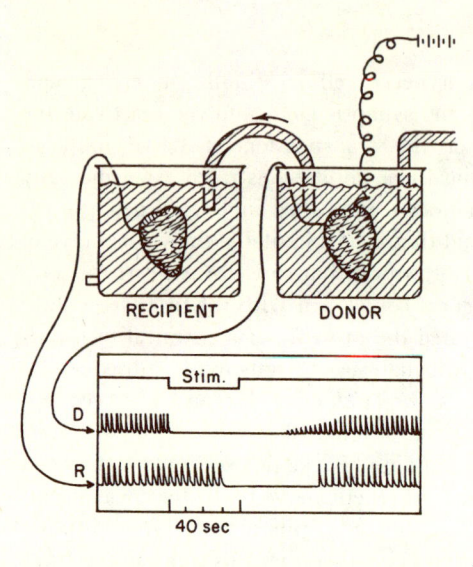

FIGURE 2. A schematic representation of Otto Loewi's classic experiment. When the vagus nerve of the donor heart is stimulated it causes a cessation in heart rate (D). The release of acetylcholine from the vagus nerve in the donor heart stimulates (by means of the bath) the recipient heart resulting in the cessation of heart rate in the recipient (R).

organism to meet emergency situations. Thus stimulation of the sympathetic system results in the expenditure of energy stores. Heart rate and blood presssure are increased. Blood flow is increased to those areas necessary for "fight or flight," in other words, the voluntary muscles. This is done at the expense of blood flow to the viscera and skin.

It is often stated that the parasympathetic system works antagonistically to the sympathetic system. This is not exactly true. They act in a more complementary fashion. For example, during stress the activity of the parasympathetic system decreases, allowing for a sympathetic dominance.

The parasympathetic system stimulates those systems associated with the restoration of the vegetative body functions. It restores energy stores to those organs necessary for the maintenance of life. It decreases heart rate and blood pressure and increases activities of the digestive system.

Although the parasympathetic nervous system is essential for life, this is not true of the sympathetic nervous system. Animals deprived of a sympathetic nervous system or an adrenal medulla (the central part of the adrenal gland that secretes epinephrine) can experience a relatively normal existence if the environment is not too stressful. However, they cannot respond properly to stress. Their body temperature does not adjust to heat or cold, nor does their blood pressure or heart rate increase under stress.

Anatomy and Physiology

The effector cells of the autonomic nervous system are innervated by a 2-neuron chain. The preganglionic neuron has its cell body within the CNS,

THE AUTONOMIC NERVOUS SYSTEM

whereas the postganglionic neuron has its cell body outside the CNS. The axon of the preganglionic neuron is lightly myelinated; however, those of the postganglionic neuron are unmyelinated. Each preganglionic neuron has an axon that terminates and synapses with postganglionic neurons. In the sympathetic nervous system the axons of the preganglionic neurons are relatively short with long axons proceeding from the postganglionic neurons. The opposite holds true in the parasympathetic system, with the preganglionic neuron synapsing close to, or even in, the effector organ.

The axon of the postganglionic neuron innervates three types of effector cells: smooth muscle cells (involuntary muscles), cardiac muscle cells, and glandular secretory cells. It is believed that the neurotransmitter substance diffuses from the axons and acts on more than one effector cell.

The neurotransmitter released by the preganglionic neuron is always acetylcholine (ACh), whether the system is sympathetic or parasympathetic. The neurotransmitter released by the postganglionic neuron is norepinephrine (NE) in the sympathetic system and ACh in the parasympathetic system. An exception to this is the release of ACh at the postganglionic synapse, innervating the sweat glands when the sympathetic system is stimulated. However, there is also adrenergic sweating from the palms, soles of the feet, and axillae during periods of stress. Adrenergic sweating is not due to NE release at the effector organ but is believed to be the result of the direct effect of circulatory epinephrine on the sweat glands of these areas (Koizumi and Brooks, 1974, p. 789).

The sympathetic and parasympathetic systems differ in the areas in which the preganglionic fibers emerge from the spinal cord. The former axons emerge from the spinal cord via the motor roots of all the thoracic and the two upper lumbar spinal nerves; however, in the parasympathetic system the preganglionic axons emerge from the spinal cord via the cranial nerves from the brain stem or from the spinal cord via the second through fourth sacral spinal nerves.

Because of these differences in emergence from the CNS, the sympathetic system is often called the *thoracolumbar* system, and the parasympathetic system is called the *craniosacral* system (see Figures 3 and 4).

The organs of the body are generally innervated by both the sympathetic and parasympathetic systems. Exceptions are the sweat glands, the pilomotor muscles of the skin, and the adrenal gland. Table 1 summarizes the effects of the autonomic system on various organ systems.

The Transmitter and Pharmacological Agents

As described in the previous section, transmission in the ANS is mediated by ACh at the preganglionic nerve endings in both the sympathetic and the parasympathetic nervous systems and at the postganglionic nerve endings in

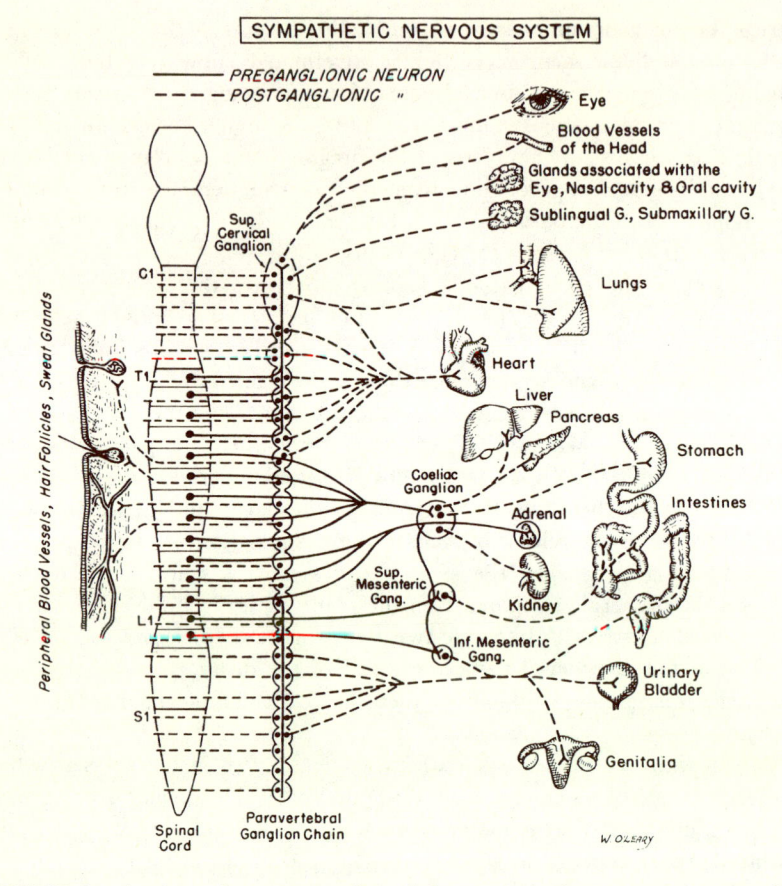

FIGURE 3. A schematic representation of the sympathetic nervous system and the organs inervated.

the parasympathetic system. This release of ACh from some fibers and NE from others led to the classification of nerves as *cholinergic* or *adrenergic,* respectively.

The term cholinergic comes from the name of the transmitter substance acetyl*choline,* and the term adrenergic comes from the name of the substance *adrenaline* (an older name for epinephrine, still used in the United Kingdom), which mimics many of the effects of NE. Thus drugs that cause the release of or mimic the effects of ACh are referred to as *cholinergic,* and those that cause the release of or mimic the effects of NE are referred to as *adrenergic.*

In addition to cholinergic and adrenergic agonists, there are two classes of compounds that act as specific blocking agents (antagonists). These are called cholinergic blockers or *anticholinergics* and adrenergic blockers or *antiadre-*

THE AUTONOMIC NERVOUS SYSTEM 51

nergics. Most drugs can be classified into one of these four types based on their actions on the ANS. Cholinergic drugs are also called *parasympathomimetic*, and adrenergic drugs are also called *sympathomimetic*. Thus if one knows whether a drug has cholinergic or adrenergic effects, one can immediately attribute many actions to it as well as have some understanding of the types of side effects the drug will cause. This does not mean that because a drug has

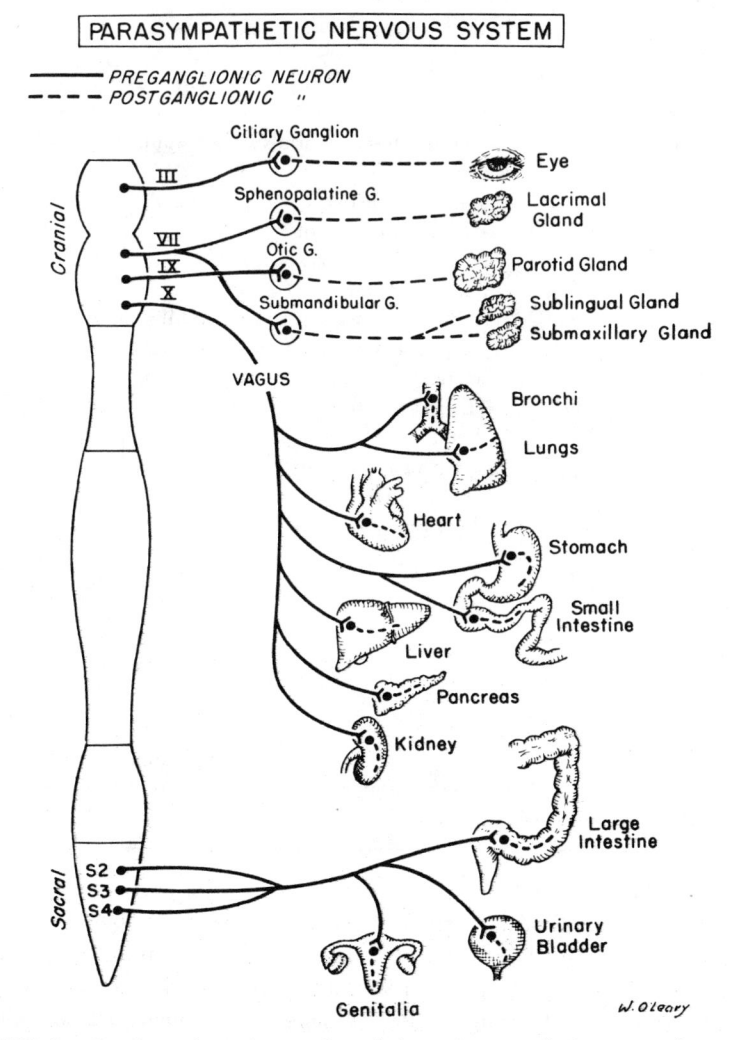

FIGURE 4. A schematic representation of the parasympathetic nervous system and the organs inervated. Note that the post synapatic neuron is often in the effector organ.

TABLE 1. RESPONSES OF EFFECTOR ORGANS TO AUTONOMIC NERVE STIMULATION

	Parasympathetic	Sympathetic
Lungs	Constriction of bronchi and bronchioles (respiration per se is controlled by the somatic NS) Increase in glandular secretion of these tubes	Dilation of bronchi and bronchioles
Digestive system	Increase in contractility, motility, and tone of digestive tract; peristalsis Relaxation of muscle sphincters (between stomach and intestine, small and large bowel, and at the anus) Increase in the secretion of the digestive glands such as the pancreas All these are directed to the digestion of food	Decrease in contractility and tone, constriction of sphincter muscles Inhibition of the secretions Increase in glucose in blood stream
Genital system	Engorgement of erectile tissue, active secretion of the accessory glands	Ejaculation of the semen by involuntary muscles of genital glands and ducts accompanied by somatic nerve stimulation of the voluntary muscles Except for the blood vessels, the ovary, testes, and uterus do not respond to autonomic stimulation
Eye and lacrimal gland	Miosis of pupil, secretion of tears	Mydriasis of pupil

adrenergic effects, all of the actions of NE will be seen, but it does tell us what effects can be attributed to the normal spectrum of actions of the drug.

ACh is also the neurotransmitter substance in the somatic, voluntary nervous system. In this system the motor fibers synapse in the spinal cord and not again until they reach the effector organs, the skeletal muscles. In the brain ACh and NE play a role in synaptic transmission; however, the exact role has not been

TABLE 1. (Continued)

	Parasympathetic	Sympathetic
Glands of nose, mouth, including salivary glands	Vasodilation, secretion of profuse watery secretion	Diminution of blood flow to glands and sparse, thick, viscous mucous secretion
Heart	Bradycardia. Decrease in blood volume expelled with each stroke and probably the constriction of the coronary arteries (arteries supply the heart muscle)	Tachycardia. Increase in blood volume. Dilation of coronary arteries
Blood vessels	Dilation of blood vessels to the digestive system. Dilation of blood vessels to the glands in the head, face (blushing). Erectile tissues of genital system	Dilation of coronary arteries, arteries of the voluntary muscles; constriction of vessels to lungs, digestive system, & skin
Sweat glands		Secretion (postganglionic transmitter is ACh, control of body temperature; adrenergic sweating due to circulatory epinephrine effects on the palms, soles, and axillae)
Pilomotor (hair) muscles of the skin		Contraction (goose pimples and piloerection)
Adrenal glands		Secretes epinephrine and norepinephrine (controlled by preganglionic cholinergic fibers of sympathetic system)

fully elucidated. In addition to ACh and NE, there are other putative neurotransmitter substances or neurohumors in the brain that play an important role in the mediation of behavior. These are discussed in Chapter 4.

Synaptic transmission of impulses involves a number of steps, and each of the steps is a potential site of drug action. When a natural impulse or an imposed experimental stimulus results in a depolarization above the threshold for a response, an action potential is generated. This action potential moves unattenuated to the nerve terminal at the end of the axon. This causes a release of the specific transmitter substance for the particular nerve cell. The transmitter substance must first be available for release, so a continual process of synthesis and storage must be maintained. When the transmitter is released by the changes in the electrical potential of the axon, it diffuses across the synaptic cleft. This results in a depolarization of the postsynaptic membrane which causes a change in the ionic balance along the length of the postsynaptic fiber and results in propagation of the impulse. In addition, there are inhibitory synapses in which the transmitter causes hyperpolarization, decreasing the probability of stimulus propagation. This depends on the nature of the receptor for the particular transmitter substance.

The transmitter substance is destroyed by enzymatic action in the case of ACh. This allows for the repeated stimulation of the nerve. With the destruction of the transmitter substance, there is repolarization of the postsynaptic membrane. At the cholinergic fibers the enzyme is *acetylcholinesterase* (AChE). The primary mechanism by which NE is inactivated is reuptake into the presynaptic terminal. Enzymes that are present in the presynaptic terminal and the synaptic cleft contribute to the metabolic inactivation of NE. Diffusion may also account for some of the termination of the action of ACh and NE at some synapses. Not only may cholinergic and adrenergic drugs cause their effects any place in the chain of neural transmission, but blocking agents may also interrupt any of the steps in the process.

Cholinergic Receptors

As previously mentioned, the preganglionic fibers in both the parasympathetic and the sympathetic parts of the ANS are cholinergic; that is, at the ganglion they release ACh. The somatic system is also cholinergic in that the transmitter released at the motor endplate is also ACh. This is schematically illustrated in Figure 5.

Research with the use of agents that mimic or antagonize some of the parasympathetic and sympathetic activity led to the concept of at least three different specific receptors for ACh. These receptors have been called *muscarinic* and *nicotinic,* and there are two separate nicotinic receptors. The naturally occurring alkaloid, muscarine, was found to mimic the action of ACh on smooth muscle, cardiac muscle, and exocrine glands (those glands that do not secrete their products in the blood stream). These actions are blocked by atropine or scopolamine without blocking ACh release in the preganglionic fiber or at the motor endplate.

When nicotine is administered, it first stimulates and then depresses the transmission at the ganglion and at the motor endplate in the somatic system.

THE AUTONOMIC NERVOUS SYSTEM

The nicotinic effect at the ganglion is selectively blocked by the drug hexamethonium, whereas the neuromuscular effects are blocked by d-tubocurarine (active component of curare) and decamethonium.

The site of action of these three types of blocking agents as well as the action of muscarine and nicotine are indicated in Figure 5. It must be remembered that there are many other blocking agents that have similar actions to those mentioned. Although the classification of cholinergic effects as muscarinic or ni-

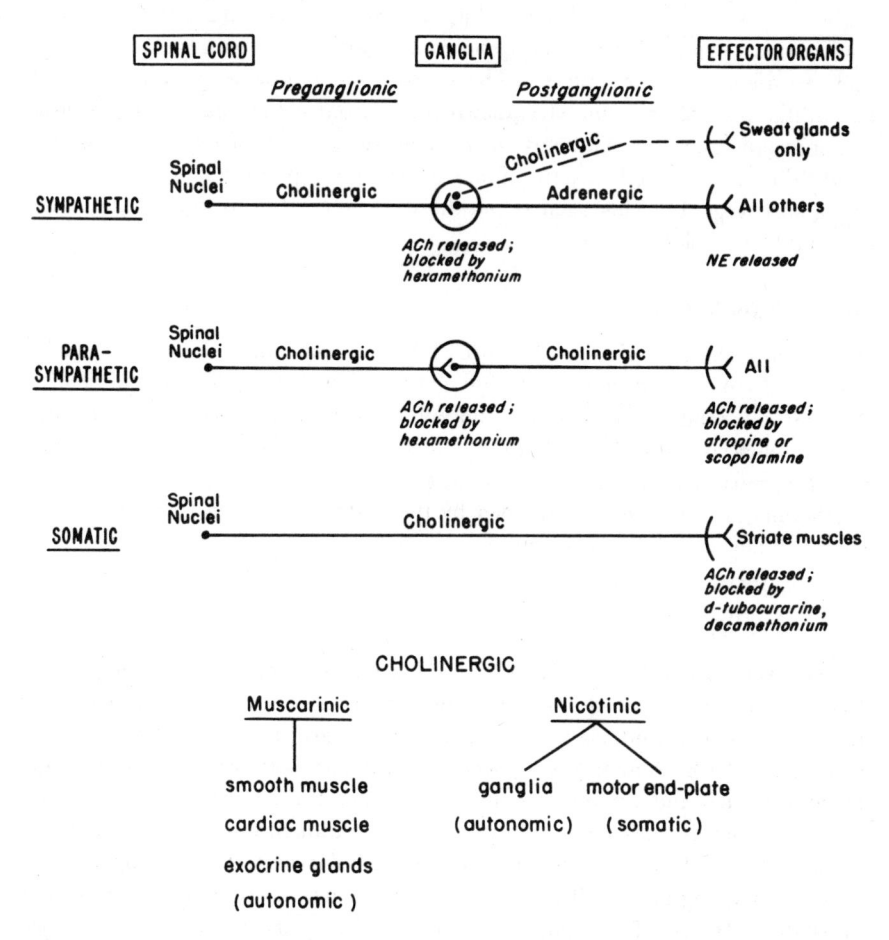

FIGURE 5. A schematic representation of the transmitter substances in the peripheral nervous system. Indicated are the presynaptic and postsynaptic transmitter substances released—the site of blockade of acetylcholine and the blocking substances. The bottom of the figure indicates which end organs are selectively blocked by either muscarinic (atropinic) or nicotinic agents.

cotinic has been used since the early part of this century, there are many aspects of cholinergic transmission that are not explained by the presence of muscarinic or nicotinic receptors alone. However, it provides a useful and common way to classify many drugs.

Adrenergic Receptors

The adrenergic system is also divided into types of receptors. These are called *alpha* and *beta* receptors. The stimulation of an alpha receptor results in vasoconstriction, pupillary dilitation, and contraction of the nictating membrane and the splenic capsule (spleen). The stimulation of a beta receptor results in vasodilitation in skeletal muscles, tachycardia, bronchial relaxation, and a positive inotropic effect on the heart (increasing the strength of muscular contraction). The drugs that block the alpha adrenergic type of response are called alpha adrenergic blocking agents, and those that block beta responses are called beta adrenergic blocking agents.

Cholinergic Drugs

ACh itself is not a useful drug because of its very brief duration of action which is caused by its almost immediate destruction by the enzymatic action of AChE. Also, ACh is relatively nonspecific and will cause both muscarinic and nicotonic effects, whereas most of the cholinergic drugs used clinically have a specificity for either muscarinic or nicotinic receptors.

Cholinergic drugs may be divided by the manner in which they cause their effects. They are either resistant to the enzymatic action of AChE or they produce their effects by the inhibition of AChE. These latter are called *cholinesterase* inhibitors.

Direct Action Cholinergic Drugs—Muscarinic. The pharmacological effects of the muscarinic cholinergic drugs are those seen when the parasympathetic system is stimulated. Most of these drugs are resistant to the enzymatic actions of AChE. Among their effects are a fall in both systolic and diastolic blood pressure and an increase in skin temperature, often accompanied by flushing which is most noticeable in the face. Although muscarinic agents will cause a drop in heart rate, this may be masked or reversed by a compensatory reflex responding to the fall in blood pressure. There is an increase in tone and peristaltic activity of the gastrointestinal and urinary tract that can cause cramps, defecation, and micturition. Gastric secretions are increased. Pupils are constricted. The exocrine glands are stimulated, and an increase in salivation is seen. Since the sweat glands of the sympathetic system are innervated by cholinergic fibers, there will be an increase in sweating. There may be feelings of bronchial constriction due to action on the smooth muscle of the bronchi plus the increase in bronchial secretions.

Among the therapeutic drugs of this class are a number of synthetic analogues of ACh. The most common are methacholine, carbachol, and bethanecol. These synthetic analogues have been used in the treatment of a variety of peripheral vascular and other diseases, although their use today is not common. Some have been used in various diagnostic procedures.

In addition to the synthetic analogues, there are a number of naturally occurring alkaloids (a complex organic molecule containing nitrogen) with muscarinic actions. The one that we have already discussed is muscarine itself. Muscarine is found naturally in certain mushrooms that cause severe poisoning if eaten. The most common is *Amanita muscaria*.

Arecoline is a muscarinic alkaloid found in the *Areca catechu* (betel nut). Its main use is in veterinary medicine where its peristaltic action on the gastrointestinal tract is used as a vermifuge (antihelminthic, an agent that expels intestinal worms or other parasites).

The only naturally occurring alkaloid with muscarinic properties that is used therapeutically is pilocarpine. Its use is primarily in ophthalmological preparations for causing miosis and reducing intraocular pressure in glaucoma by local administration to the conjunctival sac.

Cholinesterase Inhibitors. This group of drugs causes an increase in ACh at the receptor by inhibiting the enzymatic destruction of the transmitter. These inhibitors will have actions at any site in which ACh is the transmitter.

There are two types of cholinesterase inhibitors, reversible and irreversible. The most commonly used reversible inhibitors are *physostigmine* and *neostigmine*. Like pilocarpine, they are used in ophthalmological preparations. Neostigmine, in addition to the muscarinic effects, has nicotinic effects believed to be a direct action on the neuromuscular junction. Because of this latter action, it has been used for the treatment of *myasthenia gravis*. Myasthenia gravis is a chronic disease characterized by muscle weakness and is believed to be due to a disturbance of neuromuscular transmission. Although the exact cause of the disease is unknown, patients do respond to treatment with neostigmine.

The irreversible cholinesterase inhibitors are the *organophosphate anticholinesterases*. They were originally developed as potential chemical warfare agents, but their main use has been in insecticides. Because of the widespread use of these compounds in insecticides, they pose a major problem of toxicology. The duration of effect of organophosphates may be from a few weeks to a few months.

In addition to effects on the ANS and neuromuscular transmission, the cholinesterase inhibitors will cause central effects. In sufficient doses a variety of actions are seen. These are characterized by excitation followed by depression, disturbances in sleep, tremor and ataxia, hallucinations, and EEG desynchronization. Death from an overdose is usually caused by respiratory paralysis.

Cholinergic Blocking Agents

There are three types of cholinergic blocking agents: those drugs that block the muscarinic actions, those that have ganglionic blocking actions, and the neuromuscular blocking agents. As previously described, the muscarinic actions are postganglionic and parasympathetic. The ganglionic blocking agents block the transmission of ACh at the ganglia and may affect either parasympathetic or sympathetic systems. The neuromuscular blocking agents interfere with the transmission of impulses in the somatic nervous system.

Although ganglionic blocking agents and neuromuscular blocking agents are of great importance in pharmacology and medicine, they are of little importance to the behavioral scientist. However, the muscarinic anticholinergic drugs are of importance to the behavioral scientist both because of extensive study of their central effect on behavior and because of their marked actions on the parasympathetic branch of the autonomic nervous system.

The atropine type of cholinergic blocking agents antagonize the muscarinic actions of ACh as well as various parasympathomimetic agents. This action is postsynaptic; these drugs do not antagonize the release of ACh at the autonomic ganglia or the neuromuscular junction. In addition to the blocking of the parasympathetic system, some of these drugs have marked effects in the CNS.

The two most common agents of this class are *atropine* and *scopolamine*. Atropine is an alkaloid and is found in the following plants: Atropa belladonna (nightshade), Hyoscyamus niger (henbane), and Datura stramonium (jimson weed). These plants have been used for medicinal purposes for thousands of years. The active principal in these natural products is *l*-hyoscyamine and *l*-hyoscine (scopolamine).

There are a number of synthetic anticholinergic drugs of this type. Many drugs with potent anticholinergic actions in the peripheral nervous system do not readily pass the blood brain barrier, and thus there is little penetration of the drug into the brain. However, some anticholinergic agents such as atropine and scopolamine readily penetrate the brain, and, at the same time, they have marked autonomic nervous system activity. Carlton (1962; 1963), among others, has done extensive studies on the behavioral effects of atropine and scopolamine. To determine whether the observed behavioral effects seen after atropine administration were due to a central or a peripheral action of the drug, he made use of methylatropine, which seems to have activity only in the

THE AUTONOMIC NERVOUS SYSTEM

peripheral nervous system. Since methylatropine did not cause the alteration in behavior observed with atropine, he concluded that the behavioral effects obtained with atropine were of central nervous system origin.

Atropine and related compounds are competitive antagonists of ACh and other parasympathomimetic agents. Since they compete for the same receptors as ACh, the action of ACh is blocked.

These drugs are used topically to produce mydriasis in opthalmological examinations. Various natural belladonna alkaloids and synthetic preparations have been used in gastrointestinal disorders because they decrease gastric secretion and have antispasmodic actions.

Atropine and scopolamine have CNS effects. Atropine, at clinical doses, has slight stimulating actions, whereas scopolamine will cause some sedation. Atropine poisoning may cause increased motor activity, irritability, and hallucinations. Both atropine and scopolamine have been useful in the treatment of parkinsonism. The mechanism involved is not known. Some of these agents are routinely administered to block the parkinson-like side effects often seen with phenothiazine drugs (antipsychotic drugs).

These belladonna alkaloids are often used for preanesthetic medication to reduce salivation and respiratory tract secretions that might obstruct the airway. The common parasympatholytic (anticholineric) effects seen with these agents are dryness of the mouth, inhibition of sweating, blurred vision, tachycardia, and constipation.

Adrenergic Drugs (Sympathomimetic)

Most sympathetic neurons produce their effects by the release of NE. Epinephrine, which is released from the adrenal medulla during sympathetic stimulation, is the emergency hormone of this system. As can be seen in Figure 3, the adrenal gland itself is a ganglion in the sympathetic system. The preganglionic transmitter is ACh. When the adrenal medulla is stimulated by the preganglionic fibers, it secretes epinephrine (and some norepinephrine) directly into the blood stream. There are no postganglionic fibers coming from the adrenal gland. Those drugs that effect the same receptors as NE and epinephrine are called adrenergic or sympathomimetic drugs. Because of their chemical structure, both epinephrine and NE are *catecholamines*. The catecholamines, which include *dopamine,* have been implicated in various biochemical theories of both depression and schizophrenia (see Chapters 4, 5, and 6).

The basic structural formula for the catecholamines, NE, and epinephrine is given in Figure 6. Note that they differ only slightly with a methyl group present on the nitrogen in epinephrine. This slight chemical difference makes for marked changes in pharmacological activity.

The most common sympathomimetic drugs, in addition to epinephrine and

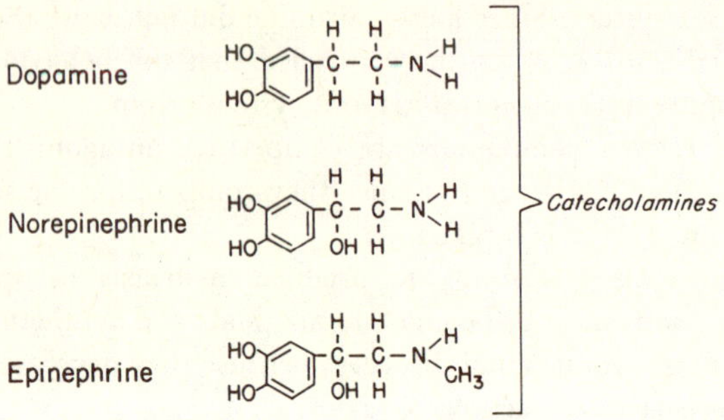

Dopamine

Norepinephrine

Epinephrine

⎫
⎬ Catecholamines
⎭

FIGURE 6. The catecholamines.

NE (levarterenol), are isopropylnorepinephrine (isoproterenol), ephedrine, and the amphetamines. However, ephedrine and amphetamine are not catecholamines. Epinephrine, NE, and isoproterenol differ chemically only with regard to substituents on the nitrogen atom.

The catecholamines combine directly with postganglionic adrenergic receptors to produce their effects. Whereas ephedrine and amphetamine may have direct effects, they also cause release of norepinephrine or epinephrine from the postganglionic neurons and the adrenal medulla. Because of the importance of amphetamine and amphetamine-like compounds in the treatment of hyperkinetic children, and because these compounds are widely abused, they will be discussed in separate chapters (see Chapters 10 and 13).

Sympathomimetic drugs can be categorized on the basis of their actions on either alpha or beta receptors. As previously mentioned, alpha receptors are generally involved with excitation of smooth muscle, however, beta receptors are associated with relaxation of smooth muscle as well as causing an increase in rate and strength of cardiac contraction.

Epinephrine. The official British name for epinephrine is *adrenaline*. It is also sold in this country under the trade name Adrenalin.

Epinephrine possesses both alpha- and beta-stimulating properties. It is found predominantly in the adrenal medulla. The actions of epinephrine are those of sympathetic nervous system stimulation. Subjectively feelings of apprehension, restlessness, and anxiety are quite common. It is used in the treatment of severe bronchial asthma because of its marked bronchodilator action, and it is also the drug of choice in serious allergic reactions, for example, anaphylactic responses to drugs, foods, or insect bites.

Epinephrine is frequently combined with local anesthetics because of its vasoconstrictor action. This decreases the speed of absorption of the local anesthetic into the general system and hence increases the duration of local action of the anesthetic and decreases its systemic toxicity. In cardiac arrest epinephrine is used in direct intracardiac injections.

THE AUTONOMIC NERVOUS SYSTEM

Since epinephrine is destroyed in the gastrointestinal tract, it is not given orally. It is usually administered parenterally, or in the case of bronchial asthma, a nebulizer (a device that delivers the drug in a fine aerosol mist) is used.

Norepinephrine (Noradrenaline, Levarterenol). NE primarily stimulates alpha receptors. It causes an increase in blood pressure as a result of an increase in peripheral resistence in the blood vessels. Clinically, it has been used in myocardial infarction to increase the blood pressure without directly stimulating the heart.

Isoproterenol (Isopropylarterenol, Isopropylnorepinephrine). This drug acts predominantly on beta receptors. Its main use is in the management of bronchial asthma and as a cardiac stimulant. It does the latter at the same time it dilates the blood vessels.

Ephedrine. The actions are quite similar to those of amphetamine (Chapter 10) with a predominance of alpha adrenergic stimulation. The primary use is in the treatment of various allergic disorders because of its decongesting (alpha stimulation) and bronchial dilating (beta stimulation) properties and more persistent duration of action than epinephrine.

Adrenergic Blocking Agents

These are drugs that block the effects of various sympathomimetic amines. Drugs that antagonize the effects of adrenergic drugs by mechanisms other than by blocking at the adrenergic receptor are not considered adrenergic blocking agents. Barbiturates will counteract the central effects of amphetamines; this is not considered to be pharmacological antagonism but simply physiological antagonism (see Chapter 1).

There are two types of adrenergic blocking agents, the alpha adrenergic blocking agents and the beta adrenergic blocking agents. The former prevent vasoconstriction and other contraction of smooth muscle caused by sympathetic drugs; the latter block the cardiac and bronchodilation effects of the sympathomimetic drugs.

These drugs have been most important as research tools in pharmacology. However, the ergot alkaloids and propranolol are of some interest to the behavioral scientist.

Ergot Alkaloids. Among the ergot alkaloids is lysergic acid diethylamide which is discussed in Chapter 12. In addition to their adrenergic blocking properties, the ergot alkaloids directly cause smooth muscle contraction, particularly in the blood vessels and uterus. The two ergot alkaloids most commonly used are *ergonovine maleate,* used primarily as a uterine stimulant in obstetrics, and *ergotamine tartrate,* used in the treatment of migraine.

Propranolol (Inderal®). Propranolol is a beta adrenergic blocking agent that is used therapeutically for the treatment of certain types of cardiac arrhythmias, angina pectoris, and hypertension. Currently it is being tested as a possible antianxiety drug. It is not clear whether or not this putative antianxiety action is a central effect of propranolol or merely a blocking of the peripheral autonomic manifestations of anxiety.

SUMMARY

Although most of the field of psychopharmacology is not primarily concerned with the various autonomic actions of drugs, an understanding of at least the basic concepts is necessary to make some sense out of the variety of side effects produced by psychoactive drugs. In addition, psychologists concerned with the field of psychosomatic medicine or the conditioning of autonomic responses or those who use any autonomic response as a dependent variable in an experiment, should be most familiar with this area. Knowledge of the ANS is necessary not only because it enables one to better understand the actions observed, but also because many of the so-called autonomic drugs can be used as tools in the design of specific experiments

REFERENCES

Cannon, W. B. and Uridil, J. E. Studies on the conditions of activity in endocrine glands. VIII. Some effects on the denervated heart of stimulating the nerves of the liver. *American Journal of Physiology*, **50**, 1921, 353–354.

Carlton, P. L. Some behavioral effects of atropine and methyl atropine. *Psychological Reports*, **10**, 1962, 579–589.

Carlton, P. L. Cholinergic mechanisms in control of behavior by the brain. *Psychological Review*, **70**, 1963, 19–39.

Goth, A. *Medical Pharmacology, Principles and Concepts.* (6th ed.). Saint Louis, Mosby, 1972, pp. 52–152.

Koelle, G. B. Neurohumoral transmission and the autonomic nervous system. In L. S. Goodman and A. Gilman (Eds.) *Pharmacological Basis of Therapeutics.* (4th ed.). New York, Macmillan, 1970, pp. 402–441.

Koizumi, K. and Brooks, C. McC. The autonomic nervous system and its role in controlling visceral activities. In V. B. Mountcastle (Ed.) *Medical Physiology*, Vol. *1*. (13th ed.). Saint Louis, Mosby, 1974, pp. 783–812.

Loewi, O. Ueber humoral uebertragbarkeit der herznervenwirkung. I. Mitteilung. Pflugers Archiv fur die Gesamte Physiologie, *189*, 1921, 239–242. Summarized in Holmstedt and Liljestrand (Eds.). *Readings in Pharmacology.* Oxford, Pergamon, 1963, pp. 190–196.

Loewi, O. Op. cit., II. Mitteilung. Pflugers Archiv fur die Gesamte Physiologie, *193*, 1921, 201–213. Op cit.

Noback, C. R. *The Human Nervous System.* New York, McGraw-Hill, 1967, pp. 105–116.

4 NEUROPHYSIOLOGY AND BIOCHEMISTRY OF THE CENTRAL NERVOUS SYSTEM

The present chapter makes no attempt to be complete. Its purpose is to give the reader some background information that will be helpful in understanding the subsequent chapters in this book.

NEUROPHYSIOLOGY

In this section we briefly review some of the anatomy and physiology of the brain that will be helpful to the reader in understanding the subsequent discussion of centrally acting drugs. There is no attempt to make this a comprehensive review, and the reader is so cautioned. Emphasis is placed on the arousal system and those parts of the brain subserving emotion. No attempt is made to cover those areas of the brain having to do with higher cognitive processes or to trace the motor and sensory pathways. For these purposes I suggest Sidman and Sidman (1965), a programmed text of neuroanatomy, and the *Foundations of Physiological Psychology* by Thompson (1967), a most readable text on physiological psychology. For an encyclopedic review of the relationship between the CNS and behavior, I suggest Grossman (1967).

Localization

There are a number of terms that are used to describe the location of structures within the brain. Some confusion arises because the terms used are based on a four-legged animal in which the top of the head is a continuous extension of the animal's back. However, in man the top of the head is at a right angle to his back. To avoid confusion (at least to some), anatomists have placed a figurative right angle bend in the human brain that puts him on the same level as his animal cousins. Figure 1 schematically shows the representation of a rat and a human brain. The head end is called *anterior, rostral,* or *cephalic,* and the tail end is referred to as *posterior* or *caudal.* The top and bottom are referred to as *dorsal* and *ventral,* respectively.

Brains are usually sectioned along one of three planes. A vertical section

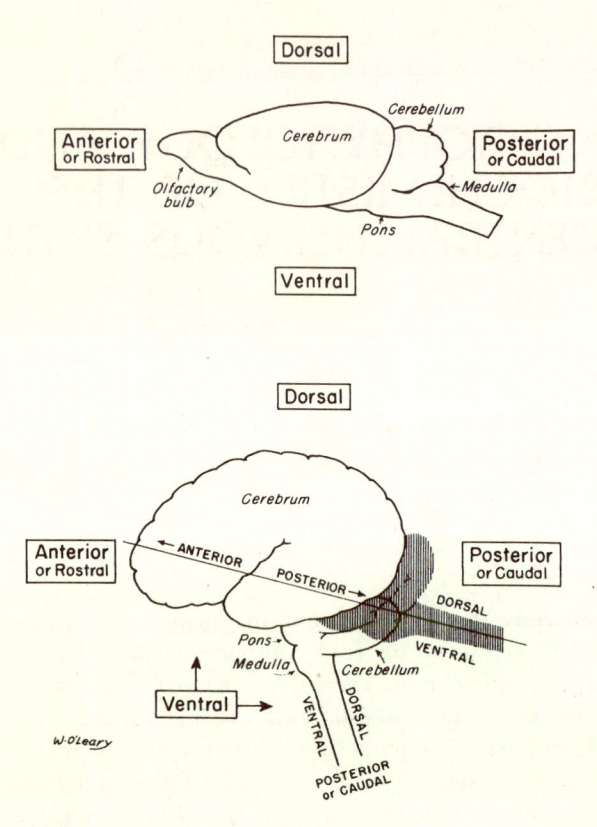

FIGURE 1. Representation of rat brain (top) and human brain (bottom) with terms used to indicate anatomical position or orientation. The human brain is reproduced with its normal bend at the level of the pons and also oriented in the same manner as the brains of lower animals (shaded portion). This allows the proper identification of the anterior-posterior poles and the dorsal-ventral surfaces.

along a rostral-caudal axis is called a *sagittal* section. A horizontal section along the same axis is called a *horizontal* section, and a section at right angles to the rostral-caudal axis is called a *coronal* section.

Anatomy

The brain may be roughly divided into five subdivisions. The names of these divisions are derived from embryological terminology. They are the *telencephalon, diencephalon, mesencephalon, metencephalon,* and the *myelencephalon*. These, along with their major components, are shown in the schematic, Figure 2.

Telencephalon. The telencephalon (the "end brain") is the part of the brain that is most developed in the higher mammals. This most rostral section of the brain includes the *cerebral hemispheres* or *neocortex*, the *olfactory bulb*, and a cell mass called the *basal ganglia*. The term, basal ganglia, usually refers to three structures: the *caudate nucleus*, the *putamen*, and the *globus pallidus*.

The cerebral hemispheres are functionally divided into the primary-sensory cortex and the motor cortex. These areas of the brain are the ultimate link of the brain with the outside world. Lesions in these areas can specifically disrupt or impair either the input of sensory information from various sensory modalities or inhibit the control of specific motor movements. The neocortex also contains the *association cortex*. As the name implies, the association cortex is concerned with the integration and elaboration of intracortical events. It is believed to be primarily involved in the development of higher behavioral functions.

The basal ganglia are the main anatomical substrate of the *extrapyramidal* system. The extrapyramidal system is to the motor system (pyramidal system) what a thermostat is to a heating system. It acts as a control system for the pyramidal system. It allows us to make fine, discrete motor movements. An example of dysfunction of the extrapyramidal system is seen in the neurological disease, parkinsonism. People suffering from this disease have an intact motor system, but there is lack of control of coordinated and fine motor movements. The extrapyramidal system is important in psychopharmacology, for parkinson-like symptoms are one of the most common side effects of antipsychotic drugs.

Diencephalon. From rostral to caudal the diencephalon is the next major

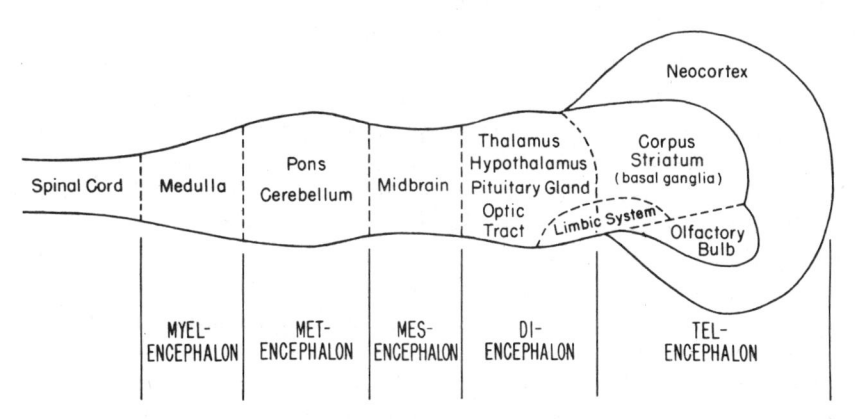

FIGURE 2. A schematic representation of mammalian brain indicating the various major subdivisions and some of their components.

subdivision of the brain. It is composed of the *hypothalamus,* the *thalamus,* and structures associated with the *limbic system.* Among the structures of the limbic system are included the *amygdala,* the *hippocampus,* and the *septum.* Other limbic structures are to be found in the telencephalon.

The diencephalon is directly involved with drive states and emotion. Lesions and/or stimulation to these areas will have marked effects on eating, drinking, sexual, and aggressive behavior. The diencephalon, along with the telencephalon, is often called the *forebrain.*

Mesencephalon. This area of the brain is also referred to as the *midbrain.* It includes the superior and inferior *colliculi,* nuclei involved in vision and audition, respectively. A major portion of the reticular formation lies in the mesencephalon.

Metencephalon and Myelencephalon. These last two areas of the brain are often called the *hindbrain,* and the mesencephalon, along with the structures of the hindbrain, is often referred to as the *brain stem.*

The metencephalon includes the *pons* and the *cerebellum.* The myelencephalon is the *medulla oblongata.* Most cranial nerves either enter or exit the central nervous system via this area.

Neuropsychology

Reticular Formation. Anatomically, the reticular formation is a net of cell bodies, fibers, and nuclei that extend from the spinal cord to the thalamus. It occupies a somewhat ventral position in the brain stem. The term *ascending reticular activating system* (ARAS) is often used in reference to these structures. It is a more functional designation that takes into account a major influence of the reticular formation on the cortex and the concomitant behavioral effects of activity within this system.

It is believed that information from effector organs is transmitted via the *spinothalamic tract* (lemniscal pathways, great afferents) to thalamic nuclei and then to the cortex. At the same time signals are relayed via afferent collaterals to the reticular formation and then to thalamic relay nuclei, and ultimately to the cortex (see Figure 3). Although the projection system to the reticular formation has been demonstrated functionally, it has yet to be anatomically identified. The ARAS seems to provide the "missing link" between the classical sensory pathways of the brain and many nonspecific behavioral phenomena, such as alertness, arousal, sleep, and attention.

The modern period of work on the ARAS stems from the experiments of Moruzzi and Magoun (1949). These investigators discovered that electrical stimulation of the reticular formation caused EEG patterns of arousal recorded from the cerebral cortex that are usually associated with behavioral arousal.

NEUROPHYSIOLOGY

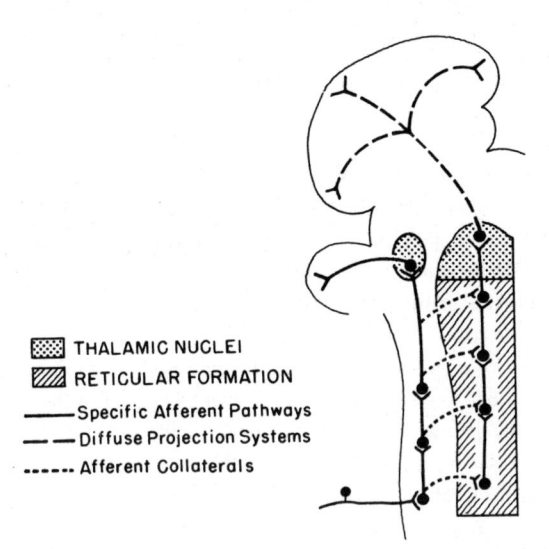

FIGURE 3. A schematic representation of the sensory pathways from periphery to cortex showing the two midbrain pathways, lemniscal and reticular (after Bradley, 1958, p. 146).

The anatomical characteristics of this area of the brain were described in 1909 by Cajal (see Thompson, 1967). Cajal described it as a ventral core of neural tissue extending from the spinal cord to the thalamus. It is composed of intermingled cell bodies and fibers having the appearance of a "reticulum" (network). It has been described as the "great net." The reticular core is surrounded by long ascending fibers and the system of the classical, lemniscal sensory pathways as well as descending motor pathways.

In 1932 W. F. Allan (see Thompson, 1967) indicated that the embryological and anatomical characteristics of the reticular formation suggest that this structure may serve the general function of inhibition, excitation, and integration of brain activity. Physiological analysis of the reticular formation began with the work of Bremer in 1935 (see Thompson, 1967; Mirsky, 1971). He transected the brain stem of the cat at the level of the midbrain (midcollicular level). This resulted in a set of irreversible symptoms that resembled deep sleep. The EEG recorded from the cortex consisted of high-voltage, relatively slow-frequency sleep spindles. Bremer called this surgical transection the *cerveau isolé* preparation. In this preparation all afferent cranial nerve input to the brain is eliminated, with the exception of cranial nerves I, II, and III (olfactory, optic, and oculomotor). Also eliminated is all efferent motor output of the brain, although some control of eye movements remains. The cranial nerves are those nerves that enter and leave the CNS at or above the level of the medulla. There are 12 such nerves (I–XII). With the exception of cranial nerve X, (the vagus nerve, which serves the heart, blood vessels, viscera), the primary function of these nerves is concerned with afferent and efferent flow to areas of the neck and head.

Bremer found only feeble evidence of EEG arousal in the cerveau isolé animal. These experiments supported the then current belief that sleep was due to the withdrawal of sensory stimulation. In order to determine the relative importance of somatic sensory input from the body in normal sleep-wake cycles, Bremer transected the brainstem of the cat at the juncture of the brain and the spinal cord (at the third cervical vertebra). He called this preparation the *encéphale isolé*. In this preparation all somatic sensory input to the brain from the body is eliminated. What remains is all input via the cranial nerves including the somatic sensory input from the face and head (cranial nerve V). Sensory stimulation of animals with the encéphale isolé preparation resulted in long lasting EEG arousal and dilatation of the pupils. The studies indicated that even without somatic sensory input from the body, sleep-wake cycles could be maintained and the EEG and limited behavioral arousal could be elicited by stimulation only from those sensory modalities subserved by the cranial nerves.

The view of Bremer was the accepted one until the experiments of Moruzzi and Magoun. Their experiments suggested that the reticular formation, and not the classical sensory pathways, was responsible for the EEG arousal seen in the *encéphale isolé* preparation animals. Moruzzi and Magoun found that in the *encéphale isolé* preparation, electrical stimulation to the reticular formation resulted in a long-lasting EEG arousal response. Animals with lesions in the classical sensory pathways exhibited a normal sleep-wake cycle. Animals with lesions in the reticular formation tended to be stuporous or somnolent, displaying an EEG usually observed in drowsy or sleepy animals.

It is believed that stimuli from the periphery lose their individual modality identification when these signals enter the reticular formation. Recent work by Groves et al. (1973) suggests that there may be specific modality nuclei in the reticular formation. This loss of modality identification, along with the previous experiments of Moruzzi and Magoun, have led to what has been described as "the classical view of the ARAS." This view holds that the reticular formation consists of a multisynaptic nonspecific system acting on the cortex via the thalamic projection system. There are projections into the reticular formation from the classical sensory pathways via collaterals. An intact reticular system is necessary for behavioral arousal. The system is necessary for conscious awareness of sensory information. It acts as a filter allowing the organism to focus attention on relevant stimuli. Subsequent experiments have challenged the interpretation of many of the early experiments. Although it is clear that sensory information does reach the ARAS, it is not clear that all the information comes from classical sensory pathways via the collaterals. Also, more recent work suggests that the anatomy of the reticular core of the brain stem is not as diffusely organized as believed. For further elaboration see Thompson (1967, pp. 428-473).

Neuropsychological Basis of Drive State. The areas of the brain that subserve drive states and emotional behavior are most important, for many drugs alter both drive state and emotional behavior. Although specific areas of the brain do not function in a unitary fashion, the diencephalon is most concerned with drive state. The experimenter must always keep in mind that experimental manipulation of the CNS either by drug or surgical procedure may alter consummatory behavior of an animal; however, this does not necessarily mean that the animal is less hungry. For example, the experimental procedure may have caused the animal to forget how to obtain food although the animal may still be hungry.

Hypothalamus. The hypothalamus seems to be intimately involved in the control of consummatory behavior. For example, lesions in the ventromedial hypothalamus lead to excessive eating (hyperphagia) and extreme obesity in the rat. Lesions in the lateral hypothalmus lead to just the opposite effect. Animals so lesioned will not eat (aphagia) or drink (adipsia). For a review of these experiments see Teitelbaum (1961).

·The hypothalamus is also implicated in sexual behavior. It exerts both neural control as well as control of the endocrine glands involved in sexual behavior. Lesions made in the anterior hypothalamus of female cats or guinea pigs result in their failure to mate. This failure to mate is believed to be due to an interference with neural control rather than endocrine control. However, lesions in the ventromedial part of the hypothalamus lead to atrophy of the ovaries. This effect can be reversed by means of estrogen treatment. In a similar fashion lesions in the male will also eliminate sexual behavior. Electrical or chemical stimulation of these centers in the hypothalamus will elicit marked increases in sexual behavior. A rat used in an experiment by Vaughan and Fisher (1962) undoubtedly achieved some kind of record with 20 ejaculations in one hour of stimulation to the anterior hypothalamus.

The hypothalamus is intimately related to the function of the pituitary gland, which is most important in the control of other endocrine glands. Also, the integrity of the hypothalamus is necessary for the control of the body temperature.

Amygdala. The amygdala is involved in a variety of emotional and motivational aspects of behavior. In animals an amygdalectomy is usually followed by loss of both fear and aggressiveness. However, there have been experimental reports in which the removal of the amygdala resulted in marked rage. Social dominance studies with monkeys indicated a drop in dominance following lesions in the amygdala. However, it has been noted that the effects of amygdalectomy on social dominance are a function of the preoperative dominance level as well as the operation itself.

Electrical stimulation of the amygdala may also cause a variety of autonomic responses. These autonomic changes may be related to rage and fear, which often accompany amygdala stimulation. However, amygdala stimulation may produce increased feeding behavior. The specific function of the amygdala has yet to be specifically elucidated, although it is clear that it plays a major role in the emotional and motivational behavior.

Hippocampus. The hippocampus, much like the amygdala, is involved in a variety of emotional and motivational aspects of behavior. There is no clear picture of its specific role. It is involved in visceral activity, immediate memory, and in some manner serves as a behavioral suppressor system. Lesions in this structure will cause an increase in undirected activity.

Intracranial Self-stimulation. Of great interest to psychologists and those interested in the effects of drugs on behavior is the fact that animals will press levers, turn wheels, and operate a variety of manipulanda in order to receive electrical stimulation to the brain. The reinforcing capability of such electrical stimulation was first described by Olds and Milner (1954). Although stimulation to a variety of areas of the brain has been found to be reinforcing, the most critical area is the lateral hypothalamus, specifically that area bordering the medial forebrain bundle. Subsequent research has indicated that there is, in addition to a positive reinforcing system, a negative system. That is, animals will operate manipulanda in order to interrupt or avoid stimulation to these areas. Although some of these "negative" areas may be intermingled with positive reinforcing sites, they are easily found clustered in portions of the reticular formation.

Self-stimulation phenomena have been demonstrated in species other than the rat. In man stimulation to these positive areas of the brain yields reports of pleasurable sensations (Sem-Jacobsen and Torkildsen, 1960). Recent studies with narcotic analgesics have related the positive and negative reinforcement systems to the opiate "high" and the analgesic action, respectively, of these drugs (see chapter 7). For a comprehensive review of intracranial stimulation, the reader is referred to Valenstein (1973).

Electroencephalogram (EEG). Many studies of the effects of drugs on the central nervous system have made use of the EEG. In man it is often the only tool we have in monitoring the level of excitation of the brain.

The EEG is a tracing of changes in voltage that are generated by the brain. Electrodes are fastened to various areas of the scalp, and activity from large areas of the cortex can be recorded. These cortical recordings also reflect activity in subcortical structures that is, however, modified by the activity of the cortex. By means of electrodes implanted subcortically, recordings have been made from specific sites within the CNS.

The EEG frequencies have been arbitrarily divided into specific bands. Greek letters have been used to designate these frequency bands. They are, from slow to fast frequency: delta, 0.5 through 3 cps; theta, 4 through 7 cps; alpha, 8 through 13 cps; and beta, 14 through 40 cps. As one goes from low to high frequency, it generally reflects an increase in the level of alertness of the subject (see Figure 4). The exception is the so-called *paradoxical sleep* in which the subject, although sleeping, gives an EEG pattern similar to that seen

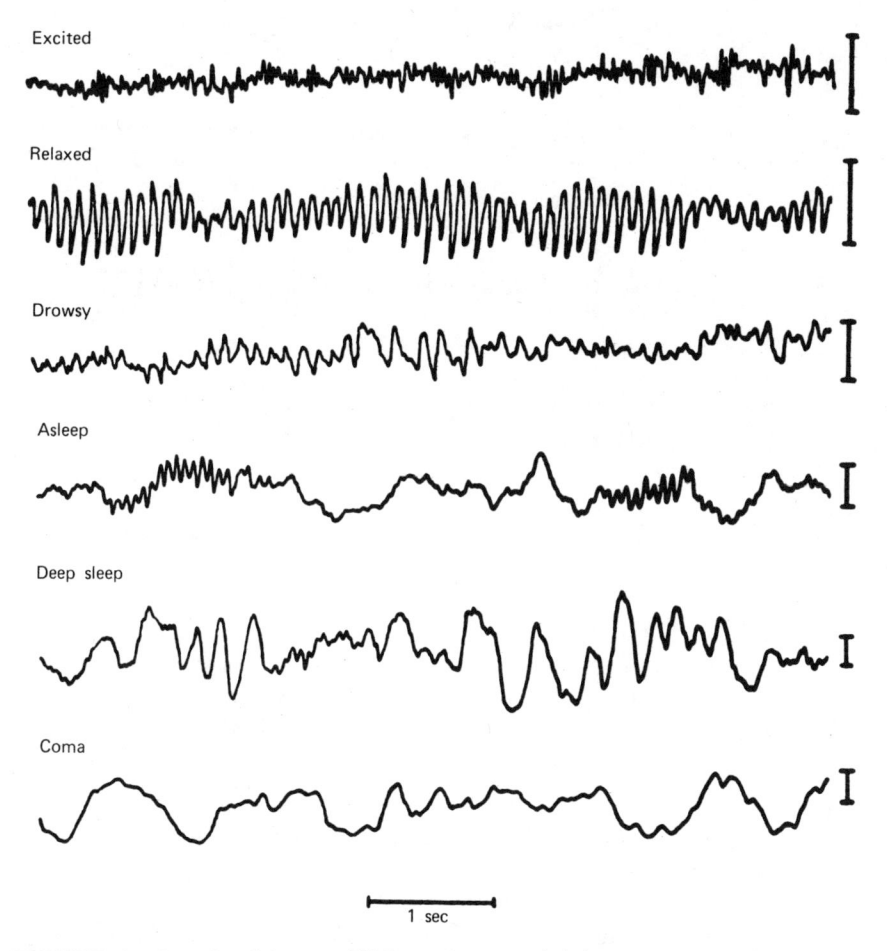

FIGURE 4. Sample of human EEG tracing recorded from the scalp. Calibration signal at right of each tracing represents 50 mV (From Penfield and Jasper, 1954, p. 188)

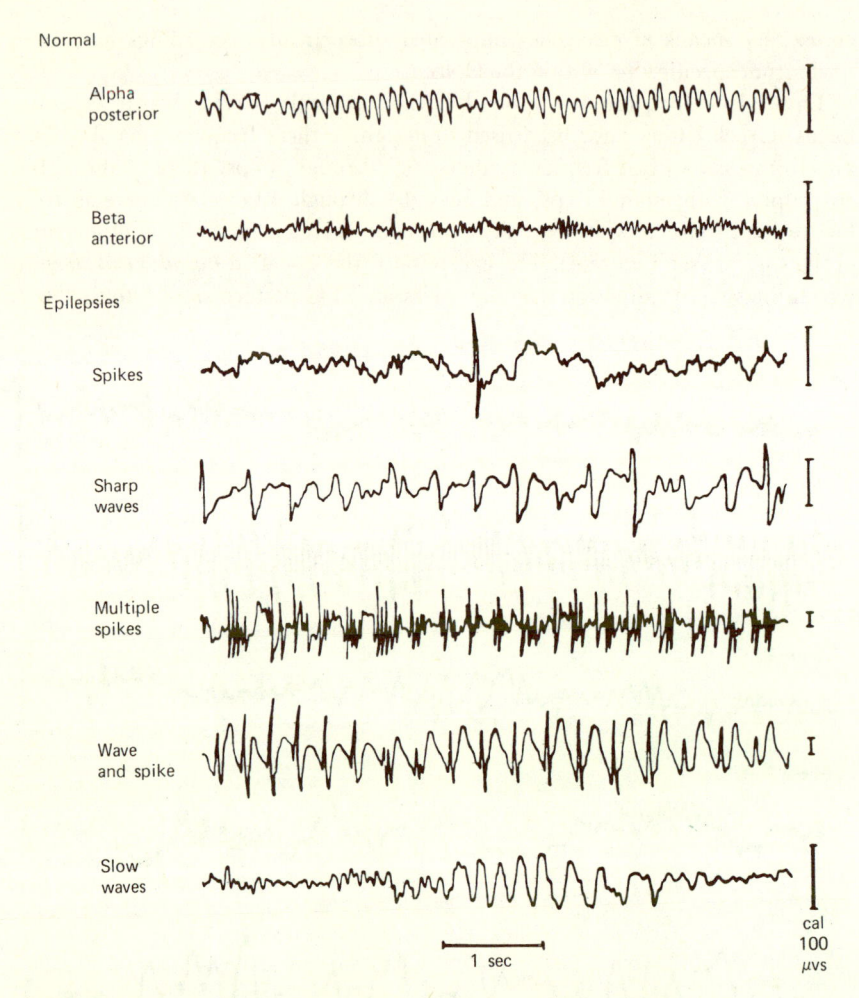

FIGURE 5. Examples of a few electrographic patterns of epileptiform discharge in comparison with normal alpha and beta rhythms. Note particularly the high voltage of the epileptiform discharges. (From Penfield and Jasper, 1954, p. 582).

during an alert phase. This EEG pattern during paradoxical sleep is usually accompanied by rapid eye movements (REM) and dreaming. Low frequency is usually accompanied by high-amplitude waves, and high frequency is usually accompanied by low-amplitude waves.

One of the major differences between pathological and normal EEG tracings is the presence of high-voltage activity in the waking state. This may be associated with the presence of "spiking" and the so-called *spike and wave* pat-

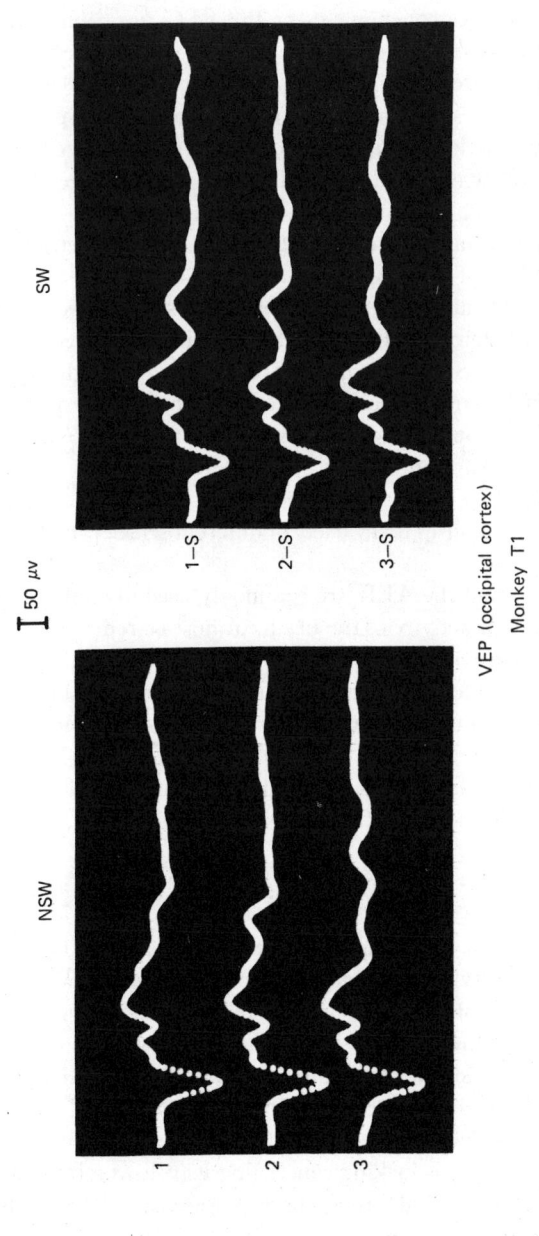

FIGURE 6. Example of the averaged visual evoked potential recorded from the cortex of a monkey. On the left the VEP is the normal and on the right is the VEP during spike-and-wave seizures (figures courtesy of Allan F. Mirsky).

tern indicative of the abnormal electrical discharge seen in petit mal epilepsy (see Figure 5).

Among the characteristic phenomena of the EEG are alpha blocking and spindling. The former is seen when an arousing stimulus is presented to a subject during an alpha phase. It reflects the alerting of the subject and the EEG changes from alpha waves to waves of a higher frequency. Spindling is seen after some of the anesthetic or hypnotic drugs. It is characterized by a burst of fast, high-amplitude waves. The envelope of these waves resembles a "spindle."

A technique that is commonly used in the study of the electrical activity of the brain is the method of *averaged evoked responses* (AER). If electrodes are properly placed over a visual, auditory, or somatosensory cortex and the appropriate modality is stimulated, there are slight shifts in voltage recorded from the appropriate cortical site. Since it is difficult to pick out a single response from the background EEG, many stimuli are presented, and the responses are then averaged by means of a computer. The subsequent wave form (AER) can be visually presented by means of an oscilloscope. The figure gives some examples of AERs (see Figure 6). The AER may be recorded from many cortical as well as subcortical sites, and responses to a variety of different sensory modalities may be studied.

Although the EEG and the AER are commonly used in studies of the effects of drugs on the electrical activity of the brain, it must be remembered that what is measured is the firing of many cells, and what is seen is the summation of these firings. Successful recordings from single neural units in the brains of animals have been done by means of microelectrode techniques. Since a single cell either fires or does not fire, the datum from these studies is the frequency of firings of a single cell. For further discussion of techniques see Grossman (1967), Thompson (1967), or Mirsky (1970, 1971).

BIOCHEMISTRY

Chemical transmission in the peripheral nervous system has been well documented. The role of acetylcholine and norepinephrine as chemical transmitter substances in the peripheral autonomic and somatic nervous system is universally accepted. However, in the central nervous system, except for acetylcholine, the role of norepinephine and other putative transmitter substances has not been conclusively proven. Even the role of acetylcholine in the CNS is based on evidence that it is a transmitter substance in the spinal cord, but complete evidence is lacking concerning its role as a transmitter in the brain. Despite the lack of final proof, there is the general belief that central nervous system transmission is mediated by chemical substances, a number of which have been found in the brain tissue.

The belief that specific chemical substances (neurohumors) are the mediators of CNS activity has been instrumental in the development of research into the biochemistry of mental illness. If there is a malfunction in the synthesis, release, or inactivation of these substances, it is very likely that behavior that is centrally mediated will in some way be altered. Many investigators hold the belief that in certain mental disorders, there is such a disturbance somewhere in the neural transmission chain, and appropriate drugs can alter the disturbance in central transmission so that normal function is restored.

Criteria for Classification as a Neurotransmitter

There are a number of accepted criteria that a substance must meet before it can be called a transmitter substance. The following are the usually accepted criteria:

1. It is necessary that the transmitter substance be in the presynaptic terminal.
2. It must be released into the synaptic cleft when the nerve is stimulated.
3. At the postsynaptic membrane the transmitter must cause a local depolarization (excitatory) or hyperpolarization (inhibitory).
4. Direct application of the transmitter to the neuron must mimic the effect of nerve stimulation.
5. There must be some mechanism for synthesis as well as removal or inactivation.
6. Specific antagonists must block the synaptic action.

The mere presence of the substance in the brain or release of the substance after stimulation is not adequate evidence that the substance is a neural transmitter.

Transmitters and Putative Transmitters of the CNS

Acetylcholine (ACh). Of the various substances that have been identified in the CNS, only ACh has been conclusively shown to be a transmitter substance in the CNS. Neurons sensitive to ACh are widely distributed throughout the brain. However, proof that ACh is a neurotransmitter in the CNS has only been demonstrated in the spinal cord.

Throughout the length of the anterior horn of the spinal cord are neurons (Renshaw cells) that are inhibitory in nature and exert their influence on motor neurons. These inhibitory ACh neurons are nicotine-like. The cholinergic neurons in the brain seem to be muscarine-like. The excitatory action of these cholinergic neurons in the brain can be blocked by atropine but cannot be greatly altered by the agonist nicotine.

Catecholamines. The term catecholamine has come to refer to those compounds containing a catechol nucleus and an ethyl amino side chain. Three catecholamines are important in psychopharmacology: norepinephrine (NE), epinephrine, and dihydroxyphenylethylamine (dopamine). Only NE and dopamine are believed to play much of a role in the CNS.

Norepinephrine. In the previous chapter the role of NE and ACh as neural transmitter substances in the autonomic nervous system was discussed. Although it is well established that NE plays an important role in the CNS and that there are extensive NE pathways in the brain, the specific manner in which NE plays a role in maintaining the integrity of the CNS is not known. Figure 8 is a schematic representation of central NE and dopamine tracts.

The highest concentration of NE is found in the hypothalamus, brain stem, and limbic system. NE is present in the reticular formation, and it is believed to be involved in neural transmission at reticular synapses. Direct application of NE to reticular tissue both excites and inhibits cells in the reticular formation.

Dopamine. Dopamine is a precursor of NE in the CNS (is converted to NE). However, it is believed to be a neurotransmitter in its own right. Highest concentrations are found in the basal ganglia, thalamus, and hypothalamus (see

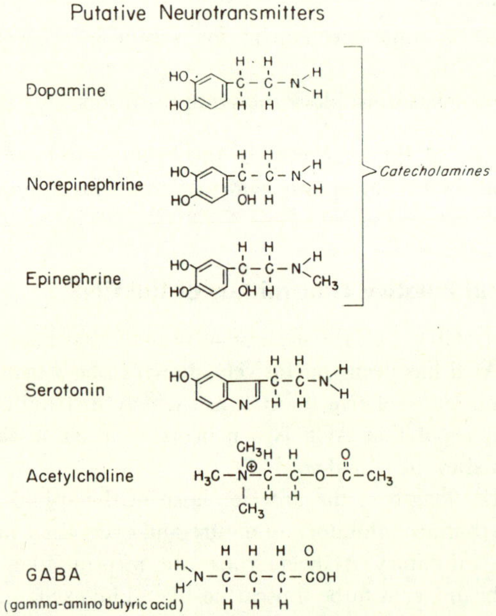

FIGURE 7. Some of the putative neurotransmitters in the CNS.

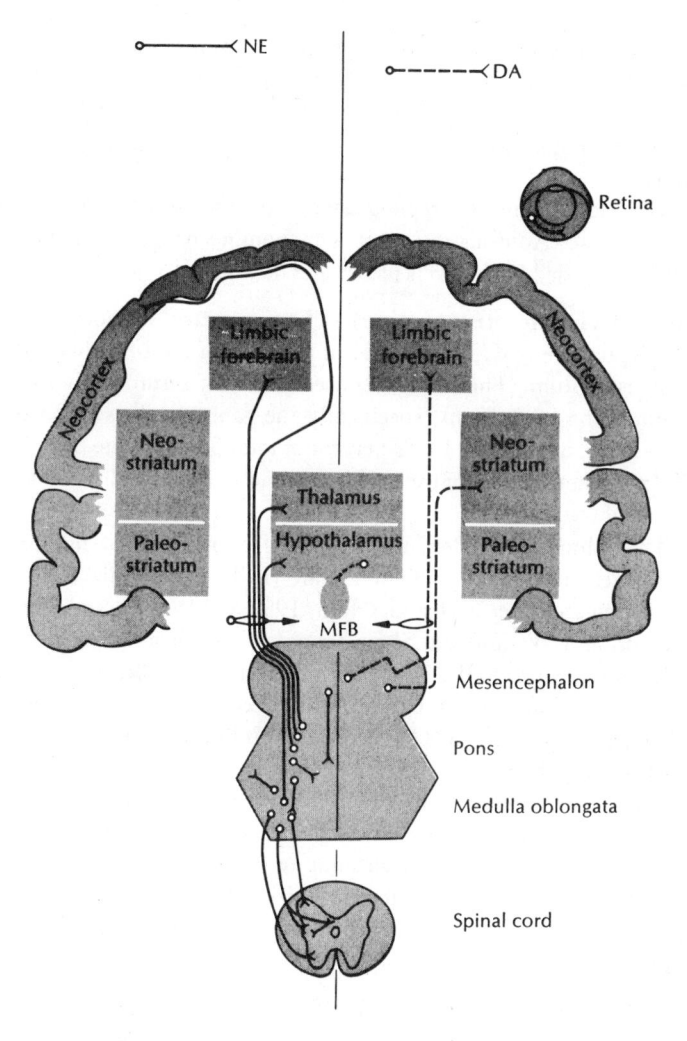

FIGURE 8. Central noradrenergic and dopaminergic tracts (after Anden et al., 1966, p. 313. In Cooper, Bloom, and Roth, 1970, p. 91).

Figure 8 for schematic representation of dopamine tracts). In the basal ganglia it is predominantly found in the caudate and putamen.

As mentioned in the previous section, the basal ganglia are involved in parkinsonism. Urinary dopamine levels of parkinson patients are greatly depressed. Since dopamine does not readily enter the brain (it does not pass the blood-brain barrier), dopamine itself cannot be used in the treatment of the disease. However, the precursor of dopamine, dihydroxyphenylalanine

(L-dopa), is readily incorporated by the brain. Administration of L-dopa results in increased dopamine levels, and it is the drug of choice in the treatment of parkinsonism. Despite the importance of dopamine in the CNS as a neurohumoral agent, it has not been conclusively demonstrated that it is a neurotransmitter.

Both NE and dopamine are degraded, at least in part, by the enzyme monamine oxidase. Administration of a monamine oxidase (MAO) inhibitor will result in increased brain levels of NE and dopamine.

Serotonin (5-Hydroxytryptamine). The putative humoral transmitter, 5-hydroxytryptamine (5-HT), is found in all parts of the brain with the exception of the cerebellum. The highest concentration of serotonin is found in the hypothalamus, the brain stem (specifically the raphé nucleus), and the limbic system. However, only about 1 to 2 percent of total 5-HT in the body is found in the CNS. In mammals most of the 5-HT is found in the pineal gland and in cells of the intestinal tract.

In 1954 Gaddum and, independently, Wooley and Shaw demonstrated that the hallucinogen, lysergic acid diethylamide (LSD), antagonized the effects of 5-HT on the isolated uterus (see Gaddum, 1957 and Wooley and Shaw, 1957). Both Gaddum and Wooley and Shaw suggested that it might have similar actions in the brain. Since 5-HT is normally present in the brain, it was believed that LSD prevented access of the 5-HT to its receptor. These findings and subsequent related hypotheses of Gaddum and Wolley resulted in a tremendous spurt of activity in laboratories all over the world. At the present time, we still do not completely understand the physiological function of 5-HT.

Serotonin is believed to be necessary for normal brain function, and it has been suggested that a lack of this neurohumor results in depression, whereas an excess results in excitation. Serotonin is degraded by MAO, and increased levels of brain serotonin are found with the administration of MAO inhibitors (see Chapter 6).

GABA (γ-Aminobutyric Acid). In 1950 GABA was identified as a normal constituent of the mammalian CNS. Except for the CNS and the retina, GABA is found only in trace amounts in other mammalian tissue. Present evidence suggests that the function of GABA in the CNS is as an inhibitory transmitter.

Summary. In addition to the substances discussed in this section, there are many other putative neurotransmitters in the CNS. Those discussed have been most extensively studied in the past; however, there are many others that may eventually be shown to be more important than those that are currently in vogue. For further discussion of these neurohumors plus others see Cooper, Bloom, and Roth (1974).

SUMMARY

No attempt has been made in this chapter to be inclusive. The main attempt was to give the reader some background and vocabulary that will allow a better understanding of subsequent chapters in this book. What should be clear to the reader at this point is that despite an apparent tremendous sophistication in biochemical and neurophysiological techniques, much is not known and often, conflicting results are reported. A complete understanding of the manner in which a drug produces its particular effect on behavior can only come when there is a much greater sophistication and understanding of the biochemistry and the neurophysiology of the brain. In addition, it will not be enough to simply understand the brain, but we must understand the manner in which environmental influences interact with the function of the CNS. Only when these interactions are fully understood can we really understand the mechanisms of drug action.

REFERENCES

Anden, N. E., Dahlström, A., Fuxe, K., Larsson, K., Olson, L., and Ungerstedt, U. Ascending monoamine neurons to the telencephalon and diencephalon. *Acta Physiologica Scandinavica*, **67**, 1966, 313–326.

Bradley, P. B. The central action of certain drugs in relation to the reticular formation of the brain. In H. H. Jasper, L. D. Proctor, R. S. Knighton, W. C. Noshay, and R. T. Costello (Eds.) *Reticular Formation of the Brain*. Boston, Little, Brown, 1958.

Cooper, J. R., Bloom, F. E., and Roth, R. H. *The Biochemical Basis of Neuropharmacology*. New York, Oxford University Press, 1970.

Ibid. (2nd ed.) 1974.

Gaddum, J. H. Serotonin-LSD interactions. *Annals of the New York Academy of Sciences*, **66**, 1957, 643–648.

Grossman, S. P. *A Textbook of Physiological Psychology*. New York, Wiley, 1967.

Groves, P. M., Miller, S. W., Parker, M. V., and Rebec, G. V. Organization by sensory modality in the reticular formation of the rat. *Brain Research*, **54**, 1973, 207–224.

Mirsky, A. F. An overview of neuroelectrophysiologic studies of centrally acting drugs. In A. DiMascio and R. I. Shader (Eds.) *Clinical Handbook of Psychopharmacology*. New York, Science House, 1970, pp. 121–136.

Mirsky, A. F. Physiological Psychology. In N. B. Talbot, J. Kagan, and L. Eisenberg (Eds.) *Behavioral Science in Pediatric Medicine*. Philadelphia, Saunders, 1971, pp. 90–161.

Moruzzi, G. and Magoun, H. W. Brain stem reticular formation and activation of the EEG. *Electroencephalography and Clinical Neurophysiology*, **1**, 1949, 455–473.

Olds, J. and Milner, P. Positive reinforcement produced by electrical stimulation of septal area and other regions of rat brain. *Journal of Comparative and Physiological Psychology*, **47**, 1954, 419–427.

Penfield, W. and Jasper, H. *Epilepsy and the Functional Anatomy of the Human Brain*. Boston, Little, Brown, 1954.

Sem-Jacobsen, C. W. and Torkildsen, A. Depth recording and electrical stimulation in the human brain. In E. R. Ramey and D. S. O'Doherty (Eds.) *Electrical Studies on the Unanesthesized Brain*, New York, Hoeber, 1960, pp. 275-290.

Sidman, R. L. and Sidman, M. *Neuroanatomy: A Programmed Text*, Vol. 1. Boston, Little, Brown, 1965.

Teitelbaum, P. Disturbance in feeding and drinking behavior after hypothalmic lesions. In M. R. Jones (Ed.) *Nebraska Symposium on Motivation*. Lincoln, University of Nebraska Press, 1961, pp. 39-65.

Thompson, R. F. *Foundations of Physiological Psychology*. New York, Harper and Row, 1967.

Valenstein, E. S. *Brain Stimulation and Motivation: Research and Commentary*. Glenview, Illinois, Scott, Foresman, 1973.

Vaughan, E. and Fisher, A. E. Male sexual behavior induced by intracranial electrical stimulation. *Science,* **137,** 1962, 758-760.

Woolley, D. W. and Shaw, E. N. Evidence for participation of serotonin in mental processes. *Annals of the New York Academy of Sciences,* **66,** 1957, 649-667.

5 ANTIPSYCHOTIC DRUGS

INTRODUCTION

In this chapter the pharmacology of those drugs used in the treatment of the psychoses is discussed. For the most part, pharmacotherapy has focused on the schizophrenic patient, with only a relatively recent use of pharmacotherapy for the manic patient. There are four major groups of drugs that are used in the treatment of the schizophrenic patient; these are the rauwolfia derivatives, the phenothiazine derivatives, the butyrophenones, and the thioxanthene derivatives. The drug that has recently been used for the treatment of manic states is lithium. The rauwolfia derivatives are primarily of interest because of their historical importance in the treatment of the schizophrenic patient; they have been replaced, for the most part, by either the phenothiazines or the butyrophenones.

The extensive use of drugs for the treatment of the mentally ill began with the use of the antipsychotic drugs (major tranquilizers). The use of these drugs revolutionized treatment methods and gave a feeling of hope to what was an increasingly depressing picture of what happened to most patients diagnosed as schizophrenic.

Until 1956 the number of resident patients in public mental hospitals was on a continuous increase. Since 1957 the number of patients in public mental institutions has been continually declining. The 1955 figure was 558,900 patients. In 1967 the figure was 426,200. This decline in absolute numbers, which has continued to the present day, has occurred even though the population of the United States has been continually increasing (see Figure 1).

The year 1956 was the first year of widespread use of the major tranquilizers. The psychotherapeutic drugs alone cannot be held responsible for this marked shift in the number of people spending time in mental hospitals. The drugs must share the credit with improvement in staff-patient ratios and introduction of new concepts, such as the "open" hospital, that could not be instituted in any major way until the advent of the psychotherapeutic drugs.

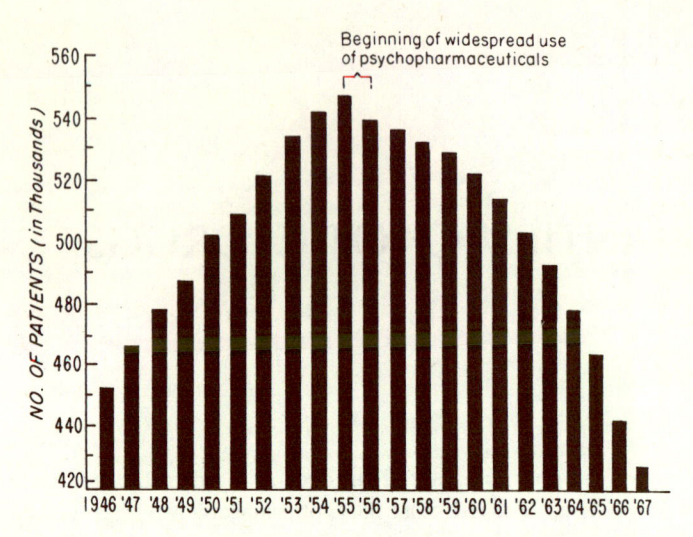

FIGURE 1. Number of resident patients in state and local government mental hospitals in the United States (based on USPHS figures) 1946–1967 (from Kline, 1968).

Although arguments could be made that the decrease in the number of patient-hospital days in this country could be attributed to factors other than the use of drugs, the evidence is strongly in favor of the psychotherapeutic drugs being the primary reason for the change that has appeared in our public mental hospitals. Today it is rare that one sees the type of florid psychotic behavior in mental hospitals that was so common only two decades ago. The Martha Washingtons and the Napoleons are not with us anymore. Also the straight jackets, hydrotherapy, and padded restraint rooms are all gone, and one seldom is overcome by the smell of human excrement when walking in the wards of a mental hospital today.

Although drugs have contributed greatly to the treatment of the major psychosis, they (at least the drugs presently used) still do not compare in therapeutic efficacy with what one sees in the chemotherapy of many physical ills. One of the major problems in treating the mentally ill is that we do not know the nature of the illness we are treating. In fact, it could be said that drug therapy in the treatment of the mentally ill is the treatment of diseases of unknown etiology by drugs of unknown actions. Hopefully this chapter can modulate such an iconoclastic view.

Many clinicians believed that the major tranquilizers were treating only symptoms, and in no way were they antipsychotic in their action. However, there is some evidence suggesting that drugs may be altering the biochemistry of the brain in such a way that they are doing more than merely depressing symptoms. Although the questions of how the drugs work and whether they alter some basic dysfunction in the brain are important, of most practical importance is the fact that they do result in clinical improvement in thousands of patients and allow them to move from the mental hospital to the community.

Ideally the antipsychotic drug should perform in the following ways:

1. Reduce agitation.
2. Reverse the presence of psychotic symptoms, for example, hallucinations, delusions, and thought disturbances.
3. Not interfere with the sensorium or motoric functioning.
4. Produce no side effects.

Unfortunately no tranquilizing drug presently on the market has all of these characteristics.

RESERPINE

Reserpine was the first of the newer drugs to be used in the treatment of the mentally ill. Although it is rarely used today, having been replaced for the most part by the phenothiazines, it does have historical importance and is still used in the field of hypertension. Reserpine is an alkaloid derived from the root of *Rauwolfia serpentina,* and it is primarily responsible for the pharmacological effects of powdered preparations made from the root of this plant. Powdered rauwolfia has been used by Hindu physicians for centuries in the treatment of a variety of conditions, including insomnia and various psychiatric illnesses. Its use in modern Western medicine was initiated by internists who were interested in its hypotensive effect and its therapeutic usefulness in the treatment of hypertension. In 1953 Wilkins and Judson at Boston University noted its beneficial effect in anxious, tense patients in the course of a clinical study of its utility as a hypotensive agent. Also, in 1954 Nathan Kline reported the results of a clinical trial at Rockland State Hospital in New York with this drug in disturbed schizophrenic patients. It was found to be useful in the treatment of the psychotic patients in doses over 5 mg/day. In doses less than 5 mg/day the effect seemed to be minimal or nonexistent.

Reserpine has effects on both the autonomic and the central nervous systems.

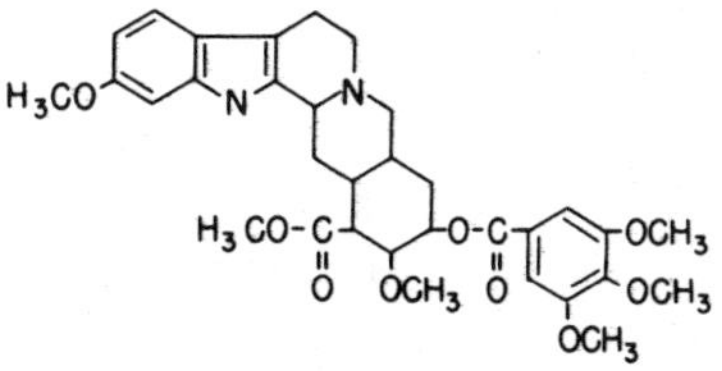

FIGURE 2. Chemical structure of reserpine.

Human subjects seem more relaxed and sedated when given reserpine. Although sleep is easily produced, patients are readily aroused after reserpine administration.

Autonomic Nervous System Effects

The autonomic effects of reserpine are primarily a decrease in sympathetic activity with a concomitant enhancement in parasympathetic activity. These effects with appropriate doses are as follows:

1. Blood pressure is decreased.
2. Pulse rate is decreased.
3. Miosis.
4. Gastrointestinal motility and hydrochloric acid secretions are increased.
5. Low doses increase respiration rate.
6. High doses decrease respiration rates.

Central Nervous System Effects

Most of the research with reserpine in the central nervous system has been concerned with its biochemical effects. This is probably because very little in the way of neurophysiological effects has been observed and because there are marked and most interesting changes in neurohumors of the brain after the administration of reserpine. The drug seems to have little effect on the EEG except for those EEG changes that are related to sedation, that is, an increase in high voltage–low frequency activity. Low doses (.05 mg/kg) show very little effect on EEG despite the occurrence of miosis and bradycardia. At higher doses (.1–.2 mg/kg) there is an increase in the alerting response to external stimuli. In man, if the dose of reserpine is increased, it will cause an EEG pattern characteristic of alertness, high frequency–low voltage, with none of the EEG characteristics associated with sleep. This finding is compatible with one of the side effects seen with this drug: reserpine may increase the severity and frequency of seizures in epileptic patients, and it may even cause seizures in subjects with no history of convulsive disorders.

In animals the drug lowers the seizure threshold to some convulsant drugs but not to others. Animals given reserpine will have convulsive seizures at lower doses of pentylenetetrazol (Metrazol); however, it does not change the seizure threshold to strychnine.

Biochemical Effects

As previously mentioned, most of the work with reserpine has been concerned with its biochemical effects. Reserpine depletes catecholamines (norepinephrine and dopamine) as well as 5-hydroxytryptamine (5-HT) from brain stores;

5-HT is also called *serotonin*. This depletion of serotonin from the brain after administration of reserpine is accompanied by an increase in the excretion of 5-hydroxyindoleacetic acid, the major metabolite of 5-HT found in the urine.

There are two major points of view concerning how reserpine produces depression in behavior. One is that the depletion of 5-HT is the primary cause of the depression, and the other is that depletion of catecholamines is the cause. Since behavioral depression can occur without depletion of 5-HT or catecholamines from brain stores, it is possible that neither of these actions is the primary cause of the behavioral effects seen after reserpine administration.

Absorption, Fate, and Distribution

The rauwolfia alkaloids are readily absorbed from the gastrointestinal tract as well as from parenteral injection sites. The manner in which these drugs are metabolized and excreted is little understood. Resperine has often been referred to as a "hit and run" drug, for long after the drug is apparently gone from the body, behavioral effects and amine depletions still persist. In experiments in which radioactive reserpine is injected into animals, the drug is found to be fairly uniformly distributed in different parts of the brain.

Toxicity and Side Effects

In man reserpine produces drowsiness, although it is not a particularly useful hypnotic drug since subjects can be very easily aroused after the administration of reserpine. The autonomic effects that are seen in man reflect the parasympathetic predominance with a depression of the sympathetic nervous system. The effects include bradycardia, increased salivation, and cutaneous vasodilation. Nausea is quite common as well as occasional vomiting. The drug will often produce diarrhea, and this has probably led to many problems in the use of rauwolfia in India where dysentery is a common occurrence. Since this drug will produce an excessive amount of gastric secretion, it might prove dangerous to the ulcer patient.

It will produce parkinsonian side effects in many patients. It has been shown to produce convulsions in people with no history of convulsive disorders and is certainly contraindicated in patients with a history of epilepsy. Although allergic reactions to the drug itself are rare, it can produce exacerbations of allergic symptoms in the allergic patient. There is fluid retention with this drug, and, in addition, patients will gain weight because of its ability to cause an increase in appetite.

Reserpine can have a marked effect on the endocrine system. It will inhibit menstruation. It is reported to produce a decrease in the sexual drive, and it will also depress fertility.

PHENOTHIAZINE DERIVATIVES

Although the compounds derived from phenothiazine form a chemically homogeneous group, they differ widely in their pharmacological properties. The parent compound, phenothiazine, had been used for many years as an antihelminthic agent in veterinary medicine. It was found that some of the phenothiazine derivatives had strong antihistaminic properties and also seemed to produce some sedative effects. Chlorpromazine was synthesized in 1950 by Charpentier and co-workers in France. The drug was first used as a preanesthetic agent prior to major surgery. Chlorpromazine alone was first used by Delay, Deniker, and Harl who, in 1952, published a paper in which they described the ability of chlorpromazine to control motor excitement in a patient. In 1952 Delay and Deninker used it to treat psychotic excitement in a group of psychiatric patients (see Swazey, 1974, pp. 82-158). The report was enthusiastic, and the use of chlorpromazine quickly spread with the first paper appearing in the English language by Lehmann and Hanrahan in 1954. (Historical overview of the discovery and development of chlorpromazine is found in Swazey, 1974.)

The initial success of chlorpromazine resulted in the synthesizing of a great number of other phenothiazine derivatives, and these were introduced into therapy with the hope that they would be superior to chlorpromazine both in therapeutic effects and in terms of reduction in the number of side effects. Despite the many additional drugs that have been used, chlorpromazine is still the drug of choice of many psychiatrists.

Chlorpromazine is marketed under various trade names: in the United States it is Thorazine; in France, Canada, England, and Italy it is called Largactil; in Germany it appears under the name Megaphan, and in South America, Ampliactil.

On the basis of chemical structure, phenothiazines may be divided into: the piperazine group, characterized by a piperazine ring in the side chain, the aliphatic group, characterized by a three-carbon straight side chain, and the piperidine group, characterized by a piperidine ring in the side chain (see Figure 3). Each group of phenothiazines differs from the other in milligram potency and propensity to cause a particular constellation of side effects. Generally speaking, one needs a greater amount of drug with the aliphatic or piperidine derivatives than with drugs of the piperazine group for producing the same clinical effect.

Although there are marked differences between drugs within a particular side-chain group, the piperazine derivatives are more likely to cause extrapyramidal side effects than the aliphatic or piperidine. The aliphatic derivatives as well as the piperidine derivatives seem to produce more sedation than do the piperazines, which are more likely to produce stimulating effects. The ali-

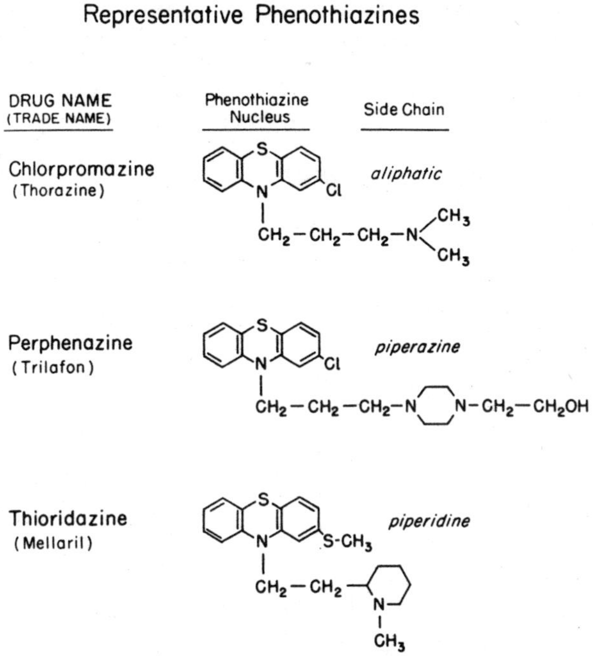

Representative Phenothiazines

DRUG NAME (TRADE NAME)	Phenothiazine Nucleus	Side Chain
Chlorpromazine (Thorazine)		aliphatic
Perphenazine (Trilafon)		piperazine
Thioridazine (Mellaril)		piperidine

FIGURE 3. Representative phenothiazines.

phatics and the piperidines are also more likely to produce changes in the blood picture, liver toxicity, hypotensive actions, and autonomic effects, as well as a photosensitivity. These are discussed in a later section.

In the following discussion of phenothiazines we concern ourselves primarily with chlorpromazine, since it is the prototype drug, and all of the phenothiazines have similar effects to a greater or lesser degree. Where marked differences exist, they are noted.

Behavioral Effects

There is marked behavioral depression seen after a single dose of chlorpromazine. In normals it seems to be characterized by an irresistible urge to sleep. In many of its aspects the behavioral effects are much like those seen in sleep deprivation. That is, although there is a tremendous drive towards sleep, it is reversible. This is quite different from what is seen with large doses of barbiturates. Some reports have suggested that this sedation is characterized by no reduction in the sensorium of the subject, but this is certainly not the case after the administration of single doses. All doses that sedate will also alter performance on various psychological tests. However, when phenothiazines are

TABLE 1. REPRESENTATIVE ANTIPSYCHOTIC DRUGS

Generic Name	Brand Name	Daily Dosage[a] Range (mg)
Rauwolfia alkaloids:		
Reserpine	Serpasil®	1–5
Phenothiazine derivatives:		
Aliphatics		
Chlorpromazine	Thorazine®	100–1,000
Promazine	Sparine®	25–1,000
Triflupromazine	Vesprin®	20–150
Piperidines		
Thioridazine	Mellaril®	30–800
Piperazines		
Trifluoperazine	Stelazine®	2–30
Perphenazine	Trilafon®	2–64
Prochlorperazine	Compazine®	15–125
Carphenazine	Proketazine®	25–400
Acetophenazine	Tindal®	40–80
Fluphenazine	Prolixin®, Permitil®	0.5–20
Butyrophenones:		
Haloperidol	Haldol®	3–50
Thioxanthene derivatives:		
Thiothixene	Navane®	6–60
Chlorprothixene	Taractan®	10–600
Lithium Carbonate		750–2,500

[a] The actual starting dose may be lower than the low dose given. Dosages as given by DiMascio, A. Classification and overview of psychotropic drugs. In A. DiMascio and R. Shader (Eds.) *Clinical Handbook of Psychopharmacology.* New York, Science House, 1970, pp. 3–15.

administered chronically to schizophrenic patients, there may be no reduction in the patient's ability to perform cognitive, perceptual, or motor tests; in fact, the more common result is some improvement in performance that correlates with the clinical improvement.

In humans as well as in animals the drug seems to have some relatively selective effects on the ability of the subject to focus attention. It must be remembered that the impairment in attention seen after the drug may have markedly different effects in normals than in schizophrenic patients. This is discussed in a later section (pp. 91–94) on putative mechanisms of actions.

Extensive studies of the effects of chlorpromazine on a simple attention test have been carried out since 1956. The test of attention that has been used, The Continuous Performance Test (CPT) (Rosvold et al., 1956), requires the subject to continually monitor a projection screen on which single letters are presented for a brief exposure time (0.1 to 0.2 sec) at the rate of one every 1.1 or 1.2 seconds. Approximately one out of six of the letters is an "X," and the subject is required to press a button or release a key whenever the "X," the critical stimulus, appears. With this type of task, subjects can make omission or commission errors. The former is failure to respond to a critical stimulus; the latter is responding to a noncritical stimulus. In many of these studies the effects of drugs on the CPT have been compared with the effects on the Digit Symbol Substitution Test (DSST) from the Wechsler Test of Adult Intelligence (Mirsky and Kornetsky, 1964). In general, the results of these studies indicate that chlorpromazine seems to cause a relatively selective impairment of the performance of subjects on an attention task as compared to a more cognitive test such as the DSST, whereas, barbiturates have the opposite type of effect. The relative effects of chlorpromazine versus barbiturates on an attention test and a cognitive test are schematically illustrated in Figure 4.

This relative selectivity of chlorpromazine on vigilance has been replicated in animal studies (Kornetsky and Bain, 1965). For these experiments a rat was required to press a lever for a food reinforcement whenever the top light of two lights was on. The top light, the critical stimulus, was randomly activated once every six times the bottom light appeared. A 0.2-second stimulus was presented every 3.2 seconds. The effects of both chlorpromazine and pentobarbital in the rat on this animal model of the CPT are shown in Figure 5. As can be seen there is an increase in omission errors, as a function of dose after chlorpromazine, with no systematic change in commission errors. The opposite is seen after the administration of pentobarbital.

Chlorpromazine also causes a selective effect on avoidance behavior in the Conditioned Avoidance Response (CAR) paradigm. In this type of procedure a

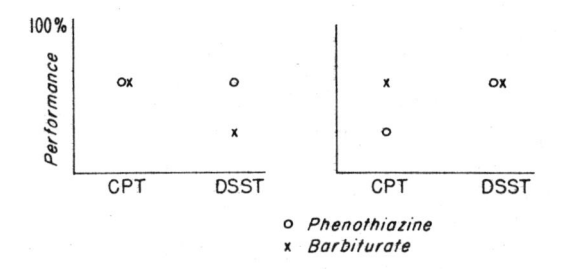

FIGURE 4. The graph on the left is a schematic illustration of the case where doses of a phenothiazine and a barbiturate that cause equal impairment of performance on the CPT differentially affect performance on the DSST with the barbiturate causing the greater impairment. The graph on the right depicts the converse situation where doses that are equipotent with regard to the DSST differentially affect performance on the CPT, the phenothiazine causing the greater impairment.

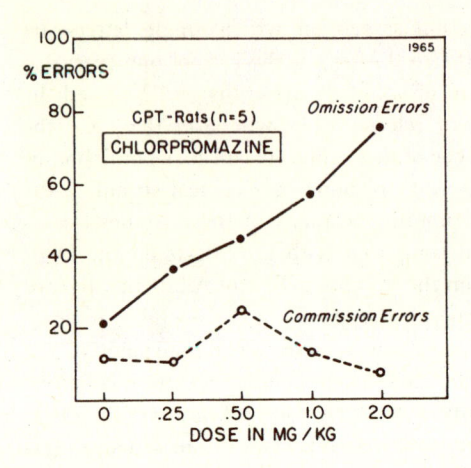

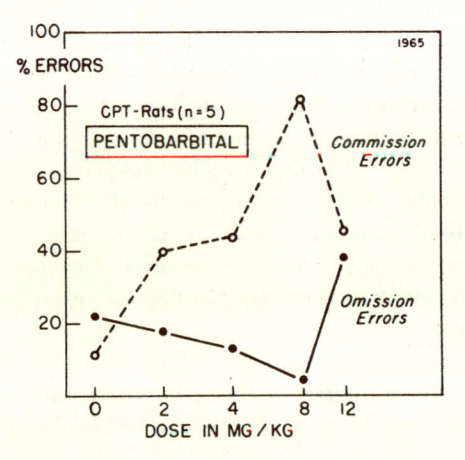

FIGURE 5. The effects of various doses of chlorpromazine (top) and pentobarbital (bottom) on CPT performance in the rat (from Kornetsky and Bain, 1965).

conditional stimulus (CS), for example, a buzzer, is usually followed by the delivery of a foot-shock, unconditioned stimulus (US), to the animal. If the animal presses a lever prior to the onset of the US, it will avoid the delivery of the foot-shock. However, if the animal does not respond to the CS, it can terminate the US by pressing the lever when the shock comes on. Thus an animal can either avoid or escape the aversive stimulation. Figure 6 shows the selective effect of chlorpromazine on the CAR behavior. As is shown, avoidance behavior can be completely inhibited at doses that do not alter escape behavior. Barbiturates and the minor tranquilizers will not alter avoidance behavior without simultaneously affecting the escape behavior. Cook and Weidley (1957) were the first to demonstrate this phenomenon, although they used pole-climbing as the operant, rather than the pressing of a lever.

These effects on the CAR have been attributed to a reduction in anxiety after the drug or simply a decrease in motor responding due to the drug. Poslun (1962) has suggested the latter; however, other experiments have suggested that it is not a simple motor retardation that causes the results with chlorpromazine (Low, et al., 1966; Lipper and Kornetsky, 1971). It is certainly hard to explain the CAR results with chlorpromazine as caused by a reduction in anxiety. Drugs that clinically are used for reducing anxiety do not have similar effects. Also, well-trained animals on the CAR paradigm do not, at least subjectively, show signs of emotionality at the onset of the CS.

Central Nervous System

In this section we describe some of the actions on the CNS and attempt to relate them to the behavioral as well as the therapeutic action of these potent compounds.

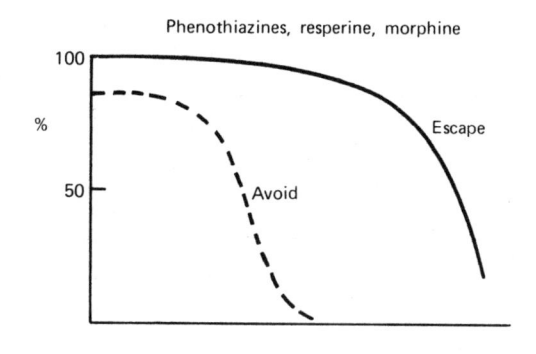

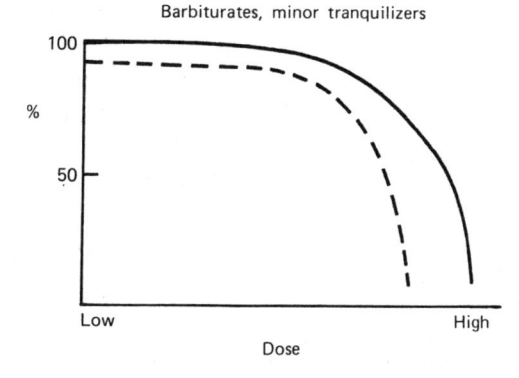

FIGURE 6. A schematic representation of various drugs on the "conditioned avoidance response" (CAR). The top indicates drugs that impair avoidance without altering escape and the bottom those that alter avoidance behavior only at doses that alter escape behavior.

The Brain Stem Reticular Formation. The work of Bradley and colleagues (as described in Bradley, 1958, 1963) as well as that of Killam and Killam (1958) and Killam (1968) has implicated the reticular formation as the putative site of the therapeutic action of phenothiazines. The work of Bradley et al. suggests that chlorpromazine raises the threshold for incoming stimuli at the level of the collaterals entering the reticular formation from the lemniscal pathways. Killam and Killam's findings have suggested that chlorpromazine enhances the filtering properties of the reticular system. Functionally, whether you accept Bradley's interpretation or the Killams', the net result is the same. Chlorpromazine reduces the output of the reticular formation in response to sensory stimuli. Figure 7 schematically indicates various sites of action of a variety of drugs. As can be seen, chlorpromazine and lysergic acid diethylamide act at similar sites but in opposite ways. Barbiturates and amphetamine form another pairing of drugs acting in opposite ways on the reticular formation.

If the role of the reticular formation is to protect the organism from a flooding of incoming stimuli, it would suggest that schizophrenic patients, or at least some schizophrenic patients, are continually flooded by afferent input. This afferent input comes from the external environment and also from the internal

Locus	Depress	Excite
1	Barbiturates	Amphetamines
2	Atropine	Physostigmine
3	Chlorpromazine	LSD-25

- Thalamic nuclei
- Reticular formation
- Specific afferent pathways
- Diffuse projection systems
- Afferent collaterals

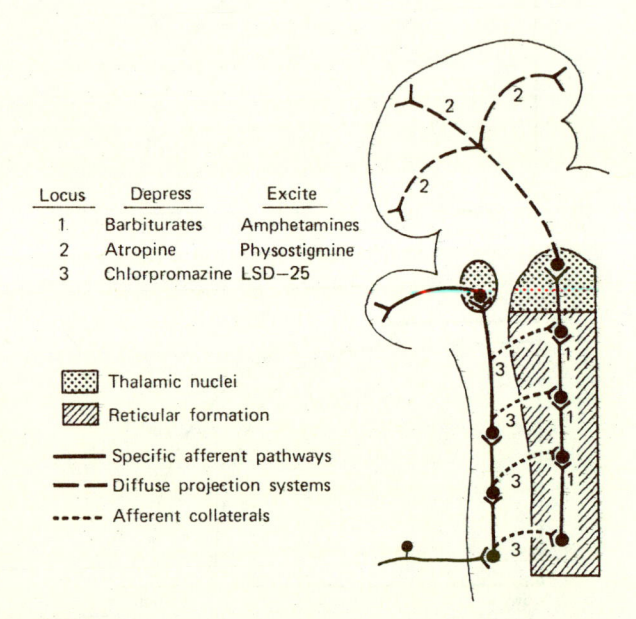

FIGURE 7. Diagram showing the suggested sites of action for certain drugs within the central nervous system: (1) the reticular formation, (2) the diffuse thalamic projection system, and (3) the afferent collaterals entering the reticular formation (after Bradley, 1958).

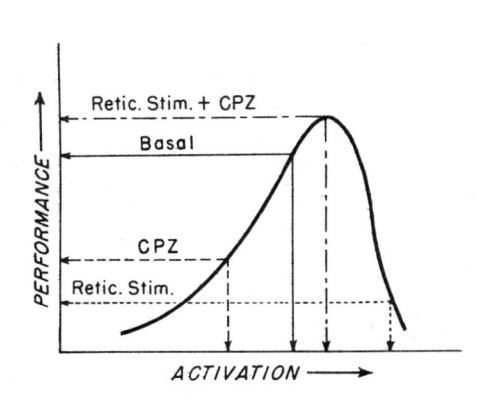

FIGURE 8. An "inverted-U" curve illustrating the postulated relationship between activation and performance. The figure indicates that chlorpromazine reduces activation from basal level, causing impairment in performance, and that reticular stimulation, by moving subjects to the descending leg of the continuum, also impairs performance. When chlorpromazine is combined with stimulation, however, the subject is moved closer to basal activation levels (from Kornetsky and Eliasson, 1969).

environment. This suggests that the therapeutic action of chlorpromazine is to reduce this flooding of sensory input back to a normal level.

Before describing some of the other CNS effects of chlorpromazine, it might be well to integrate the behavioral actions of the drug, both in animals and man, with its effect on the arousal system.

As mentioned, chlorpromazine has relatively selective effects on a simple test of attention in both animals and man. If the schizophrenic patient is continually flooded with afferent input that in some way is not gated by the reticular formation, the decrease in this sensory storm would be therapeutic. We have postulated an inverted "U" function to explain this action of chlorpromazine in patients (Kornetsky and Mirsky, 1966) (see Figure 8). In an attempt to model this inverted "U" in animals, rats were trained on a modification of the CPT. For the model to work, flooding the animals with stimuli to the reticular formation should result in errors of omission. Chlorpromazine, as previously described, will cause errors of omission; however, when stimulation is combined with chlorpromazine, the animal should make fewer errors than with either drug or stimulation alone. These results were obtained (Kornetsky and Eliasson, 1969; Eliasson and Kornetsky, 1972). As Figure 9 shows, the drug or stimulation impairs performance, but when combined, the animals perform much like after receiving saline. This type of interaction is not seen after a barbiturate and stimulation, or when the performance test is a fixed ratio procedure, or when other areas of the brain are stimulated.

Other CNS Actions. Chlorpromazine effects can be recorded by means of EEG from many parts of the brain. However, none of these actions has yet been related to its clinical effect, although it would be naive to assume that these actions are not important. Effects on the cortex seem to be minimal. EEG recorded in man from the cortex indicate that high doses will increase the oc-

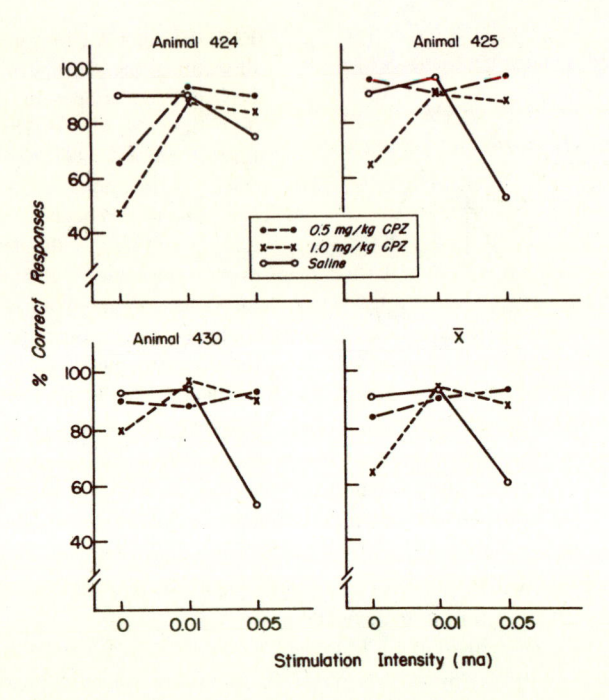

FIGURE 9. The effects of chlorpromazine on percent correct responses as a function of level of stimulation (electrodes in the mesencephalic reticular formation) for each of three animals. Mean percent correct responses are shown on the lower right-hand graph (from Eliasson and Kornetsky, 1972).

currence of theta (slow) frequencies. However, this effect may be more the result of action on the midbrain rather than on the cortex. Mirsky and Tecce (1967), in an experiment in which the EEG was recorded from both cortical and subcortical sites in monkeys performing on the CPT, found an interesting dissociation. When errors were made on the CPT after chlorpromazine, changes in the EEG activity were recorded from subcortical areas. However, when pentobarbital caused errors, the changes in EEG were predominantly seen in recordings from the cortical sites.

It is believed that the hypothalamus is affected by chlorpromazine since many vegetative functions controlled by this region are altered. Temperature reduction (hypothermia) is seen in patients treated with chlorpromazine.

The actions of chlorpromazine in the limbic system are not clearly differentiated. At very high doses spontaneous seizure activity is seen emanating from the amygdala. Of importance is the fact that chlorpromazine can lower the convulsive threshold and offers no protection against the convulsant properties of pentylenetetrazol, strychnine, or picrotoxin.

Actions on the basal ganglia are most important, for one of the major side effects of the phenothiazines is parkinsonism. This marked effect on the extrapyramidal system is the result of the blockade of dopamine in the CNS. Dopamine is the transmitter substance in neural tracts that have their cell bodies in the substantia nigra and synapse in the caudate nucleus and putamen of the corpus striatum (part of the basal ganglia). The postsynaptic blockade of dopamine in this nigrostriatal dopamine pathway results in a loss of efficiency in the extrapyramidal system's ability to function as a servo feedback system in controlling the pyramidal (motor) system. In naturally occurring Parkinson's disease there is degeneration of the nigrostriatal tract.

Chlorpromazine is a useful antiemetic agent. This action seems to be a central effect, for it directly depresses the chemoreceptor trigger zone (vomiting center), and it will not inhibit reflex vomiting caused by emetic agents, nor is it effective against nausea caused by vestibular disturbance.

Autonomic Nervous System

In the ANS chlorpromazine has strong adrenergic-blocking action and weak cholinergic-blocking activity. It causes an alpha-type adrenergic-blocking effect. The hypertensive effect of epinephrine can be antagonized. However, the blocking action of the phenothiazines on norepinephrine is not as consistent as one would see with a classic adrenergic blocking agent. The phenothiazines will block, although weakly, the nicotinic and muscarinic actions of acetylcholine. The muscarinic blocking action accounts for nasal stuffiness, dry mouth, and slight constipation as well as some mydriasis.

Chlorpromazine has weak antihistaminic effects. A phenothiazine with marked antihistaminic action is promethazine (Phenergan) which is not a useful antipsychotic drug.

The actions of chlorpromazine on the cardiovascular system are due to direct effects on the heart and the blood vessels as well as indirect effects mediated by the central nervous system and the autonomic nervous system. Hypotension, especially orthostatic hypotension (a marked fall in blood pressure resulting from a sudden transition from a less to a more upright posture), is possibly due to an inhibition of centrally mediated pressor reflexes, but the alpha adrenergic-blocking action in the peripheral nervous system contributes to this action. Drug-induced vasodilation results from both autonomic effects as well as direct effects on blood vessels. This also contributes to the hypotensive action. Following the administration of the drug, tachycardia is often seen. This is probably due to an attempt of the heart to compensate for the vasodilation and hypotensive effect.

Biochemical Mechanisms

The phenothiazines block the action of serotonin and the catecholamines, norepinephrine and dopamine, throughout the brain. It has been suggested that there is a better relationship between clinical efficacy of the antipsychotic drugs and their relative efficiency in the blockade of dopamine than in the blockade of norepinephrine or serotonin (Snyder et al., 1974). In addition to the dopamine found in the nigrostriatal tracts of the extrapyramidal system, an abundance of dopamine is found in the limbic system and the cerebral cortex.

In addition to the above actions, it has recently been suggested (Snyder, 1974) that many of the phenothiazine drugs have central anticholinergic actions because of an affinity of the phenothiazine molecule for central as well as peripheral muscarinic receptors. Those antipsychotic drugs with little affinity for muscarinic receptors and thus little anticholinergic activity cause more extrapyramidal effects than those with marked anticholinergic actions. N.B.: Prior to the use of *L*-dopa for the treatment of Parkinson's disease, the anticholinergic drugs were the drugs of choice, and they are still used to control drug-induced parkinsonism. A commonly used drug for this purpose is benztropine (Cogentin).

Miscellaneous Actions

Chlorpromazine has marked local anesthetic effects, although it has not been used for this purpose. It is the drug of choice for the treatment of intractable hiccups.

Skeletal Muscles. With acute administration, chlorpromazine depresses skeletal muscle tone in normal subjects and in patients with certain spastic conditions. It has been used to control the muscle spasms of tetanus in man; however, tolerance rapidly develops to this action. Since there may be enhanced muscle spasms after the drug effects have subsided, it is not a drug of choice in treating tetanus spasms.

The most marked motor effects of the phenothiazines are the extrapyramidal effects often seen with chronic administration, but they can occasionally be seen after a large single dose of the drug. (See previous section on basal ganglia and later section on side effects.)

Endocrine System. Chlorpromazine will reduce urinary levels of the gonadotropins, estrogen, and progesterone. It will block ovulation, it suppresses the estrous cycle and it may cause infertility; however, it is not recommended as a "morning-after-pill." The male does not escape, for chlorpromazine also decreases testicular weight. Many of these actions are probably due to effects on the hypothalamus which acts as a control for the pituitary gland which, in turn, mediates the activity of other endocrine glands. Chlorpromazine

PHENOTHIAZINE DERIVATIVES

also decreases the secretion of the adrenocorticotropic hormone (ACTH) via its action on the hypothalamus.

Absorption, Fate, and Excretion

Although chlorpromazine is often used parenterally in the highly agitated patient, the drug is readily absorbed from the gastrointestinal tract. The drug rapidly distributes to all body tissues, and 60 to 70 percent is rapidly removed from the circulation by the liver. A large number of metabolites of chlorpromazine have been isolated from human urine. The metabolites are excreted via the urine or in the feces. The phenothiazines are slow to be excreted. In mental patients who have not received chlorpromazine for six to eight months, various metabolites as well as free chlorpromazine have been found in the urine.

Side Effects and Toxic Reactions

Chlorpromazine has a relatively flat dose-response curve with a large therapeutic index. The major toxic reactions to the phenothiazines are the extrapyramidal reactions.

Extrapyramidal Effects. These are toxic reactions that are dose related, thus they are more likely to occur with higher doses. As previously mentioned they are more often seen with the piperazine derivatives than with the aliphatic or piperidine group, although they are not absent with the aliphatic or piperidine groups. These extrapyramidal actions are manifested as parkinsonism, dystonia, dyskinesia, and akathesia. Parkinsonism will manifest itself in the form of loss of associated movements, including disturbances in gait, rigidity of limbs, tremors, facial rigidity, posture disturbances, and excessive salivation. Dystonia and dyskinesia are involuntary muscle movements characterized by abrupt onset of throwing back and twisting of the head, facial grimacing and distortions, and labored breathing. These involuntary movements may take the form of staring with a fixed gaze, the eyes rotated upward and to the side. The mouth is opened wide with the tongue protruding. The patient's facial expression may suggest that he is in pain.

Akathesia, or motor restlessness, is often seen and reported by the patient as "jitters." The patient will pace the floor, and while sitting, he will constantly shift his position, tap his feet, and complain of anxiousness. The dyskinesia and akathesia are more likely to occur in the younger patient, whereas the parkinsonism is more likely to occur in the older patient. The presence of these side effects can be reduced by a reduction in the dose of the drug. Often antiparkinsonism drugs are used to control these side effects.

Another motor effect that is seen is akinesia. This is characterized by feelings of weakness and muscle fatigue. The patient will often complain of aches and pains in the muscles of the affected limbs. The patients will be apathetic and disinclined to start or spend energy to complete a task, resulting in a marked reduction in their voluntary activity. Tardive dyskinesia is a relatively recently described side effect that is most often seen in patients maintained on phenothiazines for many years. This dyskinesia is characterized by excessive head movements, uncontrolled sucking and/or smacking lip movements, and tongue thrusting.

Tardive dyskinesia is more often seen in older patients and more frequently occurs in women. Unlike other extrapyramidal side effects, the syndrome is exacerbated by reducing the dose of the drug, and it can be controlled by increasing the dose. One hypothesis concerning the cause of tardive dyskinesia is that it is due to denervation supersensitivity. This phenomenon is seen when end organs become excessively responsive to neurotransmitters after normal neural input has been inhibited. It is seen clinically after sympathetic nerves are cut, and organs respond to levels of circulating epinephrine that normally would have no effect.

Jaundice. Obstructive type of liver involvement has been observed in a small percentage of patients treated with phenothiazines. It is not felt to be a serious complication, and it has not been clearly demonstrated that there is permanent hepatocellular damage. If it becomes manifest, jaundice usually appears in the second to fourth week of therapy. It is not dose related. Patients who previously exhibited jaundice when treated with chlorpromazine often show no signs of jaundice when the drug is reintroduced. Until 1965 only fourteen fatalities directly related to chlorpromazine-induced jaundice had been reported (Jarvik, 1970).

Blood Dyscrasias. A number of changes in the cellular composition of the blood may result from treatment with phenothiazines. One of these alterations, agranulocytosis (a marked decrease in particular types of blood cells, i.e., leucocytes and neutrocytes), may be irreversible and is often fatal. Fortunately, this complication of therapy is infrequent. However, less serious alterations in cellular composition of the blood are not uncommon.

Skin Reactions. An abnormal pigmentation of the skin often appears with long chronic use of the phenothiazines, with chlorpromazine seeming to be the chief offender. This change in pigmentation is the result of a hypersensitivity to ultraviolet light, and it consists of a gray-blue pigmentation. Other skin reactions occur in a small number of cases. These are manifested as skin eruptions (urticaria).

Eye. Lens opacities, often large enough to impair vision, have been observed.

These have been found only in patients receiving chlorpromazine for many years.

Convulsive Effects. Phenothiazines lower seizure threshold. Patients with a history of convulsive disorders have exhibited grand mal seizures with high doses. Although the incidence is low, it has been reported as high as 6 percent with chronic chlorpromazine administration.

BUTYROPHENONES

The butyrophenone, haloperidol, has been used in treatment of psychosis in Europe since 1958; however, it was not introduced into treatment in this country until 1967.

Pharmacological Action

The two butyrophenones that have been used in the treatment of schizophrenia are *haloperidol* and *trifluperidol*. The former is most commonly used. Haloperidol has effects quite similar to the piperazine group of phenothiazine drugs. Thus it has many of the same side effects of this class of compounds. The most marked side effects are those involving the extrapyramidal system. Haloperidol has actions in animals quite similar to the phenothiazines. There is no evidence that the butyrophenones have any advantage over the phenothiazines.

THIOXANTHENE DERIVATIVES

The two thioxanthene derivatives used in therapy are chlorprothixene (Taractan) and thiothixene (Navane). They are well tolerated by patients, but there is again no evidence that they are superior to, or even as useful as, the phenothiazines or the butyrophenones.

LITHIUM CARBONATE

The first report of the therapeutic use of lithium in the treatment of mental illness was by an Australian psychiatrist, John F. J. Cade, in 1949 (see Gattozzi, 1970). Cade reported that lithium provided the first specific chemical treatment of mental illness; it failed to cause any interest in the United States. The reason for this was probably due to its use as a salt substitute during this period and the subsequent reports of severe toxic effects. Lithium carbonate has been available for general prescription use in the United States only since 1970. It has Food and Drug Administration (FDA) approval for use in the treatment of manic and hypomanic states.

Although lithium is effective in the treatment of mania and hypomania, there is some controversy concerning whether it is more effective than other antipsychotic medications for the treatment of manic states. The most comprehensive large-scale study of its use was conducted by the Veterans Administration (Prien et al., 1972).

The manner in which lithium produces its therapeutic effect is not known. The major problem with lithium is its potential toxicity.

Lithium is excreted through the kidneys and, if not excreted properly, abnormally high lithium blood levels will occur. Thus extreme care should be maintained in individuals with renal disease or heart disease. Even patients with no evidence of renal or heart disease may not excrete the lithium at the proper rate. The drug can disturb electrolyte balance (sodium and potassium levels), and thus should not be used with diuretics.

The most common side effect is a fine tremor of the hands. This, by itself, is not too bothersome and can be controlled by reducing the dose. Nausea and diarrhea are also early signs of lithium toxicity. Progressive toxicity leads to slurred speech, drowsiness, and if blood levels continue to rise, the patient will lapse into a coma. Occasionally, a patient on lithium will develop symptoms common in diabetes, such as manifested by the drinking of large quantities of water with concomitant passing of large volumes of urine. Blood levels should be frequently checked in patients receiving lithium.

In summary, the evidence suggests that lithium is effective in treating manic and, in some cases, hypomanic states and seems to be an effective agent in preventing relapse. It is probably not the drug of choice in treating the hypomanic state, although there is some evidence that it might be used prophylactically, once the depression has been successfully treated by other drugs (Cole, 1972).

SUMMARY

Despite the possibility of severe side effects, the phenothiazines have had more impact on the treatment of the mentally ill than any other pharmacological agent. Although some of the side effects are potentially dangerous, the incidence of severe side effects is quite low.

In a study by May (1968) phenothiazine therapy was compared to psychoanalytic-oriented psychotherapy and supportive therapy. In addition, one group of patients received psychotherapy and drugs. The results, using a variety of indexes of patient improvement, clearly indicated the superiority of drug therapy over the other therapeutic methods. In patients who do not tolerate the phenothiazines, the butyrophenones are often substituted.

Although these drugs are useful and have clearly had an impact on the treatment of schizophrenia, they are not a "magic bullet," and they are not substitutes for good clinical care. Currently, it is believed that they are antipsychotic in action; that is, they in some way alter the basic process of schizophrenia. The difficulty with drug therapy of the schizophrenic is that even if we knew that the specific cause of schizophrenia was a biochemical abnormality that could be completely reversed by a drug, we would not have a completely "normal" person even after the biochemical reversal. The drugs cannot change years of maladaptive behavior. However, by combining the drug with the proper support, the possibility of a good therapeutic outcome in the schizophrenic patient is high.

For a detailed review of the pharmacology of the antipsychotic drugs, the reader is referred to Jarvik (1970), Byck (1975), or Hollister (1973).

REFERENCES

Bradley, P. B. The central action of certain drugs in relation to the reticular formation of the brain. In H. H. Jasper, L. D. Proctor, R. S. Knighton, W. C. Noshay, and R. T. Costello (Eds.) *Reticular Formation of the Brain.* Boston, Little, Brown, 1958, pp. 123-149.

Bradley, P. B. Phenothiazine derivatives. In W. S. Root and F. G. Hofmann (Eds.) *Physiological Pharmacology.* New York, Academic, 1963, pp. 417-477.

Byck, R. Drugs and treatment of psychiatric disorders. In L. S. Goodman and A. Gilman (Eds.) *The Pharmacological Basis of Therapeutics.* (5th ed.). New York, Macmillan, 1975, pp. 152-200.

Cole, J. O. The current status of lithium treatment. *Massachusetts Journal of Mental Health,* **3,** 1972, 4-13.

Cook, L. and Weidley, E. Behavioral effects of some psychopharmacological agents. *Annals of the New York Academy of Sciences,* **66,** 1957, 740-752.

DiMascio, A. Classification and overview of psychotropic drugs. In A. DiMascio and R. Shader (Eds.) *Clinical Handbook of Psychopharmacology.* New York, Science House, 1970, pp. 3-15.

Eliasson, M. and Kornetsky, C. Interaction effects of chlorpromazine and reticular stimulation on visual attention behavior in rats. *Psychonomic Science,* **26,** 1972, 261-262.

Gattozzi, A. A. Lithium in the treatment of mood disorders. *National Clearinghouse for Mental Health Information Publications,* No. 5033, 1970.

Hollister, L. E. *Clinical Use of Psychotherapeutic Drugs.* Springfield, Charles C Thomas, 1973.

Jarvik, M. Drugs used in the treatment of psychiatric disorders. In L. S. Goodman and A. Gilman (Eds.) *The Pharmacological Basis of Therapeutics.* (5th ed.). New York, Macmillan, 1970, pp. 151-225.

Killam, E. K. Pharmacology of the reticular formation. In D. Efron (Ed.) *Psychopharmacology, A Review of Progress 1957-1967.* U.S. Government Printing Office. Public Health Service Publication, No. 1836, Washington, D.C., 1968, pp., 411-445.

Killam, K. F. and Killam, E. K. Drug action on pathways involving the reticular formation. In H. H. Jasper, L. D. Proctor, R. S. Knighton, W. C. Noshay, and R. T. Costello (Eds.) *Reticular Formation of the Brain.* Boston, Little, Brown, 1958, pp. 111-122.

Kline, N. Rauwolfia serpentina in neuropsychiatric conditions. *Annals of New York Academy of Science,* **59,** 1954, 107-122.

Kline, N. Presidential Address. In D. Efron (Ed.) *Psychopharmacology. A Review of Progress 1957-1967.* U.S. Government Printing Office. Public Health Service Publication, No. 1936, Washington, D.C., 1968, pp. 1-3.

Kornetsky, C. and Bain, G. Effects of chlorpromazine and pentobarbital on sustained attention in the rat. *Psychopharmacologia (Berlin),* 8, 1965, 277-284.

Kornetsky, C. and Eliasson, M. Reticular stimulation and chlorpromazine: An animal model for schizophrenic overarousal. *Science,* 165, 1969, 1273-1274.

Kornetsky, C. and Mirsky, A. F. On certain psychopharmacological and physiological differences between schizophrenics and normal persons. *Psychopharmacologia (Berlin),* 8, 1966, 309-318.

Lehmann, H. E. and Hanrahan, G. E. Chlorpromazine, new inhibiting agent for psychomotor excitement and manic states. *A.M.A. Archives of Neurology and Psychiatry,* 71, 1954, 227-237.

Lipper, S. and Kornetsky, C. Effect of chlorpromazine on conditioned avoidance as a function of CS–US interval length. *Psychopharmacologia (Berlin),* 22, 1971, 144-150.

Low, L. A., Eliasson, M., and Kornetsky, C. Effect of chlorpromazine on avoidance acquisition as a function of CS–US interval length. *Psychopharmacologia (Berlin),* 10, 1966, 148-154.

May, P. R. A. *Treatment of Schizophrenia: A Comparative Study of Five Treatment Methods.* New York, Science House, 1968.

Mirsky, A. F. and Kornetsky, C. On the dissimilar effects of drugs on the digit symbol substitution and continuous performance tests. *Psychopharmacologia (Berlin),* 5, 1964, 161-177.

Mirsky, A. F. and Tecce, J. J. The relationship between EEG and impaired attention following administration of centrally acting drugs. In H. Brill, J. O. Cole, P. Deniker, H. Hippius, and P. B. Bradley (Eds.) *Neuro-Psycho-Pharmacology,* Amsterdam, Excerpta Medica International Congress, Series No. 129, 1967, pp. 638-645.

Poslun, D. An analysis of chlorpromazine induced suppression of the avoidance response. *Psychopharmacologia (Berlin),* 3, 1962, 361-373.

Prien, R. F., Coffey, E. M., and Klett, C. J. Comparison of lithium carbonate and chlorpromazine in the treatment of mania. *Archives of General Psychiatry,* 26, 1972, 146-153.

Rosvold, H. E., Mirsky, A. F., Sarason, I., Bransome, E. D., and Beck, L. H. A continuous performance test of brain damage. *Journal of Consulting Psychology,* 20, 1956, 343-350.

Snyder, S. H., Banerjee, S. P., Yamamura, H. I., and Greenberg, D. Drugs, neurotransmitters, and schizophrenia. *Science,* 148, 1974, 1243-1253.

Swazey, J. *Chlorpromazine in Psychiatry: A Study of Therapeutic Innovation,* Cambridge, MIT Press, 1974.

Wilkins, R. W. and Judson, W. E. The use of rauwolfia serpentina in hypertensive patients. *New England Journal of Medicine,* 248, 1953, 48-53.

6 DRUGS USED IN THE TREATMENT OF DEPRESSION AND ANXIETY

ANTIDEPRESSANT DRUGS

Feelings of sadness are a common human experience, but for some the extent of the sadness is a pit of deep depression that is beyond the range of normal experience. The most common drug used by the general population to combat periods of sadness is not pharmacologically a stimulant but a central nervous system depressant, alcohol. Alcohol has been praised since ancient times in both story and song as the liberator from sorrow and depression. The German poet Wilhelm Bush (1832–1908) wrote:

It is the custom from ancient times
Who sorrow has,
Has also wine.

In situations of worry, depression, and tension, small doses of alcohol do seem to produce in many a temporary euphoria. This self-therapy with alcohol provides only transient relief and does not seem to have much effect on endogenous depression.

In the 1950s there was a revolution in the drug treatment of the psychotic patient, but socially regressed, apathetic, depressed patients often had their symptoms intensified by these tranquilizing drugs. The only really effective treatment of depression was electroconvulsive therapy. For milder types of depression the amphetamines were often used.

Like the antipsychotic drugs, the first of the antidepressant drugs was used for the treatment of some other disease. In 1951 isoniazid, as well as a derivative, iproniazid, was introduced in the treatment of tuberculosis. Both drugs seemed to cause some mood-elevating effects in the patients. This was especially true for iproniazid. The patients showed, in addition to elevation of mood, increase in physical activity and an increase in resistance to fatigue. It was not clear whether the improvement was due to some direct CNS action or simply the result of a decrease in their tuberculosis infection. However, it became clear that iproniazid seemed to have stimulating properties, and the action of this drug on mood was not simply due to the amelioration of the infection. In 1952 Zeller and co-workers found that iproniazid was a monoamine oxidase (MAO) inhibitor, whereas isoniazid was not. That is, it inhibited the enzyme monoamine oxidase that is responsible for the degradation of various naturally occurring catecholamines as well as serotonin (5-hydroxytryptamine, 5HT). Thus blocking MAO results in an increase in levels of serotonin as well as norepinephrine in the brain.

Since reserpine administration causes a depletion of serotonin in the brain, and iproniazid blocks MAO which results in increased serotonin levels, a theory developed that the neurohumor serotonin was central for the control of one's affective state. Thus if serotonin levels were elevated, there would be an increase in agitation, and if the levels were depressed below normal levels, then the behavioral state was one of lethargy and depression. This model was used to explain how iproniazid as well as reserpine produced their therapeutic action.

The first reported clinical use of iproniazid in depressed patients was in 1958 by Kline. Kline called the drug a "psychic energizer." It was found to be useful, not only to the hospitalized depressed patient, but also in the so-called nonhospitalized, neurotic, depressed patient. These early positive results led to the synthesis and marketing of many other MAO inhibitors as well as the later development of nonMAO-inhibitor, antidepressant drugs. Because of their marked toxicity, many of the early MAO inhibitors, including iproniazid (Marsilid), were withdrawn from the market.

MAO Inhibitors

The antidepressant MAO inhibitors can be divided into two classes of compounds: the hydrazine and nonhydrazine derivatives. Hydrazine is highly toxic to the liver. Because of this marked hepatotoxicity, compounds that were not hydrazine derivatives, yet were potent MAO inhibitors, were developed. These latter compounds were structurally related to amphetamine. Table 1 lists the various antidepressant drugs by type.

Behavioral and CNS Effects. In normal subjects very little is seen after single doses. This is not surprising since in depressed patients, a number of weeks may be needed before any discernible clinical effect is observed.

In animals there is some stimulation after single doses, but it is not marked. This is so even at doses in which there are not striking changes in brain levels of dopamine, norepinephrine, and serotonin. The MAO inhibitors cause low-voltage, fast activity in the EEG. They do appear to alter the threshold for EEG and behavioral arousal caused by stimulation of the reticular formation. These drugs do cause marked effects on the behavior of animals when combined with other drugs. If animals are pretreated with MAO inhibitors, the action of

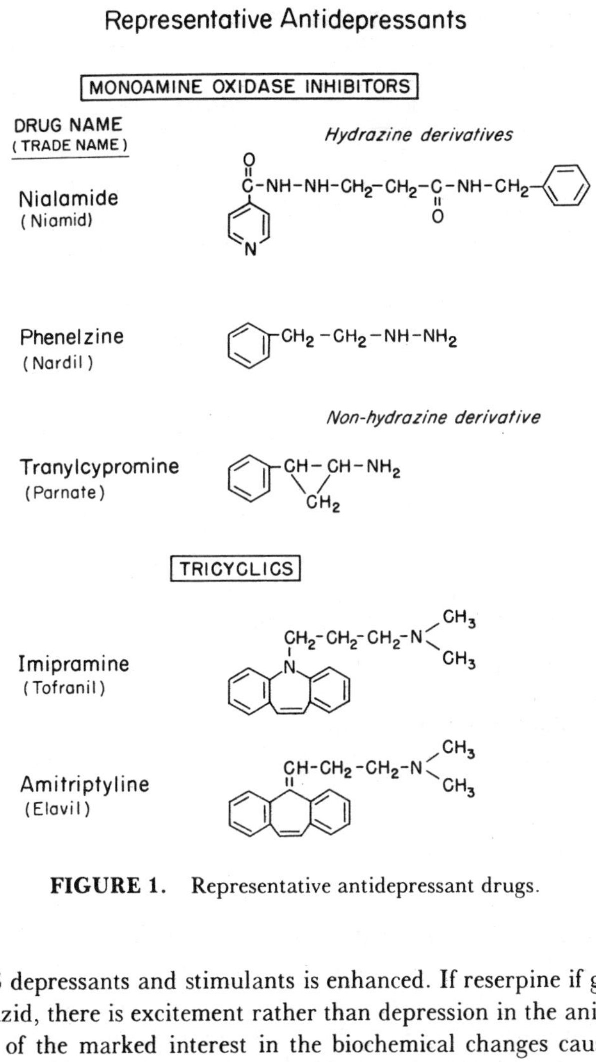

ANTIANXIETY DRUGS

Representative Antidepressants

MONOAMINE OXIDASE INHIBITORS

DRUG NAME (TRADE NAME)

Hydrazine derivatives

Nialamide (Niamid)

Phenelzine (Nardil)

Non-hydrazine derivative

Tranylcypromine (Parnate)

TRICYCLICS

Imipramine (Tofranil)

Amitriptyline (Elavil)

FIGURE 1. Representative antidepressant drugs.

many CNS depressants and stimulants is enhanced. If reserpine if given following iproniazid, there is excitement rather than depression in the animal.

Because of the marked interest in the biochemical changes caused by these compounds and the minor behavioral changes seen in animals, research has focused on the biochemical aspects, rather than the neurophysiological and neurobehavioral effects.

The MAO inhibitors are not specific for MAO but inhibit many normal enzymatic functions in the body. They interact with many drugs including the nonMAO-inhibitor antidepressants and analgesics, and they prolong the actions of all CNS depressants. Thus patients receiving MAO inhibitors should not be given other CNS drugs, and they should be warned against the use of alcohol.

TABLE 1. REPRESENTATIVE ANTIDEPRESSANT DRUGS

Generic name	Brand name	Daily dose range (mg)[a]
Monoamine Oxidase Inhibitors:		
Hydrazine derivatives		
Isocarboxazid	Marplan®	30–50
Phenelzine	Nardil®	10–75
Nialamide	Niamid®	12.5–200
Nonhydrazines:		
Tranylcypromine	Parnate®	10–30
Pargyline	Eutonyl®	25–75
Tricyclics:		
Imipramine	Tofranil®	75–150
Desipramine	Pertofrane® Norpramin®	30–150
Amitriptyline	Elavil®	75–150
Nortriptyline	Aventyl®	75–200

[a] Dosages as given by DiMascio, A. Classification and overview of psychotropic drugs. In A. DiMascio and R. Shader (eds.) *Clinical Handbook of Psychopharmacology*. New York, Science House, 1970, 3–15.

Absorption, Fate, and Excretion. The MAO inhibitors are readily absorbed by the intestinal tract. Although it is believed that these drugs do not stay in the body for a long period of time, the enzyme changes that are produced are lasting. The enzyme inhibition is believed to be irreversible, and termination of the effects occurs only with enzyme regeneration.

Toxicity and Side Effects. The MAO inhibitors, as previously mentioned, inhibit other enzymes besides MAO and thus interfere with many functions of the body. Because of the possible severity of the side effects of the MAO inhibitors, therapy with them has been confined, for the most part, to the hospitalized patient. Also because of the enzyme-inhibiting effects, they will drastically interfere with the metabolism of other administered drugs.

In addition to interacting with other drugs, MAO inhibitors may interact with components of some foods. Cheese, specifically, has been implicated as a cause of hypertensive crises in patients being treated with these drugs. It has been reported by Asatoor and co-workers (1963) that an average meal of natural or aged cheese contains enough tyramine to cause a marked rise in blood pressure. Tyramine is a sympathomimetic agent that causes a release of stored norepinephrine and thus causes a pressor effect. Because of the action of the MAO inhibitors on liver enzymes, the tyramine is not oxidized and releases excessive amounts of norepinephrine that are present in the nerve endings.

ANTIDEPRESSANT DRUGS

Cheeses that have been implicated have been cheddar, camembert, and Stilton; however, other foods high in tyramine that have produced this toxic syndrome are: beer, wine, chicken liver, yeast, coffee, pickled herring, bean pods, and canned figs (Jarvik, 1970). Deaths have been reported in patients on these drugs who have ingested moderate amounts of cheese. The syndrome includes: increase in body temperature, marked rise in blood pressure, severe headache, and in those cases in which death resulted, intracranial bleeding. In addition to tyramine, other sympathomimetic amines, such as amphetamine, that release catecholamine stores at the nerve endings, should not be taken by patients receiving MAO inhibitors (Byck, 1975).

Orthostatic hypotension commonly occurs with the use of MAO inhibitors. Although extreme blood pressure depression is not usual, slight depression in blood pressure may last for a number of days after discontinuation of the drug.

Jaundice, with accompanying liver toxicity, is common. The jaundice caused by these drugs is of the degenerative type, and a number of fatalities have been reported. The incidence of hepatotoxicity is quite low with the MAO inhibitors currently accepted for therapy. This risk is considered acceptable in the severe depressions that do not respond to the imipramine type of antidepressant (see below).

There may be *central stimulation* resulting in tremors, agitation, and insomnia. Convulsions as well as peripheral neuropathy (pathology of peripheral nerves) have resulted from therapy with the MAO inhibitors. Decrease in libido has been reported, but the level of sexual drive in the depressed patient is such that any further decrease will probably not be noticed by the partner. Unlike the amphetamines, the MAO inhibitors may produce a mild hypoglycemia with a concomitant increase in appetite and weight gain.

Nonhydrazine MAO Inhibitors. As a result of the extreme toxicity of the hydrazines, MAO inhibitors that were not hydrazines were developed. The most commonly used of this class is tranylcypromine (Parnate). Although tranylcypromine is a potent MAO inhibitor, it does not have hepatocellulartoxicity of the hydrazine type, although it will severely interact with ingested foods having a high tyramine content.

The action of this class of drugs is more rapid, probably because of its amphetamine structure. In 1964 Parnate was withdrawn from the market because of its marked interaction with many drugs or foods rich in amines. It subsequently was placed back on the market for use only in hospitalized depressed patients.

Tricyclic Antidepressants

The tricyclic antidepressants currently in use are imipramine (Tofranil), desipramine (desmethylimipramine, Norpramine, Pertofran), amitriptyline

(Elavil), and nortriptyline (Aventyl). These drugs are structurally related to the phenothiazines. They are the most widely used drugs for the treatment of endogenous depression, and except for cases that are refractory to the tricyclic group, they have almost replaced MAO inhibitors.

Behavioral and Central Nervous System Effects. In animals the effects are somewhat similar to those of the phenothiazine drugs but to a lesser degree. Unlike chlorpromazine, the tricyclic antidepressants will cause stimulation in some schedules of reinforcement at some doses in pigeons (Dews, 1962) and rats (Kornetsky, 1965).

In normal volunteers the effects are much more chlorpromazine-like than amphetamine-like. Studies by Grunthal (1958, as reported by Byck, 1975, p. 175) and DiMascio and co-workers (1964) showed that imipramine seemed to alter cognitive performance more than chlorpromazine and reduced motor performance less than chlorpromazine in volunteers.

In man, EEG studies show that the tricyclic antidepressants decrease the amount of alpha and increase the amount of theta and beta waves. They will lower the threshold for seizures in epileptics. In some patients excitement has been reported.

Autonomic Nervous System. Like the phenothiazines, the tricyclic antidepressants have a cholinergic-blocking effect of a muscarinic nature. This results in some of the side effects reported: dry mouth, constipation, urinary retention, and blurred vision.

Mechanism of Action. The mechanism of action of the tricyclic antidepressant drugs is unknown. However, there is no dearth of theories to explain the manner in which they cause their therapeutic gains. Their successful use is a beautiful example of the treatment of a disease of unknown etiology with a drug of unknown pharmacologic action. Schildkraut (1970, 1973), in reviewing the available evidence, implicates abnormalities in the monoamine metabolism in patients suffering from affective disorders. He postulates that drugs that are therapeutically useful in the treatment of depression increase one or more of the biogenic amines at the receptor sites in the brain, whereas, drugs that are effective in the treatment of mania decrease the activity of the monoamines at the receptor. Although the evidence available supports this putative model of the affective disorders, the theory is far from proven.

Absorption, Distribution, and Fate. These drugs are readily absorbed from the gastrointestinal tract. Some imipramine is excreted unchanged or in the form of an active metabolite, desmethylimipramine. In animals imipramine is found in greatest concentration in the brain, kidney, and liver.

Side Effects and Toxicity. The side effects of imipramine are similar to those seen with the other tricyclic antidepressants. The most common untoward effects are due to the anticholinergic action of the drug. These are: dry mouth, constipation, urinary retention, and tachycardia. An unexplained side effect is excessive sweating.

Weakness and fatigue, much like that seen with the phenothiazines, is not uncommon. Myocardial infarctions as well as congestive heart failure have been believed to be precipitated by imipramine. Orthostatic hypotension, headache, and muscle tremors are also seen. Jaundice, of the obstructive type similar to that seen with phenothiazines, as well as agranulocytosis has also been reported in patients receiving the tricyclic antidepressants.

The drug should not be given to patients receiving MAO inhibitors for the reasons described previously. It is believed that at least 10 days to two weeks should intervene between medication in patients going from MAO inhibitors to tricyclic antidepressants.

Tolerance does develop to many of the anticholinergic and blood pressure effects of the antidepressant drugs. However, there does not seem to be tolerance to the main therapeutic action.

Clinical Use

Of the various antidepressant drugs, imipramine has been most extensively studied. In one review of its use in newly hospitalized patients, the rate of improvement was sixty percent. However, the overall rate of improvement with a placebo was forty percent (Klerman and Cole, 1965). Cole (1970), in reviewing the efficacy of the antidepressant drugs, points out that imipramine is significantly superior to a placebo but not by a "reassuring margin." Amitriptyline is probably equal in efficacy to imipramine and, in some cases, has been found to be superior.

However, Cole states that uncontrolled studies by private psychiatrists and those emanating from outpatient clinics often report improvement rates of eighty percent or better. He suggests that the higher-reported improvement rate may not simply be due to the optimism of the therapist but that some outpatient clinics and private practitioners see more acute patients with less previous symptomatology than are usually seen in the hospital setting. Also suggested is that the greater improvement may be a function of the potentiation of the drug effect by the more highly personal nature of treatment that is available in the private practice or the outpatient clinic.

For certain types of depression success has been achieved with phenothiazines rather than the antidepressants. Cole divides depression into five types: retarded depression, agitated depression, hostile depression, anxious depression, and atypical depression. These do not conform to the usual existing nomenclature but are phenomenologically derived. In the retarded depressed patient the tricyclic antidepressant should be tried first. In the agitated depression it has been reported that thioridazine is as effective as imipramine.

Thioridazine seems to be superior to imipramine in treating the anxious depression (Cole, 1970, p. 62). For the atypical depression the British literature suggests the use of the MAO inhibitors; however, Cole believes that because of the dangers of the MAO inhibitors, the tricyclic antidepressants or the minor tranquilizers should first be tried. The atypical depression is described as the depression in patients with a severe preexisting personality disorder. Phobias and compulsive behavior are common in this group.

Summary. In general, the use of the antidepressants has been somewhat disappointing. Depression is usually self-limiting, and a therapeutic response to the antidepressant drugs usually takes several weeks. Also, there is no evidence that this class of compounds is superior to electroshock therapy for severe depression. Unfortunately, because of a history of overuse and the spectre of medieval torture, electrotherapy is not often used in this country. Drug therapy may take days or even weeks before producing a favorable outcome, and there is the danger of severe side effects. Psychotherapy is also a slow and tortuous treatment with a minimum of documented success, and the added danger of suicide is always present. When these drawbacks are compared with the rapid improvement and minimum of sequelae seen with electroshock therapy, one wonders which therapy is more medieval.

ANTIANXIETY DRUGS

Anxiety is a common experience, certainly necessary for life. The human body, by means of its autonomic nervous system, is well designed to handle the normal range of anxiety. It is a positive force in the emergency or stress situation. However, anxiety of a pathological nature is detrimental to life. I would define anxiety as pathological when it no longer serves to sustain life and only hinders the functioning of the individual.

Prior to the so-called antianxiety drugs, physicians often treated the anxious patient with phenobarbital. If phenobarbital were to be discovered today, it is most likely that it would be marketed as an antianxiety drug rather than as a sedative.

Meprobamate (Miltown, Equanil)

Meprobamate was the first of the antianxiety drugs that was developed. In the 1950s the name Miltown became part of our language and was often seen in cartoons. (There was a *New Yorker* cartoon of this period of a man standing in front of a vending machine in the subway. The vending machine is selling candy, gum, and Miltown.)

Meprobamate was originally synthesized in 1951 as a muscle relaxant that would replace mephenesin, a potent muscle relaxant that unfortunately had a

ANTIANXIETY DRUGS

TABLE 2. REPRESENTATIVE ANTIANXIETY DRUGS

Generic name	Brand name	Daily dosage range (mg)[a]
Benzodiazepines:		
Chlordiazepoxide	Librium®	10–100
Diazepam	Valium®	6–40
Oxazepam	Serax®	30–120
Propanediols:		
Meprobamate	Equanil®, Miltown®	600–1,200
Tybamate	Solacen®	750–1,200
Miscellaneous:		
Azacyclonol	Frenquel®	60–300
Benactyzine	Suavitil®	3–9
Phenaglycodol	Ultran®	800–1,200

[a] Dosages as given by DiMascio, A. Classification and overview of psychotropic drugs. In A. DiMascio and R. Shader (Eds.) *Clinical Handbook of Psychopharmacology.* New York, Science House, 1970, pp. 3–15.

very short duration of action. In addition to meprobamate's muscle relaxant properties, it seems to be useful in suppressing anxiety and within a few years was widely used for its antianxiety action, replacing phenobarbital.

Behavioral and Central Nervous System Effects. The effects of meprobamate are very similar to those of the barbiturates. Like the barbiturates, it will impair performance on psychological tests. Learning is impaired with a single 800-mg dose in man, whereas 1600 mg will impair learning, motor coordination, and reaction time (Kornetsky, 1958). Most investigators have failed to find a deficit in behavior with the usual 400-mg dose. However, Loomis and West (1958) did find some impairment on a simulated driving test with 400 mg. Laties (1959) reported that the drug decreased palmar sweating in subjects riding a ferris wheel; however, there was no concomitant subjective reduction in anxiety reported by the subjects. In animal studies the effects of meprobamate are similar to those of barbiturates. On the conditioned avoidance procedure (CAR) suppression of avoidance behavior is only manifest at doses that also suppress escape behavior.

EEG effects are similar to those of the barbiturates. Large doses result in fast activity as seen with hypnotic doses of secobarbital (200 mg). However, the slow activity seen with large doses of barbiturates is not reported, even with toxic doses of meprobamate. The drug is somewhat effective against petit mal epilepsy but may aggravate grand mal seizures. Meprobamate's action in the CNS is somewhat diffuse. It causes some slow wave activity in the basal gan-

Representative Anti-Anxiety Agents

DRUG NAME
(TRADE NAME)

Meprobamate
(Miltown)
(Equanil)

Chlordiazepoxide
(Librium)

Diazepam
(Valium)

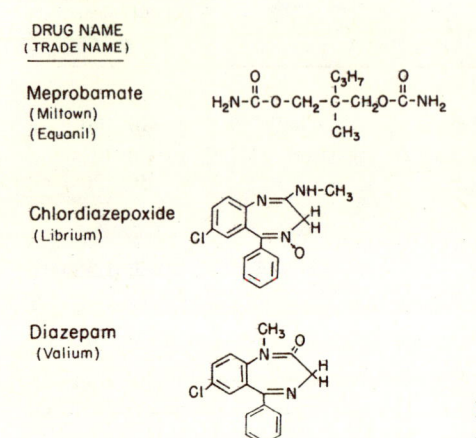

FIGURE 2. Representative antianxiety drugs.

glia and limbic system and like barbiturates, will raise the threshold for direct reticular stimulation. Kletzkin and Swan (1959) suggest a relatively greater effect on the limbic system than on the reticular system. The drug has no antiadrenergic or anticholinergic effects. Thus many of the autonomic side effects seen with the antipsychotic and antidepressant drugs are absent.

Although when meprobamate was first introduced it was believed that physical dependence was not produced, subsequent use of the drug indicated that physical dependence can be manifested with chronic administration of high doses. The withdrawal syndrome resembles that seen with the barbiturates. It consists of convulsions and/or psychosis.

Absorption, Fate, and Excretion. Meprobamate is readily absorbed from the gastrointestinal tract. Peak concentrations in the blood are reached within one or two hours. It is uniformly distributed throughout the body. About ninety percent of the drug is excreted as a metabolite and about ten percent as unchanged meprobamate. It is excreted via the kidneys.

Side Effects and Toxicity. Drowsiness is the most common side effect of this drug. The drug has a relatively flat dose-response curve, making it relatively safe for use with the suicide minded. Allergic reactions have been reported as well as a very few cases of hematological disorders. Hypotensive effects, especially in the elderly, have been observed. The danger of physical dependence is always present in subjects receiving daily doses exceeding 2400 mg.

Clinical Use. The clinical usefulness of meprobamate is debatable. Many clinicians have ceased to use it, preferring the newer benzodiazepine compounds (see below). The difficulty in evaluating the effectiveness of meprobamate or any antianxiety drug is that it is difficult to come to some meaningful definition of anxiety that is quantifiable. Laties and Weiss (1958), in reviewing the literature on meprobamate, concluded that meprobamate was no better than a placebo or a barbiturate in ameliorating anxiety in the outpatient, but seems to have some usefulness in the hospitalized patient.

Benzodiazepine Compounds

There are presently three benzodiazepine derivatives commonly used: chlordiazepoxide (Librium), diazepam (Valium), and oxazepam (Serax). All have somewhat similar actions.

The first drug of this class to appear on the market was chlordiazepoxide. Randall and co-workers in 1960 reported that it seemed to be effective in "taming" aggressive laboratory animals at doses that did not cause ataxia. These animal studies were quickly followed by clinical trials to determine the efficacy of chlordiazepoxide as an antianxiety drug.

Behavioral and Central Nervous System Effects. These compounds have sedative, anticonvulsant, and skeletal muscle relaxant properties. Their actions are similar to those of meprobamate, although they are more effective in the treatment of anxiety. At adequate doses they unselectively impair a variety of psychological behaviors. In animals, like meprobamate and the barbiturates, they only decrease avoidance behavior at doses that also decrease escape behavior. On a procedure first described by Geller and Seifter (1960) benzodiazepines seem to selectively decrease conflict behavior in animals (see Cook and Kelleher, 1963).

The benzodiazepines can be used as hypnotics, and at usual clinical doses, they do not suppress REM sleep but do markedly suppress stage-IV sleep. They cause an increase in fast activity (dose dependent) and an increase in amplitude in the EEG. Like chlorpromazine and meprobamate, they depress electrical discharge from the limbic system. They raise seizure thresholds and are used in the control of seizure activity in the epileptic (see Chapter 11).

Actions on the reticular formation are similar to those of the barbiturates, raising the threshold for EEG and behavioral arousal in response to direct electrical stimulation.

Absorption, Fate, and Excretion. Chlordiazepoxide is readily absorbed from the gastrointestinal tract. In man several hours are needed for the drug to reach peak blood levels. When the drug is discontinued, it takes several days before the drug is not detectable in the plasma. Excretion is via the kidneys and the gastrointestinal tract. Most is metabolized, but one to two percent is found in unchanged form. Diazepam has a somewhat different metabolic fate. Part of the ingested dose is excreted rapidly (as drug or metabolites), whereas the remainder is excreted more slowly, with a half-life of 2 to 8 days.

Toxicity and Side Effects. The most frequent side effect of this class of compounds is drowsiness. If the dose is high enough, ataxia is common, and in aged and debilitated patients, syncope has been observed. Skin rashes, nausea, menstrual and ovulatory disturbances, and hepatic changes have been observed. The benzodiazepines will often act synergistically with other CNS depressants, including alcohol.

Physical dependence with a withdrawal syndrome similar to that seen with barbiturates and meprobamate is seen with chlordiazepoxide. For physical dependence to develop, the dose must be far in excess of the usual clinical dose. Although some individuals have attempted suicide with chlordiazepoxide or diazepam, they have not been successful. Zbinden et al. (1961) reviewed twenty-one suicide attempts with chlordiazepoxide at doses from 0.2 to 2.25 g taken orally. Patients were drowsy but were able to talk. Respiration, blood pressure, and pulse rate were depressed. None of the attempts was successful. One side effect that might lead to problems with patients is the fact that there may be a marked increase in appetite with concomitant weight gain.

Clinical Use. The benzodiazepine compounds have been used extensively in the treatment of anxiety and alcoholism. Diazepam has been used as therapy in certain types of convulsive disorders. In the treatment of alcoholism they relieve the symptoms of alcohol withdrawal, suggesting that they may substitute for alcohol.

Because of the muscle relaxant properties of these drugs, they are often used to decrease muscle spasms; diazepam seems preferred for this use.

As a result of the extensive use of these drugs for all sorts of supportive therapy by nonpsychiatrist physicians as well as use by psychiatrists, the benzodiazepine compounds are one of the most frequently prescribed classes of drugs in the United States. For the most part, they have supplanted the use of phenobarbital or meprobamate for the treatment of anxiety.

Summary. The use of the antianxiety drugs has been excessive. It is much easier for a physician to write a prescription than it is for him to take the time to listen to the patient. Too many people are taking drugs to handle a normal anxious response. Certainly, when anxiety is pathological, the drug may be appropriate, but the statement to the doctor that "I am nervous and tense" is never enough reason to prescribe a potent pharmaceutical. These drugs are evidently effective in many cases, but there is need for a more judicious use.

REFERENCES

Asatoor, A. M., Levi, A. J., and Milne, M. D. Tranylcypromine and cheese. *Lancet,* **2,** 1963, 733–734.

Byck, R. Drugs and treatment of psychiatric disorders. In L. S. Goodman and A. Gilman (Eds.) *The Pharmacological Basis of Therapeutics.* (5th ed.). New York, Macmillan, 1975, pp. 152–200.

REFERENCES

Cole, J. O. Antidepressant drug treatment. In A. DiMascio and R. I. Shader (Eds.) *Clinical Handbook of Psychopharmacology.* New York, Science House, 1970, pp. 57–70.

Cook, L. and Kelleher, R. T. Effects of drugs on behavior. *Annual Review of Pharmacology,* 3, 1963, 205–222.

Dews, P. B. A behavioral output enhancing effect of imipramine in pigeons. *International Journal of Neuropharmacology,* 5, 1962, 361–371.

DiMascio, A. Classification and overview of psychotropic drugs. In A. DiMascio and R. Shader (Eds.) *Clinical Handbook of Psychopharmacology.* New York, Science House, 1970, pp. 3–15.

DiMascio, A., Heninger, G., and Klerman, G. L. Psychopharmacology of imipramine and desipramine. A comparative study of their effects in normal males. *Psychopharmacologia (Berlin),* 5, 1964, 361–371.

Geller, J. and Seifter, J. The effects of meprobamate, barbiturates, d-amphetamine and promazine on experimentally induced conflict in the rat. *Psychopharmacologia (Berlin),* 1, 1960, 483–492.

Harris, T. H. Methaminodiazepoxide. *The Journal of the American Medical Association,* 172, 1960, 1162–1163.

Jarvik, M. E. Drugs used in the treatment of psychiatric disorders. In L. S. Goodman and A. Gilman (Eds.) *The Pharmacological Basis of Therapeutics* (4th ed.). New York, Macmillan, 1970, pp. 151–203.

Klerman, G. L. and Cole, J. O. Clinical pharmacology of imipramine and related antidepressant compounds. *Pharmacological Reviews,* 17, 1965, 101–141.

Kletzkin, M. and Swan, K. The effects of meprobamate and pentobarbital upon cortical and subcortical responses to auditory stimulation. *The Journal of Pharmacology and Experimental Therapeutics,* 125, 1959, 35–39.

Kline, N. S. Clinical experience with iproniazid (Marsilid). *Journal of Clinical and Experimental Psychopathology,* 19, Suppl. 1, 1958, 72–78.

Kornetsky, C. Effects of meprobamate, phenobarbital and dextroamphetamine on reaction time and learning in man. *The Journal of Pharmacology and Experimental Therapeutics,* 123, 1958, 216–219.

Kornetsky, C. A comparison of the effects of desipramine and imipramine on two schedules of reinforcement. *International Journal of Neuropharmacology,* 4, 1965, 13–16.

Laties, V. G. and Weiss, B. A critical review of the efficacy of meprobamate (Miltown, Equanil) in the treatment of anxiety. *Journal of Chronic Diseases,* 7, 1958, 500–519.

Laties, V. G. Effects of meprobamate on fear and palmar sweating. *Journal of Abnormal and Social Psychology,* 59, 1959, 156–161.

Loomis, T. A. and West, T. C. Comparative sedative effects of a barbiturate and some tranquilizer drugs on normal subjects. *The Journal of Pharmacology and Experimental Therapeutics.* 122, 1958, 525–531.

Randall, L. O., Schallek, W., Heise, G. A., Keith, E. F., and Bagdon, R. E. The psychosedative properties of methaminodiazepoxide. *Journal of Pharmacology and Experimental Therapeutics,* 129, 1960, 163–171.

Schildkraut, J. Biochemical studies of drugs used in the treatment of the affective disorders. In A. DiMascio and R. I. Shader (Eds.) *Clinical Handbook of Psychopharmacology.* New York, Science House, 1970, pp. 137–148.

Schildkraut, J. Neuropharmacology of the affective disorders. *Annual Review of Pharmacology,* 13, 1973, 427–454.

Zbinden, G., Bagdon, R. E., Keith, E. F., Phillips, R. D., and Randall, L. O. Experimental and clinical toxicology of chlordiazepoxide (Librium®). *Toxicology and Applied Pharmacology,* **3,** 1961, 619–637.

Zeller, E. A., Barsky, J., Fouts, J. R., Kirchheimer, W. F., and VanOrden, L. S. Influence of isonicotinic acid hydrazine (INH) and 1-isonicotinyl-2-isopropyl hydrazide (IIH) on bacterial and mammalian enzymes. *Experientia,* **8,** 1952, 349–350.

7 NARCOTIC ANALGESICS

In this chapter the pharmacology of one of the most interesting classes of compounds is presented. The opiates and related narcotic analgesics are of interest because of some of their unique actions. These include the attenuation of pain and a degree of tolerance with repeated administration that can be matched by few if any other classes of compounds.

One of the narcotic drugs, heroin, is well known on the streets of our urban centers, and in recent years use of heroin has increased in the more affluent suburbs. The narcotic drugs receive a great deal of attention in the mass media. Actions are attributed to this class of compounds that should be attributed to society. Certainly social disorganization is not caused by the use of heroin, but certainly social disorganization can lead to heroin use.

Despite the "bad" name that opiates have obtained, they are without equal in the alleviation of pain in man. David Macht, writing in 1915, in the *Journal of the American Medical Association* stated, "If the entire materia medica at our disposal were limited to the chronic use of only one drug, I am sure that a great many if not the majority of us would choose opium. . . ." Many new drugs have been added since 1915, but it would not be far off the mark to state that most physicians would still rate the opiates as one of the most important classes of compounds at their disposal.

Opium, the raw material from which morphine is isolated, is obtained by incising the unripe seed capsule of the poppy plant, *Papaver somniferum,* which is indigenous to Asia Minor. The milky juice that is released is dried in air and forms a brown, gummy mass. After further drying, it is powdered. This powdered opium contains many alkaloids, only a few of which have clinical usefulness. Those alkaloids that are clinically useful are morphine and codeine.

Although the earliest authentic references to the use of opium are found in Greek literature of the early third century, B.C., it is believed that the ancient Sumerians (circa 4000 B.C.) may have been familiar with its properties. Their ideograph for poppies was *hulgil* ("joy plants"). Some interpretations of sections of the Old Testament suggest that opium was known by the ancient Hebrews.

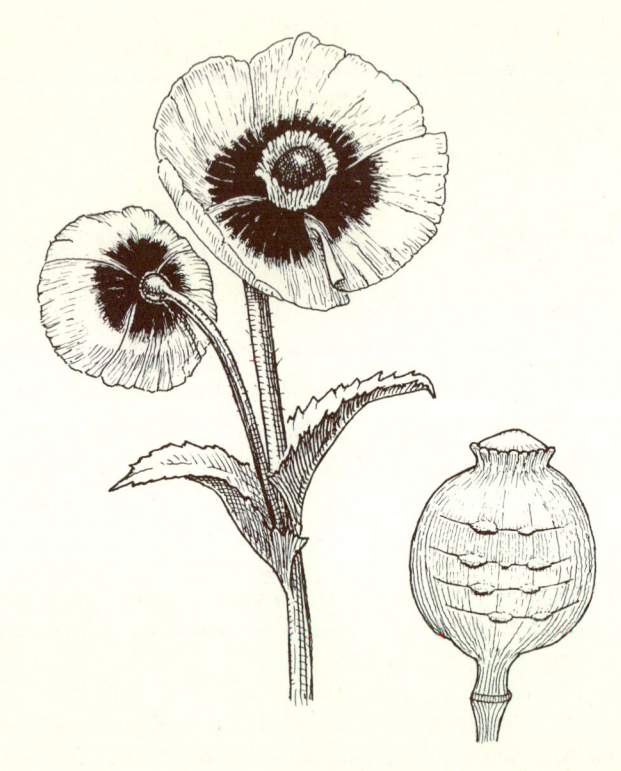

FIGURE 1. Drawing of the opium poppy (*Papaver somniferum*) on left, and on right a ripened seed pod slit to obtain the gummy exudate that contains the opium.

The word *rosh*, meaning "head," is believed to refer to the head of the poppy and the word *me-rosh*, to the juice of the poppy.

Arab physicians were most knowledgeable in the use of opium, finding it most efficacious in the control of diarrhea. It is believed that the Arabian traders introduced opium to the Orient. Here the use was primarily for the treatment of dysentery, and it was not until well into the seventeenth century that opium smoking became a problem.

Tincture of opium, called *laudanum*, dates back to the early part of the sixteenth century and still can be found as an official remedy in the United States Pharmacopeia (U.S.P.), although laudanum is rarely used today. *Paragoric*, which is camphorated tincture of opium, is still used extensively in the treatment of diarrhea, especially in children.

Morphine was isolated from opium in 1803 by a German pharmacist, Sertürner. The name *morphine* that he gave to this alkaloid comes from Morpheus, the Greek god of dreams. The invention of the hypodermic needle and syringe in the middle of the nineteenth century allowed for the parenteral use of morphine. Parenteral administration was used extensively during the American Civil War. For further discussion of the history of opium the reader is directed to Macht's interesting review published in 1915.

Heroin, which is the opiate of choice on the illicit drug market, is the diacetyl derivative of morphine. Although it is not a legal preparation in the United States, it is used as a recognized remedy in Great Britain. In addition to the naturally obtained alkaloids from opium, a number of synthetic narcotic analgesics have been synthesized. Table 1 lists the common narcotic analgesics with the approximate equipotent analgesic dose of each. Since most experimental work on the opiates has been carried out with morphine, most of the following sections describe the pharmacology of this alkaloid. However, what is true about morphine generally holds for the other narcotic analgesics. Where marked differences exist, they are discussed.

TABLE 1. REPRESENTATIVE NARCOTIC ANALGESICS

Generic name	Brand name	Dose (mg)[a]
Agonist:		
Morphine		10
Heroin (diacetylmorphine)		3[b]
Hydromorphone (dihydromorphinone)	Dilaudid®	1.5
Codeine		120[c]
Phenazocine	Prinadol®	3
Methadone	Dolophine®	7.5–10
Meperidine	Demerol®	80–100
Mixed agonist-antagonist:		
Nalorphine	Nalline®	10–15[b]
Pentazocine	Talwin®	30–50[c]
Antagonist:		
Naloxone	Narcan®	—
Naltrexone (Experimental)		

[a] Dose shown is the amount given subcutaneously that produces approximately the same analgesic effects as 10 mg of morphine administered subcutaneously. The latter is generally considered to be an optimal initial dose of morphine in the average 70-kg human. Dosages as given by Jaffe, J. H. Narcotic analgesics. In L. S. Goodman and A. Gilman (Eds.) *The Pharmacological Basis of Therapeutics.* (4th ed.). New York, Macmillan, 1970, pp. 237–275.

[b] These compounds are not in clinical use (heroin is not an approved drug in U.S. and Nalline® is used only for its antagonist properties).

[c] These compounds are generally administered orally.

Morphine and related compounds exert their major actions on the CNS and on the gastrointestinal system. Despite thousands of research papers on the narcotic analgesics, the mechanism of action of these compounds still remains a mystery. The two major uses of these compounds are for the control of pain and the symptomatic relief of diarrhea or dysentery.

ABSORPTION, DISTRIBUTION, AND EXCRETION

Morphine, although usually administered by the parenteral route, is readily absorbed from the gastrointestinal tract. However, the difference between the effective dose for oral and parenteral administration is much greater with morphine than for some of the other narcotic analgesics. Opiates are also easily absorbed from the nasal mucosa and the lungs. A common method of heroin

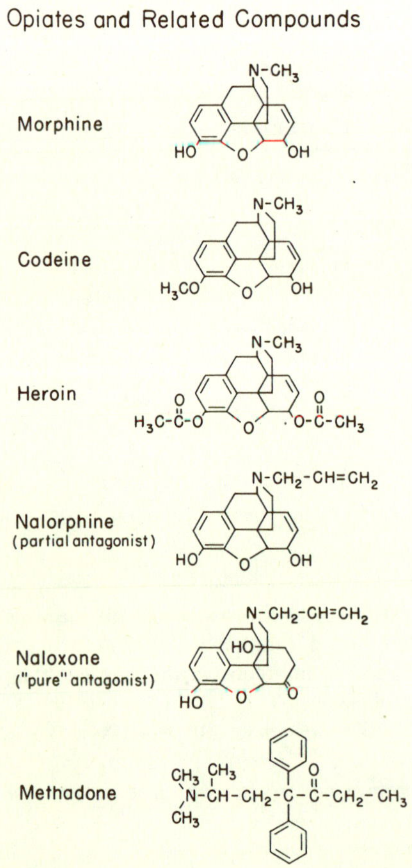

FIGURE 2. Opiates and related compounds.

CENTRAL NERVOUS SYSTEM

ingestion is "snuffing," and opium is smoked. Intravenous administration of opiates gives the most rapid onset of action and is the preferred mode of drug taking by the opiate addict. Codeine is usually administered orally, and an oral dose of codeine is approximately two thirds as effective as a parenteral dose.

The CNS, which shows a high sensitivity to morphine, accumulates only a small amount of the drug that enters the body. The concentration is much higher in such organs as the liver, lungs, and spleen. The concentration is lower in skeletal muscles, but because of the relatively large mass of muscle in the body, a major proportion of all morphine administered is found in muscle.

Within 24 hours after the last dose of morphine, tissue level is quite low. Morphine is mainly excreted by the kidneys with smaller amounts excreted via the bowel. Ninety percent of the total excretion occurs within the first 24 hours, although traces can be found in the urine 48 hours after the last dose. Heroin is changed to morphine by the body and is excreted as morphine. The peak effect of a subcutaneous dose of morphine is achieved within thirty minutes to an hour. The duration of action is approximately four to six hours. The onset of action for oral administration is somewhat delayed, and there is a slightly longer duration of effect.

CENTRAL NERVOUS SYSTEM

Morphine seems to have somewhat different effects when given to the patient in pain than when it is given to the normal, pain-free subject. In the former the effect is usually pleasant, but in the latter the effect can often be quite unpleasant. Most people addicted to opiates report that their first experience with the drug was unpleasant.

Subjective Effects

The subjective effect of a single dose of morphine in man is a feeling of drowsiness, heaviness of limbs, and warmth. There may be itching of the extremities, including the face and nose, caused by histamine release. Histamine release also causes vasodilatation. These effects are most pronounced after an intravenous administration. There may be a feeling of euphoria with a sensation of floating. In the nonpatient subject there may be dysphoria accompanied by nausea and vomiting, especially if the subject is standing or sitting.

Analgesia

The manner in which morphine relieves pain is not completely understood. It is not clear whether morphine simply relieves the subjective aspects of pain, alters the reaction to it, or actually raises the pain threshold per se. Although it is clear that morphine relieves clinical pain, it is impossible in the laboratory experiment to model clinical pain. First of all, most experimental pain is of the sharp pinching type rather than the dull continuous sensation, and it is impossible for experimental pain to have the same subjective component as clinical pain. In experimental pain the subject can terminate the experiment at will; he can, without the anxiety associated with clinical pain, make judgements concerning the intensity of the applied stimulus.

Analgesia with morphine is relatively selective in that the threshold in other sensory modalities is not altered at doses that will alleviate pain. This would support the notion that what is really relieved is the subjective anxiety-provoking aspect of the pain and not the perception itself. Many patients who receive adequate relief from pain still report the pain but state that it does not bother them. To attribute all relief of pain by morphine to a reduction in anxiety is a marked oversimplification, for many drugs that are useful in the treatment of clinical anxiety are useless as analgesics. However, the role of anxiety or anticipation does play a role in pain perception and was demonstrated a number of years ago by Hill et al. (1952) and Kornetsky (1954). In these experiments electric shock was the stimulus in the former and thermal radiation in the latter. The experiments were quite similar in that two procedures were used in both, one in which thresholds were measured under "formal" rigorous experimental procedures and one in which everything was identical to the first, except there was a more "informal" approach to the subject. In the "informal" conditions subjects were allowed to see how the apparatus worked, to explore the experimental room, and to even see the experimenter receive some of the painful stimuli. In the "formal" procedure morphine raised the threshold; however, in the "informal" procedure morphine did not significantly raise the threshold. However, the pain threshold in the "informal" nondrug condition was similar to that obtained in the "formal" drug condition (Figure 3). From these experiments and others, including Beecher's (1959) study of clinical patients, it is clear that there is a subjective component of pain that is altered by morphine, but it is also clear that this is not all that morphine does. In some of the experiments described by Hill et al. the subjective estimate of the intensity of the pain stimulus was more accurate after morphine than without the drug. In the latter condition subjects tended to overestimate the intensities. Thus morphine may alleviate pain by raising pain threshold when it is overly low as a result of anticipation, fear, and panic.

In animals, which also have been studied by means of a potpourri of techniques, morphine will raise the threshold for a response to putative painful stimuli at doses that will not disrupt other behavior. Thermal radiation to the tail or back of the animal is a common method used in the pharmaceutical industry. Also popular is a "hot plate" procedure. In this procedure an animal is placed on a constant temperature plate, and the latency of a foot-withdrawal response is measured. A procedure that allows the automatic study of analgesic

CENTRAL NERVOUS SYSTEM

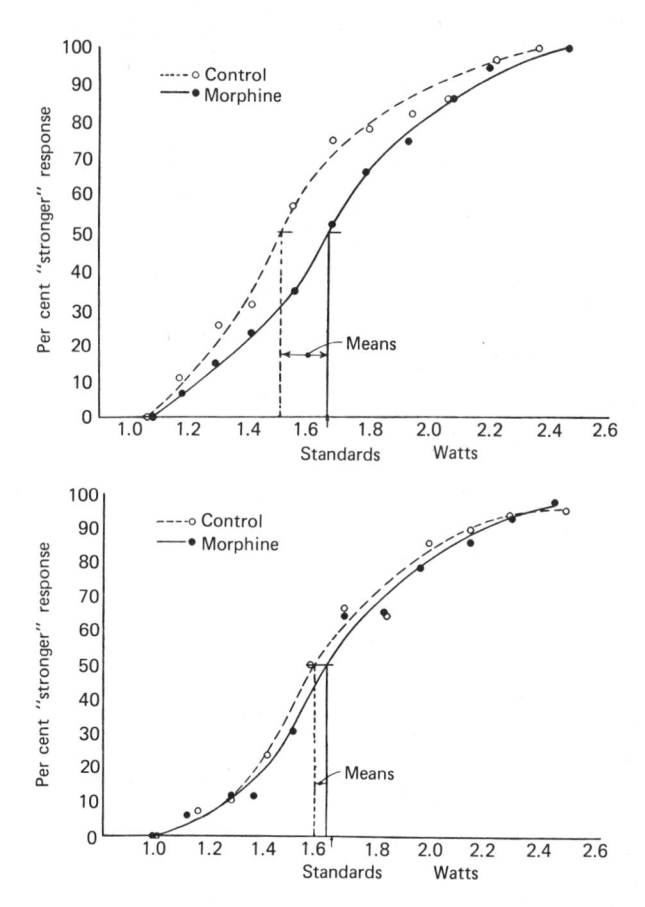

FIGURE 3. Frequency of the response "stronger" to electric shock stimuli after control or morphine conditions. Top indicates results under "formal" setting, bottom indicates results under "informal" setting. (From Hill et al., 1952.)

effects is a titration or fractional escape procedure (Weiss and Laties, 1959). In this type of technique electrical shock delivered to the animal via a grid floor is gradually increased. A response (lever press, wheel turn) terminates the shock and resets it to a lower intensity. In this way an animal maintains the shock at a "comfortable" level (Figure 4).

Sites of Action for Analgesic Effects

The specific manner in which the narcotic analgesics act in the CNS to produce their analgesic effects is not known. For extensive reviews of opiate action in

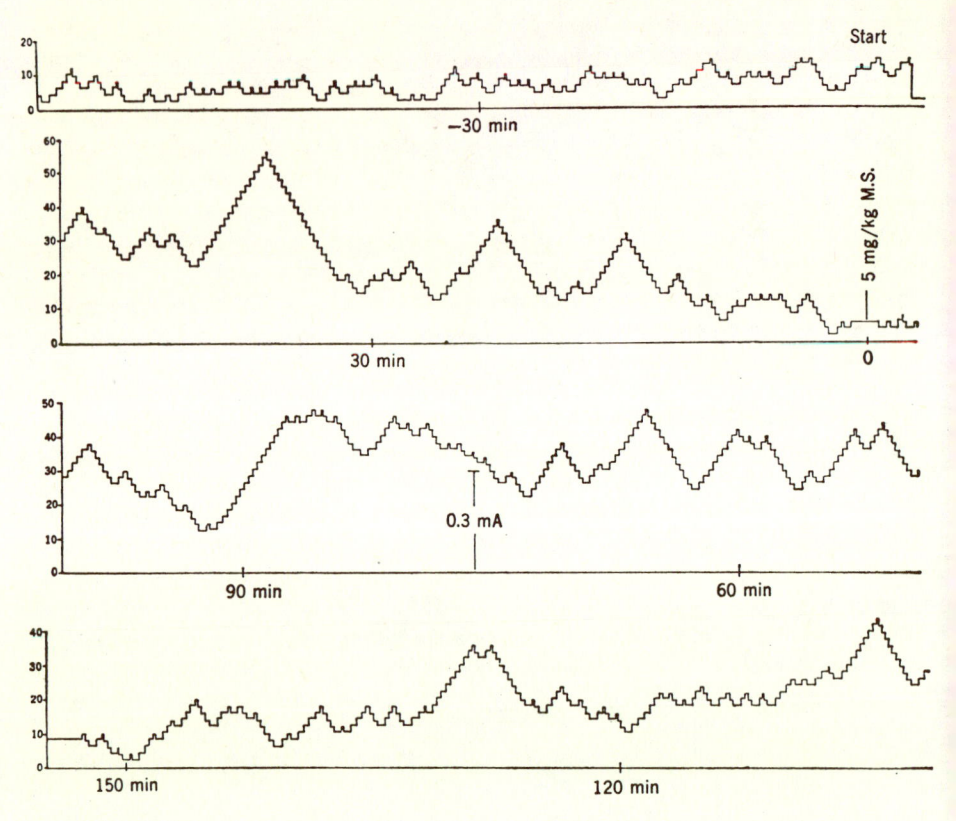

FIGURE 4. An example of the effects of 5 mg of MS per kilogram of body weight in an animal on the shock attentuation procedure. The tracing reads from right to left and from top to bottom. The vertical distance is a linear representation of the shock intensity, and the horizontal distance represents time (from Kornetsky and Bain, 1968).

the CNS, see reviews by Wikler (1950), Martin (1963), and Domino (1968). Although reduction of anxiety is an important component of the analgesic experience, it alone cannot explain analgesia since those drugs most successful in the treatment of anxiety have little or no analgesic effects. Also, the actions of morphine in the limbic system, a putative center for mediation of anxiety, is reported to be different from that observed with the barbiturates and some of the minor tranquilizers used in the treatment of anxiety.

Experiments on the effects of morphine on direct stimulation of the reticular formation have yielded inconsistent results. Some of these inconsistencies are probably related to different sites within the reticular formation where stimulation takes place and differences in species and/or dose of the drug (see Killam,

1962). Recordings of spontaneous electrical activity from the reticular formation has also given inconsistent results; however, the overall evidence suggests that narcotic analgesics cause EEG synchronization (increased amplitude and decreased frequency) from both cortical as well as subcortical recording sites. Nelsen (1970) and Nelsen and Kornetsky (1972) reported the effects of morphine on EEG amplitude in rats in which there was a bipolar recording electrode in the dorsal tegmentum region of the reticular formation and one bipolar electrode in the medial forebrain bundle (MFB). The former site is one in which electrical stimulation is aversive, and stimulation to this area will maintain avoidance behavior; the latter site has been repeatedly demonstrated to be a positive reinforcement area (Valenstein, 1973), that is, animals will press levers, turn wheels, and so on, to receive stimulation to the MFB. The results of this experiment indicated that morphine increases the amplitude of EEG waves from the negative reinforcement sites and at the same time, decreases the amplitude from positive reinforcement sites.

Behavioral confirmation of opposite changes in the positive and negative reinforcement systems was given in experiments by Marcus and Kornetsky (1974) in which thresholds for electrical stimulation to these reinforcement sites were measured before and after morphine administration. These results indicated that morphine raised the threshold in the negative sites in the reticular formation and lowered the threshold in the positive reinforcement sites in the MFB. The findings of Nelsen (1970) and Marcus and Kornetsky (1974) as well as anatomical and physiological evidence (see Casey, 1973) suggest that the analgesic action of the narcotic analgesics, at least in part, is due to the inhibition of pain transmission in the reticular formation.

The Narcotic "High"

Among the effects of many of the narcotic analgesics, especially those of which there is a great deal of nonmedical use, is the so-called narcotic "high." This phenomenon is not readily understood, although it might be related to the stimulating properties of the drugs. Many of the stimulating effects are not those that one would call pleasurable, for example, increased tone of the anal sphincter, hyperthermia, and restlessness. However, the high that is reported as pleasurable does not seem to be due to the depressant effects of the opiates. Some suggestion of the mechanisms mediating the high is given by the experiments of Nelsen and those of Marcus. Nelsen simultaneously recorded EEG after morphine administration from positive reward areas as well as from those areas that will maintain avoidance behavior. The decrease in amplitude from the positive reinforcement areas suggested that morphine caused excitation of this area. This finding was reinforced by the behavioral studies of Marcus in which it was found that morphine lowered the threshold for intracranial reinforcement to these same positive reinforcement areas.

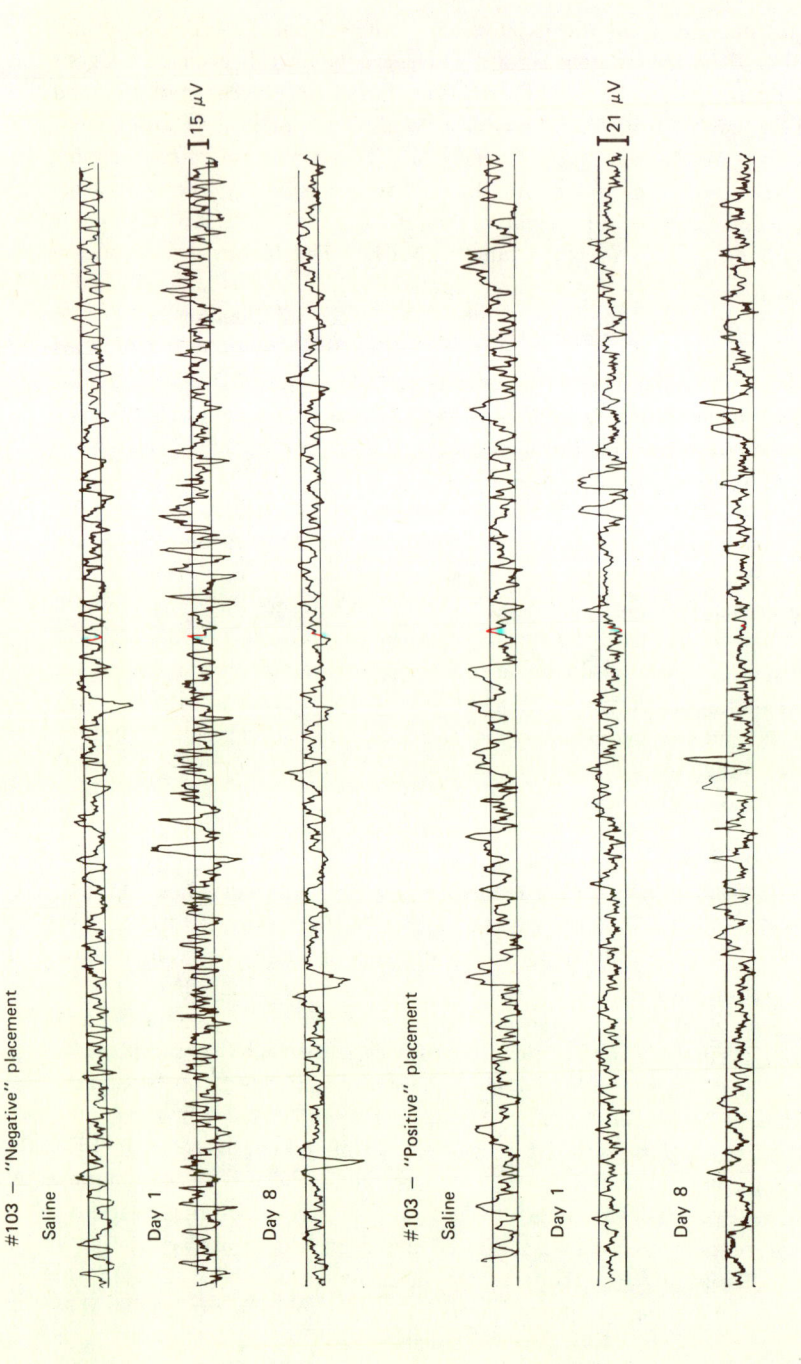

FIGURE 5. Sample EEGs from depth placements in the rat after the administration of morphine. The top three tracings are from electrodes placed in "negative" reinforcement areas of the brain; the bottom three (recorded at the same time) from "positive" reinforcement areas. Note that there is evidence of tolerance in the "negative" placement day 8 with little or no evidence for tolerance from the "positive" placement (from Nelsen, 1970).

CENTRAL NERVOUS SYSTEM

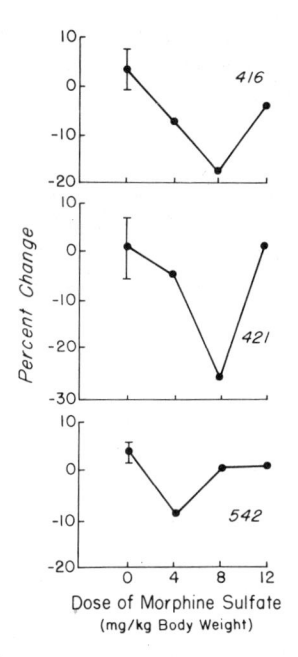

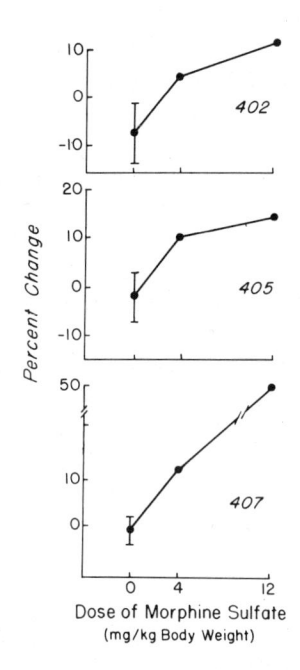

FIGURE 6. The effects of morphine on positive (on left) and negative (on right) reinforcement thresholds. The precent change variable is defined as postinjection threshold minus preinjection threshold, times 100, divided by preinjection threshold. The point at 0 mg/kg represents the mean of at least five saline days; the bars represent ± one standard deviation for the saline days (from Marcus and Kornetsky, 1974).

These experiments on the effects of morphine on the reward system in the brain suggest that the high may be due to an increase in the responsiveness of these pathways to afferent stimulation. Electrical stimulation to these positive reinforcement areas in human subjects is accompanied by pleasurable sensation (Sem-Jacobsen and Torkildsen, 1960). Since opiate reinforcement will sustain behavior, as will electrical stimulation of the medial forebrain bundle, and since morphine will lower the threshold for stimulation of the medial forebrain bundle, a reasonable hypothesis is that this area of the brain may be responsible for the narcotic high.

Pupil

Morphine has marked effects on the pupil, causing miosis. The exact mechanism of this effect is not known. It most likely is centrally mediated, for decorticate dogs do not show this effect after morphine administration. With toxic doses the miosis is greatly enhanced, so that a pinpoint pupil in a comatose individual is by itself an adequate sign that the patient is suffering from an overdose of an opiate drug. Unfortunately, the diagnosis of opiate poisoning may be confused in the final stages, for mydriasis occurs with asphyxia (cause of death in opiate poisoning).

There is some variation across species in the pupillary response. Cats and monkeys may show mydriasis. The mydriasis is not simply the result of excitatory effects of morphine, for monkeys show the dilatation of the pupil, and they do not show the behavioral excitement after morphine administration that cats do.

Tolerance does not develop to the miotic effect of opiates, so that even subjects physically dependent on and exhibiting a great deal of tolerance to many of the other actions of morphine will still exhibit constriction of the pupil after morphine administration.

Respiration

Morphine decreases respiration. After an intravenous dose maximum depression of respiration usually occurs within seven minutes. After intramuscular or subcutaneous injection the maximum effect may not be seen for 30 or 90 min., respectively. Return to normal respiration rates starts in approximately two to three hours after drug. Death from an overdose of opiates in man is usually due to respiratory arrest. The depression of respiration is due to a direct effect on respiratory centers in the brain stem.

Miscellaneous CNS Effects

The narcotic analgesics depress the cough reflex. This antitussive effect is due, in part, to a direct depressant effect on the cough center in the medulla.

Nausea and vomiting are caused by morphine and its derivatives. This unpleasant side effect is the result of direct stimulation of the chemoreceptor trigger zone (CTZ) for emesis. Nausea is less likely to occur in the recumbent patient. This suggests that the vestibular system is also affected by opiates. Although this class of compounds causes vomiting in some patients, there is a blocking of this effect to subsequent doses. Other emetic drugs are ineffective if given after morphine.

Many clinicians believe that narcotic drugs such as meperidine or codeine can be used with impunity because they are effective analgesics but do not cause the respiratory depression or emesis seen with morphine. However, in equianalgesic doses these narcotics may have equally unpleasant side effects. Thus for relief from severe pain, there is no advantage of meperidine or codeine over morphine.

AUTONOMIC NERVOUS SYSTEM

Cardiovascular Effects

There are no significant effects of opiates on heart rate or blood pressure in a supine patient. However, the narcotics do cause orthostatic hypotension; the patient who stands will show a drop in blood pressure that is great enough to cause fainting. This is the result of the marked peripheral vasodilatation that is caused by the opiates.

The vasodilatation is not believed to be centrally mediated. Part of this effect is due to the release of histamine. This vasodilatation is one of the first signs after an intravenous injection of an opiate. Almost before the needle is removed from the vein, there is an observed reddening of the face, particularly the nose; this is accompanied by itching on the face and nose as well as the extremities.

Gastrointestinal Tract (G.I.)

There is a marked decrease in the motility of the G.I. system. There is some decrease in hydrochloric acid secretion, and propulsive peristaltic activity is diminished. The tone of the anal sphincter is increased. Opium and the opiates have been used for centuries for the control of diarrhea and dysentery. However, in the patient given morphine for analgesic purposes, this is an unwanted side effect.

Other Parasympathetic Actions

The tone of the muscles of the urinary bladder is increased by opiates so that there may be an urge to urinate; however, the tone of the vesical sphincter is also enhanced, making urination difficult.

Opiates have little effect on the normally contracting uterus. However, narcotic analgesics given to the delivering mother may prolong labor and may produce adverse effects in the neonate.

TOLERANCE AND PHYSICAL DEPENDENCE

All opiate drugs will cause tolerance and physical dependence with repeated use. Tolerance which develops very rapidly to the narcotic analgesics, often limits their use for the control of pain in the patient. However, physicians have controlled severe chronic pain for extended periods by judicious management of dosage. Although it has been suggested by some writers that tolerance and physical dependence are part of the same phenomenon, there is also evidence suggesting that they are independent phenomena. That is, tolerance can be demonstrated without evidence of physical dependence. However, it is unlikely that physical dependence can exist without there being some tolerance to the opiate analgesics.

Tolerance

The rapidity with which tolerance can develop in animals is shown in Figure 7. Although numerous theories have been proposed to explain this phenomenon, tolerance is still an enigma. There is also not a single theory that adequately explains all aspects of tolerance to the narcotic analgesics.

For many years it was believed that repeated dosing with the opiates led to an altered metabolism and/or distribution and excretion. Thus the tolerant animal metabolized the drug in a different or faster manner so that there was less of the drug able to reach the CNS, or it was excreted at a much higher rate. Recent work, using chemical techniques far more sensitive than those available to earlier workers, indicates little or no difference between the tolerant and nontolerant animal with regard to metabolism, distribution, or excretion rates.

A *receptor occupation* theory, first suggested in 1933 by Schmidt and Livingston, makes the assumption that the opiate molecule exerts its action at the time of occupation of the receptor but then continues to occupy the receptor without having any continued effect. This occupation prevents additional opiate molecules from occupying the receptor, and thus the additional molecules have little effect. This type of theory may explain the rapid tolerance known as

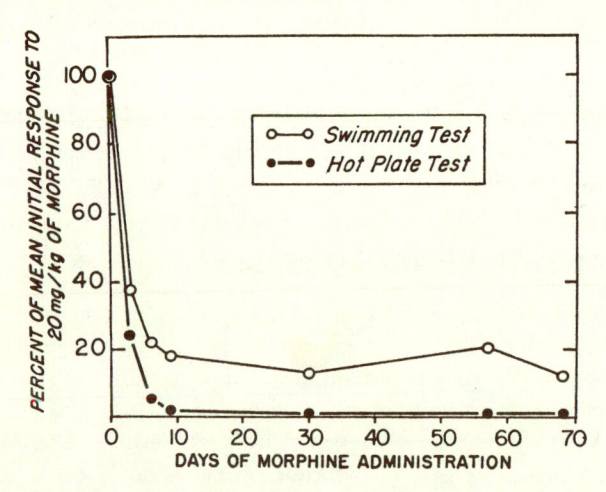

FIGURE 7. Example of the rapid development of tolerance to morphine in the rat with daily doses. Test procedure consisted of the "hot plate analgesic" testing method and speed of swimming a straight alley maze.

tachyphylaxis but does not explain long-term tolerance or tolerance that exists for months after the last dose of the opiate.

Recent work in attempting to understand the problem of tolerance has focused on the hypothesis that there must be some sort of cellular adaptation of the organism to the drug after repeated administration. The cellular adaptation may involve changes in enzymatic activity, changes in the release of certain biogenic amines, or possibly some immune response. At the present time, none of these theories has been proven, and the most that one can say for them is that they are of great heuristic value.

Physical Dependence

Physical dependence is defined by the presence of a syndrome that occurs if there is cessation in the use of a drug. An abstinence syndrome is seen after cessation of chronic use of the opiate analgesics, barbiturates, and alcohols as well as some of the antianxiety agents.

The development and severity of physical dependence is a function of the particular opiate, the dose, the frequency, and the duration of use. In the subject who is physically dependent on morphine or heroin, symptoms of abstinence will appear as early as six hours after the last dose. These early symptoms consist of feelings of weakness soon followed by the specific signs of abstinence: yawning, lacrimation (eyes tearing), rhinorrhea (runny nose), and perspiration. After approximately 24 hours there will be restlessness, twitching of muscles, back and leg pain, hot and cold flashes, and chills. Characteristically, there is movement of the legs. Patients seem to be continually trying to find a comfortable position. It is believed by some that the term "kicking a habit" comes from the continual leg movements of the withdrawing patient.

Accompanying these signs of withdrawal are various changes in autonomic functioning. There is an elevated body temperature and an increase in rate and depth of respiration. Blood pressure is elevated, and there is dilatation of the pupils. The syndrome peaks after about 48 hours of abstinence. Nausea, itching, vomiting, and diarrhea are common. There is rapid loss of weight; this is a result of both the lack of food intake and the marked dehydration of the patient. These symptoms begin to subside after approximately 72 hours, and the patient is, for the most part, symptom free in 5 to 10 days. However, there may be residual signs and symptoms lasting for several weeks. The closest experience to withdrawal that the nonaddict has experienced might be a severe case of the flu, accompanied by nausea, diarrhea, and muscle twitching.

The physiological basis of dependence and tolerance is not known. Among the popular theories is one that simply states that with repeated use of the narcotics, various homeostatic mechanisms are set at different levels. When the drug is withdrawn, there is a rebound effect so that those functions previously depressed are elevated, for example, decreased motility of the gastrointestinal tract after opiates is reversed to an increase in motility during withdrawal.

Another theory is the *dual-action theory* (Seevers and Woods, 1953). This theory is one that tries to explain both tolerance and physical dependence. This theory makes use of the observation that opiates have both depressant and excitatory actions, depending on the location of the receptor-drug combination. Theoretically, the opiate interacts with some intracellular sites to cause excitation, whereas the interaction at extracellular sites causes depression. Tolerance develops as fewer extracellular sites become available as a result of repeated exposure to the drug. When administration of the drug is terminated, the extracellular receptors responsible for depression are freed of the drug very rapidly; however, those responsible for excitation (intracellular) are freed more slowly. This results in an expression of the stimulating effects that were previously masked by depressant actions.

None of these theories or, for that matter, any of the theories of tolerance or physical dependence fit all the data. Tolerance and physical dependence can develop, for example, in the spinal cord, which does not have a functional system concerned with homeostatic regulation. The dual action theory is inadequate to explain the tolerance or physical dependence seen in animals months after the last dose of the drug. For a discussion of theories of tolerance and physical dependence, see Cochin (1974); Shuster (1971); and Way (1974).

In 1962 Weeks published a paper demonstrating that morphine could be used as a reinforcer and that physical dependence could be self-maintained in the rat. Rats prepared with an indwelling intravenous catheter would press a lever to receive a fixed amount of morphine. This experimental demonstration of the reinforcing properties of morphine has led to extensive work on the use of drugs as reinforcers and has allowed for an experimental model of the addiction liability of drugs. For a review of the technique, the reader is referred to Schuster and Johanson (1974).

Meperidine (Demerol)

This is a synthetic narcotic agent that was developed as a substitute for morphine. It has actions similar to those of morphine, with a slightly less constipating effect at equianalgesic doses. Although meperidine is often used with the belief that it is less addicting than morphine and that it has far fewer side effects, this is unfortunately not true. At equianalgesic doses meperidine seems to have almost all the side effects of morphine with about equivalent addiction liability. It is not particularly effective when given orally and it is not a good cough suppressant (antitussive agent). It does not cause constriction of the pupils. It is the narcotic analgesic that is most commonly taken by physicians and nurses who have become narcotic abusers.

Codeine

Codeine is an effective analgesic for the relief of mild to moderate pain. Also, it is an effective antitussive agent. Although it can be given parenterally, the usual mode of administration is oral. For the relief of mild to moderate pain, equipotent doses of codeine and morphine that produce comparable side effects can be obtained. However, such a statement cannot be made for the control of severe pain.

Methadone

Methadone is primarily known for its use in the treatment of opiate addiction; however, its first use was as a synthetic substitute for morphine, and it is an effective oral analgesic. It was synthesized in Germany during World War II. Although methadone is not a natural alkaloid, its pharmacological action is very similar to that of morphine. It is usually given by mouth and seems to have an extended duration of action. Methadone has been used in the treatment of withdrawal from opiates since the late 1940s, and since the early 1960s in "methadone maintainence" programs. In the substitution-withdrawal technique patients physically dependent on heroin are switched to methadone. The methadone is then slowly withdrawn. This type of withdrawal leads to less severe withdrawal symptoms than those seen during slow withdrawal from heroin or morphine. See Chapter 12 for further discussion of methadone as a treatment method in opiate addiction.

NARCOTIC ANTAGONIST

The history of the development of the narcotic antagonist is a very good example of how the significance of an early observation in the laboratory was missed. It was in 1915 that the first report appeared in the literature concerning an opiate antagonist. Twenty-five years later the morphine-antagonizing properties of nalorphine were described independently by two laboratories. However, it was not until 1951 that the clinical significance of these findings was described (see Martin, 1971).

In 1953 Wikler et al. reported that nalorphine given to subjects physically dependent on morphine, heroin, or methadone, immediately precipitated the abstinence syndrome. This report was immediately followed by a report that this drug, that ex-addicts did not like, was also analgesic in patients with postoperative pain. This suggested that a narcotic analgesic had finally been found that had no addiction liability. Unfortunately, nalorphine and many of the newly synthesized antagonists caused tremendous dysphoria and occasionally hallucinations in patients. The search has continued for new antagonists that would be useful analgesics without the unpleasant side effects.

For the chemically minded it has been found that the substitution of the N-methyl group in most of the narcotic analgesics results in a drug with narcotic-antagonistic effects. Substitution can be with an allyl group, as with the earliest antagonists, but may be with other groups such as methallyl, propyl, isobutyl. Nalorphine (n-allylnormorphine) was the first of these common antagonists.

The first clinically useful antagonist, nalorphine, not only had antagonist effects but also agonist activity. Only one of the antagonists thus far synthesized has no known intrinsic (agonist) activity: this is *naloxone*. However, there is the possibility that *naltrexone* may be similar to naloxone.

The pharmacology of the mixed agonist-antagonists is of interest because they have many of the actions of morphine without marked addiction liability. Although tolerance to the agonist activity does develop, there is no evidence of tolerance to the antagonist activity. Physical dependence does develop, however, the withdrawal syndrome is less severe than that seen with morphine withdrawal.

When an opiate antagonist is given to the physically dependent patient, an acute withdrawal syndrome is seen. This syndrome is similar to that seen after abrupt withdrawal from opiates, except that the withdrawal signs are seen in 5 to 15 minutes after a subcutaneous injection. The duration of the withdrawal signs is equivalent to the duration of the action of the antagonist. In the case of nalorphine it is about two hours.

The antagonists are most useful in cases of overdose with narcotic analgesics. In patients with marked respiratory depression due to an overdose of a narcotic drug, the action of a subcutaneous injection is most dramatic and seen within a few minutes.

At the present time only one of the antagonists seems to be useful as an analgesic. This is *pentazocine*. Pentazocine was developed for the purpose of obtaining a narcotic analgesic with little or no abuse potential. In early screening studies postaddicts, given the opportunity to continue taking this drug, preferred to give it up. However, there has been some evidence of compulsive use of pentazocine, and physical dependence can be demonstrated. Despite this, it is believed that the abuse potential is not particularly great for this drug.

SUMMARY

As mentioned, the narcotic analgesics are a most interesting class of compounds that became more interesting with the introduction of the opiate antagonists. Despite extensive use of the opiates and the problems of abuse, we still do not understand their mechanism of action. In recent years there has been renewed interest in the narcotic analgesics, probably due to the increase in the number of people abusing these drugs. Although most investigators are interested in the abuse of the narcotic analgesics, it is only one facet of the effects of a most interesting class of compounds.

REFERENCES

Beecher, H. K. *Measurement of Subjective Responses.* New York, Oxford University Press, 1959, pp. 157–190.

Casey, K. L. Pain: A current view of neural mechanisms. *American Scientist,* **61,** 1973, 194–200.

Cochin, J. Factors influencing tolerance to and physical dependence on narcotic analgesics. In S. Fisher and A. M. Freedman (Eds.) *Opiate Addiction: Origins and Treatment.* Washington, D.C., Winston 1974, pp. 23–42.

Domino, E. F. Effects of narcotic analgesics on sensory input, activating system and motor output. In A. Wikler (Ed.) *The Addictive States.* Baltimore, Williams and Wilkins, 1968, pp. 117–149.

Hill, H., Kornetsky, C., Flanary, H., and Wikler, A. Effects of anxiety and morphine on discrimination of intensities of painful stimuli. *The Journal of Clinical Investigation,* **31,** 1952, 473–480.

Killam, E. K. Drug action on the brain stem reticular formation. *Pharmacological Reviews,* **14,** 1962, 175–223.

Kornetsky, C. Effects of anxiety and morphine on the anticipation and perception of painful radiant thermal stimuli. *Journal of Comparative and Physiological Psychology,* **47,** 1954, 130–132.

Kornetsky, C. and Bain, G. Morphine: Single-dose tolerance. *Science,* **162,** 1968, 1011–1012.

Macht, D. I. The history of opium and some of its preparations and alkaloids. *The Journal of the American Medical Association,* **64,** 1915, 477–481.

Marcus, R. and Kornetsky, C. Negative and positive intracranial reinforcement thresholds: Effects of morphine. *Psychopharmacologia (Berlin),* **38,** 1974, 1–13.

Martin, W. R. Analgesic and antipyretic drugs. I. Strong analgesics. In W. S. Root and F. G. Hofmann (Eds.) *Physiological Pharmacology,* Vol. 1, *The Nervous System—Part A.* New York, Academic, 1963, pp. 275–312.

Martin, W. R. Opioid antagonists. *Pharmacological Reviews,* **19,** 1971, 463–521.

Nelsen, J. M. Single dose tolerance to morphine sulfate. *Electroencephalographic correlates in central motivational systems.* (Doctoral dissertation, Boston University) Ann Arbor, Michigan, University Microfilms, No. 70-22425, 1970.

Nelsen, J. M. and Kornetsky, C. Morphine-induced EEG changes in central motivational systems: Evidence for single dose tolerance. *Fifth International Congress of Pharmacology.* 1972, p. 166.

Schmidt, C. F. and Livingston, A. E. The relation of dosage to the development of tolerance to morphine in dogs. *Journal of Pharmacology and Experimental Therapeutics,* **47,** 1933, 443–471.

Schuster, C. R. and Johanson, C. E. Behavioral analysis of opiate dependence. In S. Fisher and A. M. Freedman (Eds.) *Opiate Addiction: Origins and Treatment.* Washington, D.C., Winston, 1974, pp. 77–92.

Shuster, L. Tolerance and physical dependence. In D. H. Clouet (Ed.) *Narcotic Drugs.* New York, Plenum. 1971, pp. 408–423.

Seevers, M. H. and Woods, L. A. The phenomena of tolerance. *The American Journal of Medicine,* **14,** 1953, 546–557.

Sem-Jacobsen, C. W. and Torkildsen, A. Depth recording and electrical stimulation in the human brain. In E. R. Ramey and D. S. O'Doherty (Eds.) *Electrical Studies on the Unanesthesized Brain.* New York, Paul B. Hoeber, 1960, pp. 275–290.

Valenstein, E. S. History of brain stimulation: Investigations into the physiology of motivation. In

E. S. Valenstein (Ed.) *Brain Stimulation and Motivation: Research and Commentary.* Glenview, Illinois, Scott, Foresman, 1973, pp. 1–43.

Way, E. L. Some biochemical aspects of morphine tolerance and physical dependence. In S. Fisher and A. M. Freedman (Eds.) *Opiate Addiction: Origins and Treatment,* Washington, D.C., Winston, 1974, pp. 99–120.

Weeks, J. R. Experimental morphine addiction: Method for automatic intravenous injections in unrestrained rats. *Science,* **138,** 1962, 143–144.

Weiss, B. and **Laties, V. G.** Titration behavior on various fractional escape programs. *Journal of the Experimental Analysis of Behavior,* **2,** 1959, 227–248.

Wikler, A. Sites and mechanisms of action of morphine and related drugs in the central nervous system. *Pharmacological Reviews,* **2,** 1950, 435–506.

Wikler, A., Fraser, H. F., and **Isbell, H.** N-allylnormorphine: Effects of single doses and precipitation of "Abstinence Syndromes" during addiction to morphine, methadone or heroin in man (post-addicts). *Journal of Pharmacology and Experimental Therapeutics,* **109,** 1953, 8–20.

8 HYPNOTICS AND SEDATIVES

The sedative and hypnotic drugs are centrally acting depressants. They are used predominantly for their ability to cause sedation, sleep, and anesthesia. In addition, they are extensively used as anticonvulsants. In the past they were often used to treat the anxious patient; however, this use has declined since the introduction of the minor tranquilizers.

The problem of definition of the term sedation is difficult when one strays from common parlance and tries to define it in some operational, meaningful way. The *Random House Dictionary of the English Language* gives the following definition: "Sedative (adj) Tending to calm or soothe. Med. allaying irritability or excitement; assuaging pain; lowering functional activity. (n) A sedative agent or remedy."

In common usage a state of sedation refers to a subjective state that is characterized by diminished responsivity to external stimuli and at least partial equanimity in regard to various psychological stresses. This state of sedation can cause a readiness for sleep. Obviously, drugs are not the only thing that will produce this subjective state in man. Anything from a warm bath to sexual activity or a vigorous game of tennis may result in a sedative effect.

The term *hypnosis*, or the noun hypnotic, is much easier to define, not only in common parlance but in terms of some objective, measurable, operational terms. Thus a hypnotic is a drug that produces sleep or at least something resembling natural sleep. We can measure sleep in both animals and man. We can determine such things as the duration of sleep, the time of onset, and with the electroencephalogram, we can even measure depth of sleep and the presence or absence of dreaming.

The sedative hypnotics are used extensively for insomnia. Unfortunately, any drug that will cause sedation or hypnosis will also impair the subject's ability to perform necessary motor, intellectual, and perceptual tasks. If these drugs are taken just prior to retiring, with the subject taking his or her capsule and then hopping into bed to await the envelopment of sleep, it does not matter that the sensorium is impaired. It does not matter that fine control of motor movements, and perception are impaired. However, if taken during the day when hypnosis is not desired, the accompanying dangers are obvious.

The various hypnotic agents resemble one another in the manner in which they affect various functions, so that most of what is said concerning the most common of the hypnotics, the barbiturates, is true for all of the various hypnotic agents.

THE BARBITURATES

Barbituric acid is formed by condensing malonic acid and urea. Credit for the first preparation of barbituric acid is given to Adolph von Beyer in 1865. At that time he was a 29-year old research assistant. According to legend, von Beyer visited a tavern frequented by artillery officers to celebrate his synthesis of the new compound. It happened that the artillery officers were celebrating the Day of St. Barbara, their patron saint. Thus the name was a synthesis of Barbara with urea. Barbituric acid itself is not a CNS depressant. The first hypnotic barbituric acid derivative was introduced in 1903 by Fischer and von Mering. This compound, barbital, was given the trade name Veronal. Barbital has been largely superceded by the more short-acting barbiturates in current medical use.

The second oldest barbiturate is *phenobarbital*, which was introduced in 1912 and marketed under the trade name of Luminal. Although in succeeding years more than 2500 barbiturates have been synthesized, phenobarbital is still one of the most useful of the class of compounds.

The barbiturates are usually classified according to their duration of action

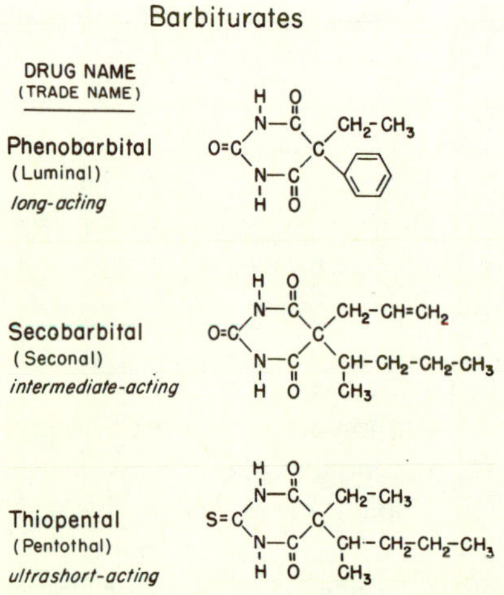

FIGURE 1. Representative barbiturates.

TABLE 1. REPRESENTATIVE HYPNOTICS

Generic name	Brand name	Dose[a] (hypnotic)
Barbiturates:		
Ultrashort Acting		
Thiopental	Pentothal®	(Intravenous
Hexobarbital	Evipal®	anesthetics)
Short Acting		
Secobarbital	Seconal®	100 mg
Pentobarbital	Nembutal®	100 mg
Intermediate Acting		
Amobarbital	Amytal®	100–200 mg
Butabarbital	Butisol®	
Long Acting		
Phenobarbital	Luminal®	100 mg
Barbital	Veronal®	
Miscellaneous Agents		
Chloral Hydrate		1–2 gms
Glutethimide	Doriden®	0.5 gms
Methyprylon	Noludar®	200–400 mg
Methaqualone	Quaalude®	150–300 mg

[a] Average hypnotic doses for adults are given for the more commonly prescribed preparations. Doses as given by Sharpless, S. K. Hypnotics and sedatives. In L. S. Goodman, and A. Gilman, (Eds.) *The Pharmacological Basis of Therapeutics*. (4th ed.). New York, Macmillan, 1970, pp. 98–134.

(see Table I). Except for this difference, they are quite similar with some exceptions which are discussed below. The difference in duration of action is a function of differences in distribution, metabolism, and excretion.

Absorption

Barbiturates are usually prepared as their sodium salt, for example, pentobarbital sodium, and are administered orally. However, in most experiments with animals the drug is given parenterally. In anesthetic preparations the ultrashort-acting barbiturates are given intravenously. Also, thiopental (Pentothal) given intravenously had extensive use in psychiatry as a method of producing psychological catharsis and was used extensively for "war neurosis" during World War II (Grinker and Speigel, 1945).

The sodium salts of barbiturates are completely absorbed from the gastrointestinal tract. Effects can be observed within 30 min after ingestion. This does not mean that all the drug is absorbed within 30 min after ingestion. In cases of accidental poisoning unabsorbed drug can be removed from the stomach hours after the drug was taken.

Since barbiturates are absorbed readily from the colon, rectal administration by means of a suppository is occasionally used. In addition to the above-mentioned uses of the intravenous method of administration, they are occasionally used in controlling *status epilepticus*.

Distribution

Barbiturates diffuse to all tissues and fluids in the body. In sufficient doses the drug can be found in the milk of the nursing mother. Barbiturates given to the pregnant woman easily diffuse through the placenta so that if used during delivery as an anesthetic, the newborn will show the depressant effects of the barbiturate.

The ultrashort-acting barbiturates, because of their higher lipid solubility, reach maximum concentration in the brain almost immediately. Those barbiturates that are less lipid soluble (the long-acting barbiturates) are slow in penetrating the blood-brain barrier, so that even after intravenous injections it may take 15 min for the central depressant effect to be maximum.

Metabolism and Excretion

The barbiturates' action is terminated by means of physical redistribution, metabolism, and renal excretion. These processes reduce the concentration in the blood and thus reduce the amount of drug in the CNS. The rapid redistribution of thiopental, not rapid metabolism, accounts for its ultrashort-acting CNS effects. The drug rapidly diffuses from the brain to other tissues where it is slowly metabolized. Most of the barbiturates are transformed by the liver to inactive metabolites. However, a greater percent of unchanged barbiturates is found in the urine of subjects after the long-acting barbiturates, with barbital almost completely excreted in unchanged form. For a more detailed discussion of the above section, the reader is referred to Sharpless (1970) or Harvey (1975).

Central Nervous System Effects

The barbiturates are ubiquitous in their action in the central nervous system. The general effect throughout the CNS is one of depression with the degree of depression a function of not only the particular barbiturate used and the psychological and physiological state of the organism, but also the social setting. Of most importance is the particular state of excitability of the CNS at the time the drug is taken. A bartiturate taken just prior to retiring will have a different effect than a barbiturate taken primarily for its intoxication properties at a social gathering.

EEG. Studies in man (Brazier, 1954) and animals (Mirsky and Tecce, 1967) using surface and depth electrodes for recording EEG indicate that the action of barbiturates seems to be on cortical structures at lower doses, and that as the dose is increased, there is a spread to the more subcortical areas of the brain. At low doses of intravenous administration or after oral administration the barbiturates first cause an increase in fast activity called "barbiturate activation." This activation is first seen in recordings from frontal areas and then spreads to parietal and occipital areas. This effect coincides with a decrease in alertness and often a feeling of well-being. As the dose is increased there is an increase in high-amplitude slow waves (2 to 8 cps). These are similar to what is seen during natural sleep. If the dose is exceptionally high, there will be occasional brief periods of electrical silence.

Sleep. The major use of the short- or intermediate-acting barbiturates is to produce sleep. As mentioned, some of the EEG effects resemble those seen in natural sleep. However, sleep is not a simple continuum going from relatively low-amplitude, high-frequency to high-amplitude, low-frequency EEG. Although the physiology of sleep is far from fully understood, it is known that during natural sleep, there are cyclic alternations between the deep stage IV sleep and a highly activated sleep in which the EEG shows an increase in high-frequency waves and the presence of rapid eye movements (REM) accompanied by dreaming. It has been found that all mammalian species as well as many submammalian species have REM during sleep. Subjects deprived of sleep for an extended period of time show only a slight increase in sleep time when finally allowed to sleep. However, after sleep deprivation, there is a significant increase in the incidence of REM sleep. It is as if the body must have a certain amount of REM sleep and if deprived of it, must catch up on the REM sleep that was missed.

Barbiturate-facilitated sleep shows a decrease in the amount of REM sleep, and to the extent that REM sleep is necessary, as believed by some, sleep induced by barbiturates is not adequate. Chronic barbiturate use results in tolerance to this effect on REM sleep with irregularity in the usual REM cycles (Oswald, 1968).

Cortical and Subcortical Structure. The barbiturates seem to act on almost all levels of neural functioning in the brain. However, it is believed that its effect on the reticular system accounts for the hypnotic action of this drug. The experiments of Moruzzi and Magoun (1949) demonstrated the importance of the reticular system as a modulator of sleep and wakefulness. The reticular formation is a neural net of pathways and synapses coursing through the brain stem from the medulla to the thalmus and hypothalamus. Subsequent experiments with barbiturates indicate that these drugs will raise the threshold for direct electrical stimulation of this area of the brain at doses that have only little effect on transmission via direct sensory pathways (Bradley, 1958). See

Chapters 4 and 5 for further discussion of the role of the reticular formation in modulating both behavior and the effects of drugs.

Anticonvulsant Action. All of the barbiturates have anticonvulsant activity; however, phenobarbital has anticonvulsant activity at doses that are nonsedative and nonanesthetic. Phenobarbital is used for the control of seizures in grand mal epilepsy. It is not the anticonvulsant of choice in acute cases of seizures as occur in *status epilepticus* or seizures precipitated by toxic doses of some drugs. As mentioned previously, phenobarbital may require as long as 15 min to be effective, even after intravenous injections (see Chapter 11).

Autonomic Nervous System (ANS)

The effects of the barbiturates on the ANS are either slight or nonexistant in usual therapeutic doses. However, in doses large enough to cause anesthesia the action on the ANS can be quite drastic. The central regulation of the ANS is altered, body temperature falls, respiration is markedly depressed, and there is a significant decrease in both systolic and diastolic blood pressure. Ganglionic transmission is depressed. The overall picture appears to be anticholinergic in nature, but there is some doubt if this effect is a direct anticholinergic action.

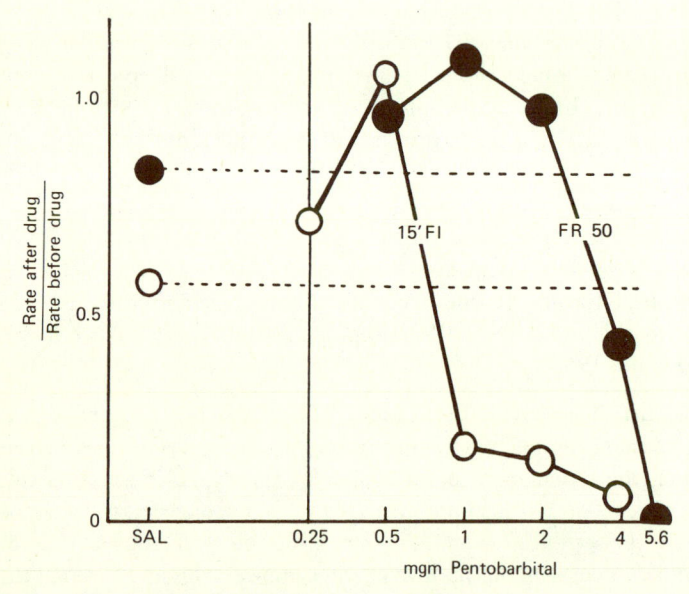

FIGURE 2. Effect of pentobarbital on pecking behavior of pigeons. Log dose-effect curves. Each point represents the arithmetic mean of the ratios for the same four birds at each dosage level on each schedule. Open circles: mean effects, birds working on 15' FI. Solid circles: birds working on FR50 (from Dews, 1955).

Behavioral Effects

The barbiturates cause marked impairment in most psychological performance tests. These effects are, of course, dose related. There are doses that yield therapeutic results with a minimum of behavioral deficits (i.e., phenobarbital in the treatment of epilepsy). Although there are some reports in the literature indicating that under some conditions behavior can be facilitated, it can be generally concluded that under most conditions performance is not facilitated. An example from the experimental literature is the report of Dews (1955) in which pigeons were trained on a multiple fixed interval–fixed ratio (FI–FR) schedule. After low doses of the barbiturate, performance as measured by the total responses increased while animals were on the FI segment of the schedule, and at the same dose their response rate decreased while on the FR segment of the schedule (see Figure 2). Hill, Belleville, and Wikler (1957), in a unique study of the effects of pentobarbital or morphine on morphine-reinforced reaction time (RT) in post-opiate addicts, demonstrated that under certain conditions a dose of pentobarbital that will normally slow RT may actually improve RT. They rewarded the postaddicts for participating in the experiment in three ways. A fixed amount of morphine was given for participating in the experiment in two of the groups. In one of these groups the morphine was given one week prior to the experiment, whereas in the other it was given after the experiment was completed. In the third group the amount of morphine reinforcement was a function of the speed of the RT response of the subject. As expected, pentobarbital impaired RT the most when reinforcement was given prior to the test, less when given after the test, and actually improved performance when reinforcement was contingent on speed of response (see Figure 3).

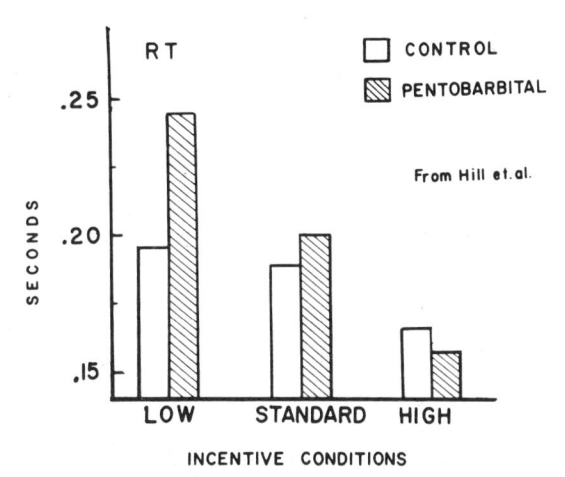

FIGURE 3. Effects of pentobarbital on reaction time (RT) under three levels of motivation (from Hill et al., 1957).

Barbiturates can have relatively long duration of effects. In a study by Kornetsky, Vates, and Kessler (1959) effects of pentobarbital given at 7:00 p.m. were observed the next morning, 12 to 14 hours after they were administered. This "hangover" effect has also been reported by Goodnow et al. (1951) and more recently by McKenzie and Elliot (1965), 10 to 22 hours after the drug was taken. Since most hypnotics are taken at bedtime, the presence of impairment in functioning the next morning can be potentially dangerous.

Tolerance, Physical Dependence

Tolerance development to the effects of barbiturates is of two types. Repeated doses result in the activation of those enzymes in the liver responsible for detoxification. Thus increased doses are needed to produce the same tissue concentration. There also seems to be an adaptation of the central nervous system to the presence of the drug so that even with adequate tissue levels, there is less of a hypnotic effect. Despite the tolerance that develops, it is never complete, and there does not seem to be a significant increase in the lethal dose.

Marked physical dependence can develop to the barbiturates. Except for a few scattered reports, mainly in the German literature, it was believed prior to the late 1940s, that true physical dependence did not occur with these compounds. However, in 1950 Isbell and co-workers reported the results of an experimental study that clearly demonstrated that physical dependence does occur in human subjects and that the barbiturate withdrawal syndrome was of such severity that life could be endangered. Subjects taking large doses chronically resemble their alcoholic counterparts in many respects, for example, slurred speech, confusion, ataxia, and so on. Twelve to sixteen hours after the last dose, many of the manifestations of chronic intoxication subside. After this the patients begin to complain of vague feelings of anxiety and increasing weakness. Twenty-four to thirty hours after the last dose, anxiety becomes severe and weakness so great that the patient can barely stand or walk. There is an increase in tremor and fasciculations of isolated muscle groups. Vomiting may occur and may become severe.

Clonic-tonic seizures are manifested in some patients as early as 16 hours after withdrawal but may occur four days after the last dose. From the third to the seventh day, a severe psychosis may appear, marked by visual and auditory hallucinations. This is usually preceded by insomnia of 24 to 48 hours. Not all patients will have seizures or psychosis, but if the duration of chronic administration is long enough and the dose sufficient, all patients will have either seizures or psychosis or both. Fraser et al. (1958) have reported that as little as 400 mg of phenobarbital or secobarbital a day for three months is sufficient to cause paroxysmal EEG changes in about 30 percent of subjects. If the dose is increased to 600 mg a day for as little as one or two months, 50 percent of the subjects will have withdrawal signs of insomnia, anorexia, and tremor, with concomitant EEG changes. Ten percent may have seizures. Above 600 mg a day the probability increases greatly for the development of psychosis. Patients receiving phenobarbital for the symptomatic relief of seizures may show many of the signs of withdrawal if the drug is abruptly withdrawn. Abrupt termination of barbiturates in someone taking large dosages for long periods of time may be fatal. The usual method of treatment is by means of slow withdrawal.

MISCELLANEOUS HYPNOTICS

Bromides

Bromide has been largely supplanted in modern medicine by other less toxic medications. It is still occasionally used in the treatment of epilepsy and those cases that are refractory to other medications. Bromide was a very popular medicinal in the latter half of the last century in the treatment of epilepsy and various nervous diseases. It is a highly toxic drug, though it is difficult to develop an acute intoxication as a result of its irritability to the gastrointestinal tract. It is excreted very slowly, a half life of 12 days, so that large amounts can accumulate with small daily doses that will reach toxic proportions. Toxic effects of bromides (bromism) include a psychosis with delusions and hallucinations along with many of the manifestations of intoxication.

Methaqualone (Quaalude, Sopor, Parest)

Methaqualone is a sedative hypnotic that became quite popular as an abuse substance during the early part of this decade. Among its pharmacological properties, in addition to its sedative-hypnotic action, are anticonvulsant, antispasmodic (decrease in motility of the gut), local anesthetic, and weak antihistaminic actions. Transient paresthesias (burning, tingling, or formication sensations of the skin) have been reported preceding the onset of sleep after hypnotic doses. Also, persistent paresthesias lasting for months or years have been related to methaqualone use. However, the specific role of methaqualone in causing this persistent neuropathy is still inconclusive.

Although the primary effect of this compound is sedation or hypnosis, occasionally subjects report restlessness and anxiety. Hangover is common after clinical use of methaqualone, despite a half life shorter than those characteristic of the short-acting barbiturates.

Marked central nervous system depression is the first sign of an overdose, although restlessness and excitement may be seen. With high doses delirium and convulsions may occur. If the dose is sufficient to cause coma, the accompanying respiratory and cardiovascular depression is less than that seen in coma caused by barbiturate overdose. Coma has been reported after a dose of 2.4 g and death after 8 g (Harvey, 1975). Methaqualone has been a drug of choice in suicide, like the barbiturates. Many of the fatalities have occurred in people who have also ingested alcohol. Abrupt withdrawal from chronic methaqualone use may cause convulsions.

Among those who use methaqualone for nonmedical purposes, it is believed that the drug has aphrodisiac properties, improves interpersonal relationships, and causes a "high" without an associated drowsiness. There is little scientific evidence to substantiate these claims.

Chloral Hydrate

Chloral hydrate is a very good hypnotic that acts much like the barbiturates. It owes its activity to the fact that in the body it is metabolized to trichloroethanol, an aliphatic alcohol. One possible advantage over the barbiturates is that at low doses it does not suppress REM sleep.

The effects of an overdose of chloral hydrate resembles those seen with barbiturates. However, unlike the barbiturates, there may be marked constriction of the pupil. Because of this a patient in a coma due to chloral hydrate could be misdiagnosed as being in coma from an overdose of opiates. An agonist–antagonist such as nalorphine would make the chloral hydrate patient worse. Naloxone, however, would have no adverse effect and would aid in making the differential diagnosis (see Chapter 7). Chloral hydrate will produce both tolerance and physical dependence similar to that seen with the barbiturates.

Paraldehyde

This drug has been used in medicine since 1882. It has been generally believed to be a very safe hypnotic; however, in recent years the safety of this drug has been questioned because of reported pathological changes in various organ systems.

The drug can only be administered orally in a liquid form, and it imparts a disagreeable odor to the breath as well as having an unpleasant taste. This probably accounts for it generally not being used by the ambulatory patient. It has had its main use in the treatment of abstinence from other hypnotics or alcohol; however, as mentioned, as a result of recent reported toxic effects from paraldehyde intoxication, its use is being curtailed.

Glutethimide (Doriden) and Methylprylon (Noludar)

These compounds were introduced as nonbarbiturate hypnotics that supposedly had none of the toxic effects or the addiction liability of the barbiturates. Unfortunately, neither of these compounds has fulfilled the hopes of the manufacturer in this regard in that tolerance and physical dependence will develop to both compounds. It would seem that neither of these drugs offers any special advantage over the barbiturates but may be useful alternative medications.

Nonprescription Hypnotics

Almost all of these drugs contain antihistaminics as their active ingredient. They are marketed for their soporific effect rather than their antihistaminic actions. Most of these drugs that can be bought without a prescription contain *methapyrilene*. Although these drugs cause sedation at low doses, they can have cental excitatory effects at high dose levels. Unfortunately, little is known concerning the central action of these compounds.

SUMMARY

Many other drugs not classified as hypnotics have soporific effects. This is especially true of those agents called *minor tranquilizers* (Chapter 6). Drugs are often classified by their use rather than action. Thus antihistamines that have sedative and hypnotic effects have this aspect of their action minimized by the manufacturer, unless they are marketing the drug as a hypnotic.

All of these drugs are potentially dangerous. All have the potential for causing physical dependence, except those that are antihistamines or the bromides that have marked toxic effects that are as severe as the withdrawal syndrome seen with the barbiturates.

REFERENCES

Bradley, P. B. The central action of certain drugs in relation to the reticular formation of the brain. In H. H. Jasper, L. D. Proctor, R. S. Knighton, W. C. Noshay, R. T. Costello (Eds.) *Reticular Formation of the Brain.* Boston, Little, Brown, 1958, pp. 123–149.

Brazier, M. A. B. The action of anesthetics on the nervous system. In E. D. Adrian and H. H. Jasper (Eds.) *Brain Mechanisms and Consciousness.* Springfield, Charles C Thomas, 1954, pp. 163–199.

Dews, P. Studies on behavior. I. Differential sensitivity to pentobarbital of pecking performance in pigeons depending on the schedule of reward. *Journal of Pharmacology and Experimental Therapeutics,* **113,** 1955, 393–401.

Fraser, H. F., Wikler, A., Essig, C. F., and **Isbell, H.** Degree of physical dependence induced by secobarbital or phenobarbital. *Journal of the American Medical Association,* **116,** 1958, 126–129.

Goodnow, R. E., Beecher, H. K., Brazier, M. A. B., Mosteller, F., and **Tagiuri, R.** Physiological performance following a hypnotic dose of a barbiturate. *Journal of Pharmacology and Experimental Therapeutics,* **102,** 1951, 55–61.

Grinker, R. R. and **Speigel, J. P.** *Men Under Stress,* Philadelphia, Blakiston, 1945.

Harvey, S. C. Hypnotics and sedatives. In L. S. Goodman and A. Gilman (Eds.) *The Pharmacological Basis of Therapeutics*. (5th ed.). New York, Macmillan, 1975, pp. 102–123.

Hill, H. E., Belleville, R. E., and **Wikler A.** Motivational determinants in modification of behavior by morphine and pentobarbital. *American Medical Association Archives of Neurology and Psychiatry,* **77,** 1957, 28–35.

Isbell, H., Altschul, S., Kornetsky, C., Eisenman, A. J., Flanary, H. G., and **Fraser, H. F.** Chronic barbiturate intoxication: An experimental study. *American Medical Association Archives of Neurology and Psychiatry,* **64,** 1950, 1–28.

Kornetsky, C., Vates, T. S., and **Kessler, E. K.** A comparison of hypnotic and residual psychological effects of single doses of chlorpromazine and secobarbital in man. *Journal of Pharmacology and Experimental Therapeutics,* **127,** 1959, 51–54.

McKenzie, R. E. and **Elliot, L. L.** Effects of secobarbital and *d*-amphetamine on performance during a simulated air mission. *Aerospace Medicine,* **36,** 1965, 774–779.

Mirsky, A. F. and **Tecce, J. J.** The relationship between EEG and impaired attention following administration of centrally acting drugs. In H. Brill, J. O. Cole, P. Denikar, H. Hippius, and P. B. Bradley (Eds.) *Neuropsychopharmacology*. Amsterdam, Excerpta Medica International Congress, Series No. 129, 1967, pp. 638–645.

Moruzzi, G. and **Magoun, H. W.** Brain stem reticular formation and activation of the EEG. *Electroencephalography and Clinical Neurophysiology,* **1,** 1949, 455–473.

Oswald, J. Drugs and Sleep. *Pharmacological Reviews,* **20,** 1968, 273–303.

Sharpless, S. K. Hypnotics and sedatives. I. The barbiturates. In L. S. Goodman and A. Gilman (Eds.) *The Pharmacological Basis of Therapeutics*. (4th ed.). New York, Macmillian, 1970, pp. 98–120.

9 ALCOHOL

To produce alcohol we need a few basic ingredients; these are sugar, water, yeast, and a mild degree of warmth. When these occur together, it is almost impossible for alcohol not to be produced. Thus it is highly likely that alcohol was present in the earliest civilizations. These beverages have been used as nutritious foods and valuable medicines as well as sacred liquids for religious ceremonies. It is most likely that alcoholic beverages were available to the American Indians long before Columbus arrived in the Western Hemisphere. The early settlers in Virginia brought alcohol with them. Approximately 12 years after their arrival in Virginia, excessive use of alcohol was such that a law was passed stating that any person found drunk for the first time was reported privately to the Minister, the second time publicly, the third time required to "lye in halter" for 12 hours as well as to pay a fine. At the same time that this was going on, the Virginian assembly passed legislation encouraging the introduction of wines and distilled spirits in the Colony. It was not that drinking was unacceptable, but drinking to excess was.

In the Massachusetts Bay Colony brewing came to be next in importance to milling and baking. In Massachusetts, as in Virginia, occasional drunkenness was punished by whipping, fines, and confinement in the stocks. The early Puritans did not prohibit the use of alcoholic beverages; however, they were emphatic in urging moderation in drinking.

The temperance movement sprang up in England during the Industrial Revolution. Its early aim was simply moderation. The movement allowed drinking of wine and beer but not distilled spirits. The temperance movement gradually changed until temperance meant total abstinence. The temperance movement was instrumental in the passage of the eighteenth Amendment to the Constitution of the United States, which prohibited the manufacture and sale of all alcoholic beverages. The eighteenth Amendment lasted from 1920 to 1933. There was a great deal of argument concerning this early experiment in the control of drinking of alcoholic beverages. Some individuals felt that it reduced substantially the amount of drinking in the United States. Others, however,

Ethanol

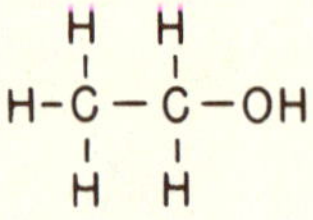

```
  H   H
  |   |
H-C - C -OH
  |   |
  H   H
```

FIGURE 1. Ethanol (ethyl alcohol).

argued that the great experiment curbed only the moderate drinker and brought new and dangerous glamour to drinking and intoxication. Those against the Prohibition Movement claimed that it destroyed public respect for law enforcement officers and brought crime, violence, and general corruption.

In all major alcoholic beverages the chief ingredient is ethyl alcohol, known also as ethanol or simply alcohol. Concentrations vary with the type of preparation, for example, about 4% by volume in beers, 12% in table wines, 20% in cocktails or dessert wines, 20 to 55% in liqueurs, and 40 to 50% in distilled whiskeys. In addition, the beverages contain a variety of other chemical constituents. Some come from original grains, grapes, or other fruits; others are produced from the chemical processes of fermentation; still others may be added as flavoring or coloring.

A critical factor in analyzing the effects of drinking is not the amount of alcohol drunk or the amount that reaches the stomach but the amount that enters the bloodstream and the speed with which it is metabolized. Beers, wines, and distilled spirits may vary markedly in the rate in which the alcohol they contain is absorbed in the blood. In general, the higher the concentration of alcohol the more rapid the absorption, and the higher the concentration of nonalcoholic components the slower the absorption.

There are certain components of alcoholic beverages, known as fusels, that are relatively more toxic than ethyl alcohol. They usually occur in low concentration and thus are usually not considered much of a hazard.

Absorption, Metabolism, and Excretion

Alcohol is rapidly absorbed from the stomach, small intestine, and colon. It also can be absorbed, if it is vaporized, by means of the lungs.

Many factors modify the absorption of alcohol from the stomach. At first absorption is rapid, then it decreases to a very slow rate, although gastric concentration still may be high. Absorption will vary as a function of the volume, the character, the dilution of the beverage, the presence of food, the period of time taken to ingest the drink, as well as various individual peculiarities. Most foods in the stomach tend to retard absorption, milk being especially effective. Beer exerts its own retarding action much like that of food. After absorption alcohol is fairly uniformly distributed throughout all tissues and fluids of the body.

The exact blood concentration of alcohol necessary to cause intoxication will vary from individual to individual. Thus two people with the same blood concentration may vary greatly in their degree of intoxication. At the present time a blood alcohol concentration of 0.10% (100 mg%, 100 mg per 100 ml of blood) is considered sufficient for a person to be considered legally drunk in most states of the United States. A blood alcohol concentration of 0.20% is associated with mild to moderate intoxication. All individuals with an alcohol concentration of 0.4% will be most markedly drunk. Fatal concentrations are somewhere between 0.5% and 0.8%. The rapid ingestion of 4 oz of 90-proof whiskey on an empty stomach will give a blood alcohol concentration of about 0.10%.

Alcohol is detoxified by the liver by means of oxidation, yielding carbon dioxide and water. In addition, it converts to 7 calories per gram. Rate of metabolism is slow, approximately a little over one ounce of whiskey per hour (10 ml of alcohol). Thus the alcohol in 4 oz of whiskey could require 5 to 6 hours to be oxidized in the average person. Ninety to 98% of alcohol that enters the body is completely oxidized.

The metabolism of alcohol differs from most substances in that it is a linear function of time, and it is only slightly raised by increasing the concentration in the blood. This rate is proportional to body weight and probably liver weight.

Central Nervous System and Behavior

The CNS is markedly affected by alcohol more than any other system in the body. Although alcohol is believed by some to be a stimulant, there seems to be little doubt that stimulating properties are slight; like the general anesthetics and hypnotics, it is a depressant of the CNS. Alcohol has been used in the past as an anesthetic, especially prior to the introduction of the common anesthetics; however, an effective anesthetic dose is very close to the lethal dose.

The effects of alcohol as measured by the EEG in both animals and humans are a decrease in frequency and an increase in amplitude. These EEG effects indicate a predominance of depressant actions, although some investigators do report a slight stimulating effect at low doses. Data from electrophysiological studies in animals indicate that after the administration of alcohol, the first effect is a depressant action on certain cortical sites as well as the polysynaptic structures of the reticular formation. These areas have a highly integrative role in the function of the brain. The loss of integrative control after alcohol allows for the unrestrained activity of other areas of the brain, giving rise to the apparent feeling of stimulation. There is enhancement of spinal reflexes as they become freed from central inhibitory control. However, as the dose of alcohol is increased, there is a marked general depression of all functions. This depression of the higher integrative function of the brain results in impairment in mental and motor processes, and what is observed is what is called intoxication (see

Ritchie, 1975). After ingesting intoxicating amounts of alcohol insight is dulled and confidence seems to abound. In some individuals the personality becomes expansive and speech, at least to the speaker, becomes eloquent and brilliant.

Almost all studies on the effects of alcohol on behavior (see Walgren and Barry, III, 1970, pp. 275-400) indicate that the drug will impair performance with the degree of impairment being a function of dose. Certain tasks seem to show a greater level of impairment than others. Studies of monocular focusing, tracking, and binocular coordination show a great deal of impairment at even low doses and as dose increases, the level of impairment also increases. Reaction is more drastically impaired when the task becomes more complex or the subject is required to simultaneously attend to some concurrent activity. This type of performance is most important in driving a vehicle. Of a total of five million arrests for all causes in the United States in 1965, 250,000 arrests were for driving while intoxicated (Brecher et al., 1972, p. 261). In a study of fatal automobile accidents it was reported that among the drivers who were probably responsible for their accident, 73 percent had been drinking, and of these, 46 percent had blood alcohol concentrations of 0.25% or higher (Ibid, p. 263).

Most studies on the effects of alcohol on complex intellectual tasks show that alcohol will cause significant impairment. However, there have been some reports of improved performance after low or moderate doses on tasks involving extremely difficult and unfamiliar problems. This may be the result of the subjects' willingness after ethanol to try new and difficult approaches to the problem. Despite impaired performance, many subjects under the influence of alcohol estimate that their performance is not impaired, and in fact, they believe that it is improved.

For a detailed review of the effects of alcohol on the CNS and behavior, see Walgren and Barry, III (1970, pp. 275-400) and Kissin and Begleiter (1972).

Organ System Effects

Moderate amounts of alcohol have only slight effects on the circulatory system. Blood pressure and the force of contraction of the heart are not significantly changed by alcohol ingestion except when levels of intoxication are quite high. Cardiovascular abnormalities have been observed in some chronic heavy drinkers. Some of these abnormalities are believed to be the result of an indirect effect of malnutrition and vitamin deficiency. However, chronic excessive alcohol intake has a direct pathogenic effect on the myocardium (see Ritchie, 1975, p. 139).

Alcohol has little direct effect on blood vessels, but because of central vasomotor depression, there is vasodilatation of the cutaneous blood vessels giving the drinker a feeling of warmth plus a flushing of the skin. Chronic effects of this are sometimes seen in the reddened bulbous nose of some heavy drinkers.

There is no laboratory or clinical evidence that moderate doses of alcohol will dilate coronary arteries. Patients suffering from angina report relief after the ingestion of moderate amounts of alcohol. It is believed that this pain relief is due to central depressant actions and not due to an increase in coronary circulation.

The drinking of alcoholic beverages to increase body warmth is not indicated, although folklore does recommend alcohol as a method to keep warm. Despite the transitory feeling of warmth after moderate amounts of alcohol due to enhanced cutaneous and intestinal blood flow, there is an increase in heat loss due to sweating. Large amounts of alcohol may depress central temperature-regulatory mechanisms resulting in a marked fall in body temperature. The increase in the number of cocktail bars at ski resorts with a concomitant increase in alcohol use by skiers might suggest that there may be some other compensatory value to the drinking of alcoholic beverages that skiers have found. Nonskiers who believe that no person in his right mind would ski have quipped that you have to drink to ski, or if you are drinking, you are not skiing.

Actions of alcohol on the gastrointestinal tract will vary as a function of the amount and type of food present in the stomach as well as the presence or absence of gastrointestinal disease. Gastric secretions are stimulated by alcohol. Because of this increase in gastric secretions plus the fact that strong alcoholic drinks (40% or greater by volume) are irritating to stomach mucosa, alcoholic beverages are not recommended for the peptic ulcer patient. The presence of food in the stomach will decrease this irritation.

Alcohol can cause an accumulation of fat in the liver. The manner in which the hepatic accumulation of fat is related to cirrhosis of the liver, common in alcoholics, is not clear. The question remains as to whether the cirrhosis is due to a deficiency of essential nutrients that are absent in the diet of alcoholics or whether it can be produced in man by chronic, excessive use of alcohol in the presence of an adequate diet.

The old story of the man in the barroom who continually pours his served glass of beer down the toilet and when queried, states that he does not wish to be a "middle man," attests to the strong diuretic action of alcohol. The large amount of liquid that is usually ingested with alcoholic beverages contributes to this increased flow of urine; however, alcohol itself has a marked diuretic action. This diuretic action is proportional to the blood alcohol concentration and is most pronounced when the blood alcohol level is rising. Except for the inconvenience, there seems to be no deleterious effect of alcohol on the kidneys.

Carpenter and Armenti (1972, p. 510), commenting on the effects of alcohol on sexual behavior, found a certain sameness in most reviews and textbooks. There seems to be a fair amount of unanimity that there is little information on the effects of alcohol on human sexuality and that William Shakespeare is still the chief authority on the subject. Most reviews quote the conversation between

Macduff and the porter from *Macbeth* (Act 2, scene 3). Since no discussion of the effects of alcohol on sexual function would be complete without the quotation, I also include it. Macduff is inquiring why the porter is still in bed.

Macduff: Was it so late, friend, ere you went to bed,
That you do lie so late?
Porter: Faith, sir, we were carousing till the second cock:
and drink, sir, is a great provoker of three things.
Macduff: What three things does drink especially provoke?
Porter: Marry, sir, nose-painting, sleep and urine.
Lechery, sir, it provokes and unprovokes; it
provokes the desire, but it takes away the performance:
therefore, much drink may be said to be an equivocator
with lechery: it makes him and it mars him; it sets
him on and it takes him off; it persuades him and
disheartens him; makes him stand to and not stand to;
in conclusion, equivocates him in sleep, and giving him
the lie, leaves him.

Although there have been a number of experiments with animals, there do not seem to be any but indirect studies of the effects of alcohol on sexual behavior in humans (see Walgren and Barry, III, 1970, pp. 180–181; and Carpenter and Armenti, 1972, pp. 509–525). In animals alcohol causes a prolongation of erection time, an increased latency to the first mount, intromission, and ejaculation; however, the animals require fewer intromissions to achieve ejaculation. At a blood alcohol level that abolished the ejaculation reflex, dogs still showed interest in receptive females but were incapable of completing copulation.

The estrous cycle of female animals is disturbed by alcohol administration; however, there is little or nothing in the literature concerning the sexual response of female animals after the administration of alcohol.

Human studies have focused on the sexual content of the response of male subjects taking personality tests after the administration of ethanol. These studies do not shed much light on the problem, and they also only deal with the response of males. Much like the experiments in animals, the human studies have concentrated on the effects of alcohol on the sexual response of the male. Maybe most scientists do not believe that a female's sexual behavior can be altered by alcohol!

Hangover

The hangover, although common and unpleasant, is rarely dangerous. It occurs in the moderate drinker when occasionally he drinks a little too much as well as in the excessive drinker after prolonged drinking bouts. The exact mechanism that produces the hangover is not known at the present time, although the evidence suggests that it is an abstinence phenomenon. The symptoms occur during the decreasing phase of the blood alcohol levels and may manifest themselves when there is little or no alcohol present in the body. The symptoms of a hangover include headache, vertigo, nausea, tremor, pallor, and sweating. Gastric distress and thirst are the most common symptoms. There is a change in the individual's water balance, and hypoglycemia may be quite marked.

Hangovers have been blamed on the mixing of different alcoholic beverages or the drinking of esoteric concoctions. However, a hangover can be caused by drinking any alcoholic beverage, including pure ethyl alcohol. There is no specific treatment for hangovers except alcohol itself. Thus if one starts drinking, a hangover can be precluded by never stopping. Since this is usually not possible, many popular remedies are used that have no scientific basis. The following are believed by some to be effective in treating a hangover: raw eggs, oysters, chili peppers, steak sauce, or vitamin preparations.

Tolerance

Tolerance to ethanol has been demonstrated in both animals and man. The degree of tolerance seen with alcohol does not compare to the tolerance seen after chronic use of the narcotic drugs. There are evidently three types of tolerance to ethanol, tissue, metabolic, and behavioral tolerance. In tissue tolerance there is a change in the CNS and organ response to the drug. In metabolic tolerance there is faster degradation of alcohol. And in behavioral tolerance there is a psychological adaptation to the tissue effects of alcohol so that the subject will manifest less effects of the alcohol.

Physical Dependence

It is quite clear that chronic ingestion of alcohol produces a state of physical dependence. The intensity of the withdrawal syndrome depends on the degree of intoxication and its duration. The mildest form of withdrawal would be a hangover. At the other extreme are seizures, sometimes called fits and delerium tremens. These usually develop only after very heavy intoxication for periods in excess of two weeks, although there is some evidence that sustained heavy drinking is not necessary (Mello, 1972). See the section on Alcoholism.

The withdrawal syndrome begins to manifest itself within a few hours after the last drink; tremulousness appears along with nausea, weakness, anxiety, and perspiration. The individual begins to seek alcohol. There may be cramps and vomiting. The tremor becomes so marked it may be difficult to lift a glass. The subject may begin to hallucinate, at first only when eyes are closed, but later even with the eyes open. Initially, insight is retained, and the subject remains oriented despite the presence of hallucinations. This is sometimes called *acute alcoholic hallucinosis*.

As the syndrome progresses insight is lost. The subject becomes weaker and more confused and disoriented and agitated. He may become terrified by his hallucinations. They become vivid, and in this stage, which appears around the third day of withdrawal, there is severe delerium.

Hypothermia is quite common, and exhaustion and cardiovascular collapse may occur. Although grand mal seizures may appear, they are less common than in barbiturate withdrawal, and they usually precede the onset of the frank delerium.

The alcohol abstinence syndrome is self-limiting. If the patient does not die, recovery usually occurs within 5 to 7 days without treatment. The fact that there is real physical dependence to alcohol was determined in 1954 when Isbell et al. published a paper on an experimental study of "rum fits" and delirium tremens.

Alcoholism

Although alcoholism has been a biological and social problem for centuries and despite the recent focus on abuse of other drugs, the problem of alcoholism has not received the attention that it warrants. The magnitude of the problem far outweighs the problem of opiate addiction. Not only are there more alcoholics than the narcotic users (it is estimated that there are between 8 and 10 million alcoholics in the United States alone), but the chronic use of large amounts of alcohol is much more dangerous to the individual than the chronic use of narcotic drugs. Physically and mentally, the alcoholic is worse off than the chronic narcotic user. The only advantage that the alcoholic has over the narcotic user is that the laws governing alcohol use are much less punitive than the laws governing the use of the opiates.

There have been a number of suggestions as to the cause of alcoholism. Among some proposed have been genetic factors, specific vitamin deficencies, hormone imbalances, and even allergies.

Obviously, the factors contributing to alcoholism are quite complicated. It is not simply overexposure to alcohol that causes alcoholism, for we would then expect the highest rates of alcoholism to be found among groups with the highest per capita intake of alcohol. No such relationship can be found. High alcohol intake with a high rate of alcoholism has been reported in France; also a high rate of intake but a low rate of alcoholism has been reported in Italy and Greece. Many people have suggested personality as the primary variable accounting for alcoholism. However, there is no alcoholic personality.

In the 1960s Mendelson and Mello, at Boston City Hospital, embarked on a series of systematic studies of alcoholic subjects in an attempt to determine the variables that contribute to the maintenance of chronic alcohol use (see Mello, 1972). They argued that attempting to reconstruct the putative precipitating constellation of events in the development of the disease was probably not a particularly effective way to modify the process of the disease. They pointed out that alcohol addiction is probably a function of many diverse factors in both the individual and his environment and that an attempt to delineate these would be of very little value in helping to alter the drinking behavior of the alcoholic. Instead they suggested that ". . . if the spontaneous initiation, perpetuation and cessation of a drinking spree were found to be correlated with a constant pattern of behavioral and biological variables, then manipulation of these variables could result in the modification of drinking behavior." (Mello, 1972, p. 223).

To carry out these experiments Mello and Mendelson studied small groups of alcoholic subjects on a research ward for drinking periods that varied from 7 days to 3 months. In some of the studies alcohol was given at fixed doses and intervals. In other studies the subject was allowed to determine the volume and frequency of his own alcohol intake. In the experiments in which the subject controlled the alcohol intake, simple tasks were used that allowed the subject to earn tokens that could be exchanged for alcohol. The Boston City Hospital group of investigators made use of operant conditioning procedures in their studies of the time course of alcohol intake in chronic alcoholic subjects. Their findings were most interesting, and many of their experiments gave results that were contrary to common expectation. They found that subjects did not try to regulate their drinking behavior to maintain a constant blood alcohol level.

Withdrawal signs and symptoms were significantly more severe in the subjects on free-choice schedules than those on a rigid program of drinking. A most surprising finding was that no subject who was allowed unlimited access to alcohol attempted to drink himself into oblivion. There was no evidence of compulsive, uncontrollable drinking patterns following an initial achievement of a high blood-alcohol level. Subjects would work for and drink relatively small amounts of ethanol (1 to 2 oz), indicating that the alcoholic was capable of exercising some control over his own drinking behavior. Figure 2 indicates the drinking and operant work behavior of a single alcoholic subject in the Mello, Mendelson studies.

Mello challenges the concept of craving and points out a number of clinical and research observations that are contrary to the notion that ingesting of ethanol by an alcoholic will inevitably trigger a sequence of compulsive drinking that results in a "loss of control." Clinical observations have indicated that some alcoholics can drink socially without reverting back to their previous compulsive drinking behavior.

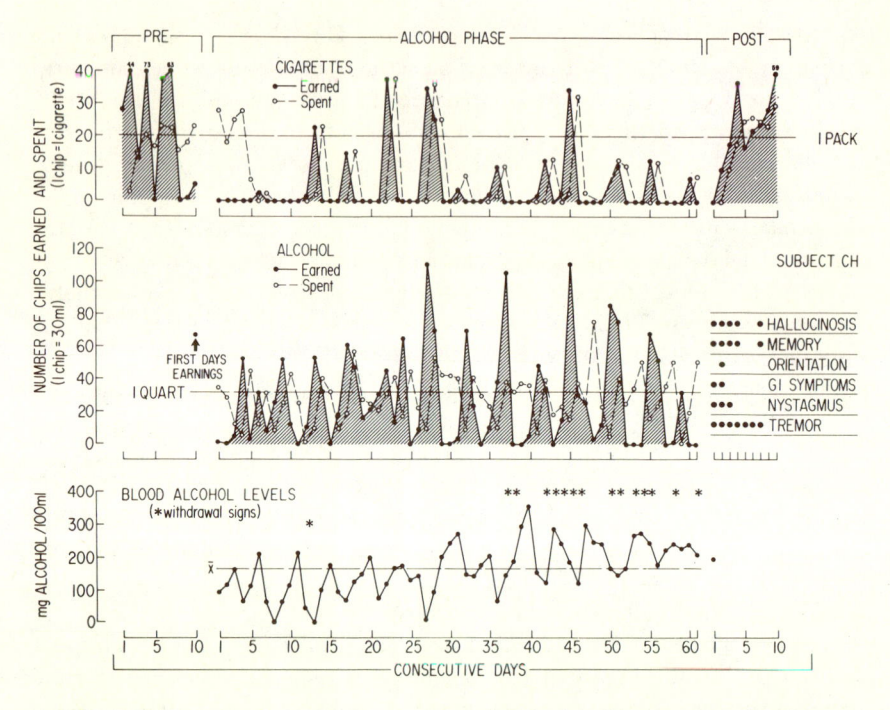

FIGURE 2. Earning and spending pattern of a single subject working for cigarettes and alcohol during a 60-day alcohol-available period. Tokens earned for alcohol were not interchangeable with tokens earned for cigarettes. Pattern of earning (closed circles, shaded area) and spending (open circles) for cigarettes is shown in the top row. Pattern of earning (closed circles, shaded area) and spending (open circles) for alcohol is shown in the middle row. Average daily blood alcohol levels are shown on the bottom row. The diagram to the right of the middle graph shows the occurrence of withdrawal symptoms during the 10-day abstinence period (from Mello and Mendelson 1972).

The Alcoholic Beverages

In all alcoholic beverages the amount by percent of ethyl alcohol varies with the type of preparation. When certain natural materials such as honey, fruits, and grains are mixed with water and left in the sun, fermentation takes place. Because of the simplicity of producing alcoholic beverages, their use appeared very early in the history of man. The earliest beverages were beers or wines. The type of beverage made by early civilizations depended greatly on the type of climate and the availability of the natural product.

Beer. Beverages made from fermented grain mashes were extensively used in ancient Egypt. The climate of the Nile Valley favored the use of grains so that beer, rather than wine, was more commonly brewed by the ancient Egyptians.

ALCOHOL

Since control of fermentation is always a problem in the making of an alcoholic beverage, the early Egyptians probably learned from experience to handle the yeast necessary to convert the grain carbohydrate to alcohol. It is believed that they grew one variety of yeast by using the same wood-mashing instrument. In the crevices of these instruments the microorganisms would grow that produced the necessary enzymes for proper fermentation of the grain mash. Sediment from the brewing process was saved and added to new batches of mash. Although the making of modern beers makes use of many refinements, the basic methods are the same now as they were in ancient Egypt.

Today's beers may differ in color, aroma, and flavor; however, most are made by fermentation of barley malt, although other grains may be used. The dried blossoms of the female *Humulus lupulus* vine (hops) are added during the brewing of beer. The hops give beer its pungent or bitter taste.

There are various types of beers. The most widely consumed is *lager* beer named from the German word *lager* that means "to store" or "to rest." Most American lagers are light in color and resemble *pilsner* beer, which originated in Pilsen, Czechoslovakia. Dark-color beer is produced by the use of roasted or carmelized malt or sugar. The alcoholic content of lager beer ranges from 3 to 6% by volume.

In the making of *ale* a different fermenting process and yeast are used than are used for making lager. Ale is more highly flavored with hops than lager, and the alcoholic concentration varies from 3 to 8%.

Stout and *porter* are dark English beers. Porter has a strong malt flavor and only a mild flavor of hops. The alcoholic concentration of porter is about 6% by volume. Stout has a strong malt flavor plus a strong bitter hops taste. It has an alcoholic concentration of 4 to 8%. The British drink, *half-and-half*, is a dilution of stout with a less potent ale or lager.

Beers contain a low concentration of a number of essential nutrients as well as a significant amount of energy-producing sugars. Since the amount of ethyl alcohol is relatively low in beer, the rapid ingestion of large amounts is necessary to produce intoxication. Small amounts of alcohols, sometimes called *fusel oils,* are present in beer.

Table Wines. The making of wine is about as old as the making of beer. Wines vary as a function of the type of grape, the soil of the vineyard, climate, and method used in crushing and fermentation. Most table wines, including sparkling wines and champagnes, contain about 12% alcohol by volume. Kosher wines may contain sufficient added sugar to push by the alcohol concentration to 20%. Table wines contain hundreds of organic compounds. For a listing and concentration of the most important chemical components of wine, the reader is referred to Leake and Silverman (1971, p. 587).

Dessert and Cocktail Wines. These are ordinary wines in which alcohol has been added to raise the alcohol concentration to 20%. They are also known as "fortified wines." The added alcohol is brandy or neutral spirits made from wine. The most common beverages of this type are sherry, port, madeira, muscatel, and vermouth. The alcohol concentration of vermouth is slightly lower than for the other cocktail wines, about 17 to 18% by volume.

Because of their relatively high alcohol content and the availability of inexpensive brands, this class of beverage is often the choice of the alcoholic.

Liqueurs. Nearly all liqueurs are sweet and have a sugar content as high as 50%. Alcohol concentrations range from 20 to 55%. Liqueurs, also called cordials, were originally used as medicinal preparations and were developed during the Middle Ages. Because of their high alcohol content, liqueurs were not made until the Arabic art of distillation became known. These early liqueurs were made from mixtures of herbs that were selected for their putative medicinal properties. Even today the specific recipes of some liqueurs are well-guarded secrets of the makers. Among some of the most common liqueurs are Benedictine, Chartreuse, Creme de Cacao, Kirsch, Cointreau, and Drambuie.

Distilled Spirits. Alcoholic beverages with alcohol concentrations greater than that found in wine awaited the art of distillation and came relatively late in the history of man. The art of distillation was discovered during the golden age of Arabic culture. Distilled spirits are made from fruits, grains, potatoes, molasses, as well as any other source of fermentable sugar.

Brandy was probably the first beverage of distilled spirits to be made commercially. It was first known as *aqua vitae* ("water of life"), and the name brandy comes from the Dutch word *brandewijn,* meaning burned or distilled wine. Brandy is distilled from fermented mash of grapes, although it can be made from other fruits. The term "brandy" by itself usually refers to the product made from grapes. The common brandies made from other fruits are apple brandy (apple jack), plum brandy (slivawitz), and cherry brandy (kirschwasser). Each brandy has a characteristic taste, depending on the basic fruit. If the pits of the fruit are allowed to remain in the fermenting mash, cyanide derivatives may be released during fermentation, and clinically insignificant amounts will be found in the final product. Brandies have 40 to 50% ethanol by volume.

Whiskey is made from grain. The grain mash is fermented to produce a strong beer (5 to 10% alcohol), and then the beer is distilled and aged in oak barrels. Current opinion is that whiskey making began in Ireland about the twelfth century, although legend has it that it all started with St. Patrick in the fifth century. This is unlikely, for the distillation art was not developed until many centuries later.

The two most common United States whiskeys are bourbon and rye. Bourbon whiskey is distilled from a mash of grain containing not less than 51% corn and is usually aged a minimum of four years in new charred-oak barrels.

Rye whiskey is distilled from a mash of grain containing not less than 51% rye grain. *Corn* whiskey is made of mash of grain with a minimum of 80% corn. These whiskeys are bottled with an alcohol concentration of 40 to 50% by volume. *Canadian* whiskeys are a blend made from rye, corn, and barley, and, of course, they are made in Canada.

Scotch whiskeys are made from a malt of barley that has been dried over a peat fire. The malt whiskey is then blended with scottish grain whiskey, which is similar to American neutral spirits. Straight *malt* whiskey is the whiskey made only from the pure barley malt. Scotch is stored in used charred-oak barrels that are imported from the United States and Canadian whiskey makers. The ethanol content of scotch whiskey is 40 to 45% by volume. *Irish* whiskey, as might be expected, is made only in Ireland. It is a blended whiskey containing barley malt as well as grain whiskey. Coal is used for drying the malt in a manner that does not allow the smoke from the fire to reach the malt. Irish whiskey contains 43% ethyl alcohol by volume.

Rum is made in almost every part of the world where sugar cane is grown. Rum is made from molasses, although fresh sugar cane juices can be used. The mash from the molasses fermentation is distilled, giving a colorless liquid that darkens with aging. It is aged in either charred or uncharred barrels. The dark rums are usually the result of extractives from the barrel and the addition of caramel. The alcohol content of rum will vary from 40 to 75% by volume.

Gin is a tasteless alcohol distillate that is flavored by a second distillation with juniper berries and other plant products. It is believed that gin was originally developed in the seventeenth century, either to make raw alcohol more palatable or to utilize the putative diuretic action of juniper oil. Gin is made from any fermentable carbohydrate. It is usually not aged but bottled immediately after the second distillation. The alcoholic concentration of gin is usually between 35 and 50% by volume. During the great prohibition experiment in the U.S. "bathtub gin" was in favor. This was made by the direct addition of flavoring to the raw alcohol. It, of course, lacked the subtlety conferred by a second distillation, but it did not lack in potency. Also, depending on the last user of the bathtub, unique and probably unreproducible flavors were made with each batch.

Vodka is essentially pure alcohol and water. Originally, vodka was distilled from a potato mash, but at the present time, many other carbohydrate sources are used. Vodka is made by filtering the distilled ethanol through charcoal. Filtering was first used to remove contaminants from distilled ethanol. The concentration of ethanol in vodka is 40 to 50% by volume.

The alcoholic content of a beverage is often expressed on a *proof* scale in English-speaking countries. The British proof scale designates 100 proof as a concentration of ethanol of 57.15% by volume at 15.56°C. The American proof scale allows for a somewhat easier conversion to percent concentration by volume; a 100-proof beverage is a concentration of ethanol of 50% by volume at 15.56°C. Percent by volume is temperature dependent; however, except when great accuracy is required, it is not necessary to adjust the proof level because of variation in temperature.

Chemical Composition of Alcoholic Beverages

The various alcoholic beverages differ in their chemical components, although the major constituent responsible for their psychological effects is the ethyl alcohol. However, as previously indicated, there are many substances in alcoholic beverages other than ethyl alcohol, including methyl, propyl, and isopropyl alcohols.

The term *congener* is often incorrectly used when applied to constituents of alcoholic beverages. The literal meaning of the term congener is "of the same kind"; however, it has taken on the connotation that all components of an alcoholic beverage other than ethyl alcohol are congeners and that all congeners are toxic or undesirable. The pejorative interpretation of the term congeners, or the use of the term to connote constituents, is incorrect. The components of alcoholic beverages include substances such as glucose, fructose, acetic acid, lactic acid, carbon dioxide, at least five members of the vitamin B family, as well as other essential elements.

The higher *alcohols,* which include propyl and butyl as well as others, are found in small amounts in all alcoholic beverages. These higher alcohols are sometimes called *fusel oils* are are more toxic than ethyl alcohol. Since they occur in such low concentrations in alcoholic beverages, they are not considered to be a hazard. It is generally assumed that higher concentrations of fusel oils are found in raw, unaged, or "bad" beverages, and they account for most of the objectionable taste, disagreeable aroma, and untoward physiological effects of alcohol. Like many myths surrounding the preparation and drinking of alcohol the belief about the fusel oils is not supported by careful and analytical data. As an example, the aging of whiskey, which increases the palatability of many whiskeys, also increases the concentration of fusel oils. In general, the highest concentration of fusel oils is found in bourbon, with the lowest concentration found in gin and vodka.

Methyl alcohol, which is highly toxic, is found in small amounts in most alcoholic beverages with the largest concentration in brandies made from fruits other than grapes. Methyl alcohol is also called methanol or *wood alcohol.* It is used as a solvent, antifreeze, or fuel. If large amounts of methanol are ingested, blindness or death will usually result.

For a detailed discussion of the constituents of all alcoholic beverages, the reader is directed to Leake and Silverman (1971).

SUMMARY

Alcohol is the only intoxicant that is socially and legally acceptable for use in most cultures. In fact, it is often considered unacceptable by some if one does not drink in certain ceremonial or social occasions. This acceptance provides work for thousands in the manufacturing of beverages and in the medical and helping professions, not to mention the automobile repair industry and those who are involved in research and writing about alcoholism. The use of alcohol and the problems of its abuse could almost be considered an international resource.

The important thing to remember is that alcohol is a drug, and like all drugs there are positive and negative aspects. It is a drug not used to any great degree by the medical profession to treat disease but a drug that is used by many to assuage depression, anxiety, and in some situations to give courage.

REFERENCES

Brecher, E. M. and the **Editors of Consumer Reports.** *Licit and Illicit Drugs.* Boston, Little, Brown, 1972.

Carpenter, J. A. and **Armenti, N. P.** Some effects of ethanol on human sexual and aggressive behavior. In B. Kissin and H. Begleiter (Eds.) *The Biology of Alcoholism, Vol. 2, Physiology and Behavior* New York, Plenum, 1972, pp. 509-543.

Isbell, H., Fraser, H. F., Wikler, A., Belleville, R. E., and **Eisenman, A. J.** An experimental study of the etiology of "rum fits" and delerium tremens. *Quarterly Journal for the Study of Alcohol,* **15,** 1955, 1-33.

Kissin, B. and **Begleiter, H.** *The Biology of Alcoholism. Vol. 2, Physiology and Behavior.* New York, Plenum, 1972.

Leake, C. D., and **Silverman, M.** The chemistry of alcoholic beverages. In B. Kissin and H. Begleiter (Eds.) *The Biology of Alcoholism, Vol. 1, Biochemistry.* New York, Plenum, 1971, pp. 575-612.

Mello, N. K. Behavioral studies of alcoholism. In B. Kissin and H. Begleiter (Eds.) *The Biology of Alcoholism, Vol. 2, Physiology and Behavior.* New York, Plenum, 1972, pp. 219-291.

Mello, N. K. and **Mendelson, J. H.** Drinking patterns during work-contingent and noncontingent alcohol acquisition. *Psychosomatic Medicine,* **34,** 1972, 139-164.

Ritchie, J. M. The aliphatic alcohols. In L. S. Goodman and A. Gilman (Eds.) *The Pharmacological Basis of Therapeutics.* (5th Ed.). New York, Macmillan, 1975, pp. 138-151.

Wallgren, H. and **Barry, H., III.** *Actions of Alcohol. Vol. 1, Biochemical, Physiological and Psychological Aspects.* New York, Elsevier, 1970.

10 THE AMPHETAMINES

The amphetamines belong to the general group of sympathomimetic amines. In general, the effects of these in the peripheral nervous system resemble the response seen when adrenergic nerves are stimulated. Evidence for the use of a sympathomimetic drug can be found as early as 5000 years ago. In China the herb *ma huang* (Ephedra vulgaris) has been used continuously during this time for many medicinal purposes, including the treatment of respiratory disease (Leake, 1958). Approximately 75 years ago ephedrine was isolated from *ma huang*; however, it was believed to be too toxic a compound and it was not used clinically. In 1925 ephedrine was rediscovered by Chen and Schmidt who introduced its use to Western medicine (Levy and Ahlquist, 1965).

Ephedrine was a big improvement over epinephrine, the prototype of the sympathomimetic amines, in the treatment of bronchial asthma. In attempting to make a synthetic substitute for ephedrine, Gordon Alles synthesized amphetamine in 1927. Alles' work led directly to the use of amphetamine in inhaling devices, which caused vasoconstriction of nasal mucosa, and for the symptomatic relief of respiratory infections. The drug was given the trademark name of Benzedrine by Smith, Kline, and French Laboratories, and the Benzedrine inhaler was introduced in 1932. At that time it was included in *New and Nonofficial Remedies* under the nonproprietary name of *amphetamine*.

The central nervous system stimulating effects of amphetamine were first described by Alles (1933). He noted that it antagonized the hypnotic effect of anesthetics in animals and that it had insomnia-producing effects in man. Therapeutic use of the central stimulating effects of amphetamine was first reported by Prinzmetal and Bloomberg in 1935.

This group of drugs consists primarily of three phenylisopropylamines: amphetamine, the racemic mixture of levo- and dextro-1-phenyl-2-aminopropane; dextro-amphetamine, the pure dextro-isomer; and methamphetamine, which is dextro-1-phenylmethylaminopropane. Of the three, the racemic form has the most potent peripheral actions and the least CNS stimulating effects.

THE AMPHETAMINES

$\text{C}_6\text{H}_5-\text{CH}_2-\underset{\underset{\text{CH}_3}{|}}{\text{CH}}-\text{NH}_2$

Amphetamine   **FIGURE 1.** Amphetamine.

Amphetamine is available as the sulfate and as amphetamine phosphate. Although usually given by the oral route, the amphetamines are available in injectable form. When taken orally, its effects are usually detectable within 30 minutes and may last four hours or more.

Absorption, Fate, and Excretion

The amphetamines are readily absorbed from the gastrointestinal tract as well as from parenteral sites of administration. Since the drug is so readily absorbed by the mucous membranes of the alimentary canal, the parenteral route is usually not recommended. Large amounts of the drug are excreted unchanged in the urine within 24 hours after oral ingestion. Excretion of the unchanged drug continues for as long as three days after ingestion. The fate of the unexcreted amphetamine is not completely understood. Studies in animals indicate great species differences in absorption and excretion.

Sympathomimetic Effects

The amphetamines fall in the broad class of compounds called sympathomimetic amines and share many of their classic effects, albeit to a lesser or greater degree, depending on the biological system affected. In general, when the sympathetic nervous system is activated, there is a dilatation of the pupils, rise in blood pressure, increase in heart rate, constriction of blood vessels with concomitant blanching of the mucous membranes, variability in cardiac output, relaxation of intestinal muscles, decrease in coagulation time of the blood, and increase in blood-sugar level. Since the amphetamines affect both alpha and beta receptors, many but not all of these effects maybe seen after the amphetamines. As with all drugs, it is important to recognize that the effects are dose-related and that an effect not present after a low dose may very well be manifested after high doses.

The amphetamines have marked hypertensive effects on both systolic and diastolic blood pressure. There is an increase in pulse pressure, and although heart rate is often increased, the opposite effect on heart rate has been observed. With large doses cardiac arrhythmias may be observed. In usual therapeutic doses there is no increase in cardiac output and little change in cerebral blood flow. Respiration rate is increased by high doses but seems to be little affected by small therapeutic doses.

The sympathomimetic amines characteristically have a marked effect on smooth muscle. Although the bronchial muscle is relaxed after amphetamine administration, the effect is not as pronounced as it is with some of the other sympathomimetic amines and is not sufficient to be of any therapeutic value. There is a contractile effect on the urinary bladder sphincter that may be great enough to cause pain and difficulty in micturation. This action has resulted in amphetamine being used in the treatment of enuresis. However, the effect on the enuretic child may be due also to some of the central effects of the drug on the disturbed child. The effect on the gastrointestinal tract will vary with the state of motility of the gut. If enteric activity is at a high level, the amphetamines may cause relaxation and a reduction of enteric motility. If there is already relaxation of the gut, the amphetamines may cause the opposite effect. There is usually an increase in tone of the uterus, but this varies. The racemic form of the drug seems to have more potent sympathomimetic effects than the dextro-isomer. This is especially true with respect to the cardiovascular effects (see Innes and Nickerson, 1975, for further discussion of amphetamine and other sympathomimetic amines).

Skeletal Muscles

The amphetamines cause increased tone and contractility of the skeletal muscles. This effect may be partially due to the sympathomimetic actions, although there is evidence for a direct action on skeletal muscles (Leake, 1958). It is very likely that the central effect contributes to the increased muscle tone.

Central Nervous System (General Effects)

The central nervous stimulating effects of the amphetamines are well known and documented. The dextro-isomer is more potent than the racemic form in causing central excitation. As a result of its action in stimulating the medullary respiratory center, the drug is effective in reversing depression caused by barbiturates, anesthetics, and other respiratory depressants.

In animals there is seen an increased motor activity, and hypersensitivity to stimuli, and wakefulness. In man an effective dose produces wakefulness, decreased feelings of fatigue, alertness, and an increase in mood often accompanied by loquaciousness and euphoria.

Performance Enhancement

There have been two good reviews of the effects of amphetamines on performance. The first was published in 1962 by Weiss and Laties and the second in 1967 by the same authors.

Although it is clear that the amphetamines will improve all types of performance impaired for such reasons as boredom or fatigue, it is not clear that they can enhance performance above that seen with the interested, motivated, unfatigued subject. Smith and Beecher (1959, 1960) studied trained athletes and found enhancement in both swimming speed and running speed. Although it could be argued that these are fatiguing sports events and the drug was simply improving a fatigued performance, these investigators found that performance in field events was also improved after amphetamine. Although a weight thrower expends a great deal of energy, the effort is brief and the amphetamine induced enhancement is not likely to be due to an antifatigue effect.

In all of these experiments by Smith and Beecher, the facilitory effects were very small but statistically significant; however, a slight improvement was manifested in almost all the subjects. The mean percent improvement in the swimming time was only 1 percent. In terms of competitive athletics this small an improvement can be very significant. World records have been broken on the basis of less than 1 percent improvement in performance. When these investigators used untrained volunteers as their subjects, they found that the amphetamines did not significantly enhance the performance. They attributed this lack of significant effects to the tremendously increased variability in performance found in the untrained subject.

Although amphetamines may often impair the performance of the well-functioning motivated subject (Kornetsky, 1958), the performance of the same subject can be markedly improved over the impaired performance caused by sleep deprivation (Kornetsky, Mirsky, Kessler, and Dorf, 1959).

In all the experiments where there is enhancement of performance, the facilitation is slight. Laties and Weiss point out that if performance can be improved by amphetamine, independent of a simple effect on fatigue and boredom, it can also be improved by careful manipulation of the variables that control behavior.

Effects on Appetite

The appetite-depressant effects of amphetamine were first described by Nathanson in 1939 and have since been well documented. The weight loss seems to be almost completely the result of a reduction in food intake. Change in basal metabolism, digestive processes, or water balance does not seem significant enough to cause the loss of weight seen after chronic use of the drug. This suggests that the anorectic effects are probably due to the action of the amphetamines on those centers of the brain directly involved with appetite control. Although the exact mechanisms are not clear, some reasonable hypotheses have been proffered. Lesions in the ventral medial nucleus of the hypothalamus in rats result in hyperphagia, whereas electrical stimulation results in a decrease in food intake. One hypothesis suggests that amphetamine acts by stimulating this nucleus; however, Stowe and Miller (1957) found that amphetamines still have an anorectic effect in rats with bilateral lesions of the ventral medial nucleus. Since electrical stimulation of the lateral portions of the hypothalamus results in hyperphagia, Stowe and Miller concluded that the diminished appetite was the result of blocking the lateral areas rather than excitation of the medial centers. This inhibitory action is in agreement with the findings of Marrazzi and Hart (1953) that amphetamines inhibit synaptic transmission in the midbrain.

Spinal Cord

Monosynaptic and polysynaptic transmission are facilitated in the spinal cord by amphetamine. The drugs improve reflex activity in the decerebrate cat, and they improve posture and righting reflexes in animals with injured spinal cords.

Analgesia

It has been reported that the amphetamines have some intrinsic analgesic activity in both animals and man. They may enhance the analgesic action of narcotic analgesics and, at the same time, antagonize the respiratory depression caused by these drugs. Despite this slight analgesic action, the drug is not used for the relief of clinical pain.

EEG Effects and Action on the Arousal System

The amphetamines produce an "aroused" type of EEG. The EEG is characterized by low voltage and fast activity accompanied in the intact animal by behavioral arousal (Killam, 1962). The effect of the amphetamines on arousal suggested to many workers that the stimulating effects were due to direct stimulation of the reticular formation.

Experimental evidence supporting the notion of a direct stimulation of the reticular formation by the amphetamines is given by a number of workers. Bradley and Key (1958), using the *encéphale isolé* preparation (transection at cervical 3) in cats, studied the effects of amphetamine on behavioral and EEG arousal produced by direct electrical stimulation of the reticular formation or by auditory stimuli. Under either condition the threshold for both the behavioral and EEG arousal was reduced after amphetamines. When they measured the evoked response from the auditory cortex caused by clicks, they found that amphetamine had very little effect. A change in the arousal threshold to peripheral and direct stimulation of the reticular formation without a change in the cortical evoked response, suggest that the site of action of the amphetamines is directly on the reticular formation rather than the sensory-cortical pathways (lemniscal) or the collaterals to the reticular formation.

Boakes, Bradley, and Candy (1972), in a study of the effects of d-amphetamine on single neurons in the brain stem of rats, found that the amphetamine mimicked the excitatory and inhibitory actions of norepinephrine. They further found that the d-amphetamine did not have actions on neurons that are unaffected by norepinephrine. These results suggest that the alerting effects of amphetamine are due to the release of norepinephrine from presynaptic sites in the brain stem reticular formation.

Further support for the involvement of the reticular formation is given by the failure of amphetamine to cause behavioral or EEG arousal in animals with a *cerveau isolé* preparation (Bradley and Elkes, 1957) (transection at the level of the colliculi) that interrupts pathways from the midbrain to the cortex.

In lesion studies in which most of the mesencephalic reticular formation was destroyed, Killam (1962) found that amphetamine failed to cause EEG arousal. These experiments suggest that the behavioral and EEG arousal caused by amphetamine is directly mediated by action on the brain stem reticular formation.

Biochemical Effects

The current view concerning the biochemical basis for the central action of amphetamine is that it causes the release of newly synthesized catecholamines, both norepinephrine and dopamine, at the presynaptic terminal. In addition, amphetamine blocks the reuptake of the transmitter and hence interferes with its inactivation. There is also a possibility that amphetamine has a direct effect on the postsynaptic receptors, mimicking the action of the catecholamines.

It is believed that the central stimulating properties are primarily due to the effects of amphetamine on the noradrenergic system, whereas the stereotyped behaviors seen with chronic and acute use of the drug in animals and man (see section on chronic use) are due to effects on dopaminergic neurons (see Snyder et al., 1974).

Amphetamine is a competitive inhibitor of monoamine oxidase (MAO). However, it is not believed that this inhibition plays a major role in the central stimulating effects of amphetamine.

Other Pharmacologic Actions

There have been reports of occasional increases in blood-sugar levels after amphetamine use, but the more general finding is that such changes do not occur. With chronic use there may appear in some patients a transitory rise in erythrocytes and in polymorphonuclear leukocytes. These changes do not seem to be significant, and levels return to normal when administration of the drug is discontinued. Kidney function seems unaffected after either large, single doses or chronic administration (Leake, 1958).

Toxicity

Acute toxic effects of amphetamine usually consist of a greater magnitude of its usual pharmacologic actions. Except in highly susceptible people, toxic actions are usually the result of excessive doses. An overdose results in restlessness, tremor, hyperactive reflexes, irritability, insomnia, confusion, anxiety, and occasionally hallucinations and delirium. Cardiovascular effects include dangerous increases in blood pressure (systolic and diastolic), arrhythmias, and angina; occasional hypotension, dry mouth, nausea, vomiting, and diarrhea accompanied by abdominal cramps have been reported. Fatal doses usually result in convulsions and coma. The main pathologic findings in deaths due to overdose of amphetamines are cerebral hemorrhages. Most people can easily tolerate doses of d-amphetamine up to 15 mg, although hypersensitivities have been reported with doses as low as 2 mg. Doses above 20 mg may cause marked hypertensive effects in some subjects.

Chronic Effects

Chronic use of the amphetamines and related compounds can cause a psychoticlike state in man that is very similar in its manifestations to acute paranoid schizophrenia. This drug-induced psychosis is quite different from the toxic delirium that may be seen after only one or two large doses of amphetamine (Snyder et al., 1974). For example, unlike one experiencing a toxic psychosis, the chronic user will still be oriented with regard to time, place, and person. Because of the similarity of the amphetamine psychosis to ideopathic paranoid psychosis, the drug-induced state has been proposed as an experimental model for schizophrenia. The amphetamine psychosis, in contrast to the amphetamine delirium, usually appears in subjects who have gradually increased their dosage over several months. However, the time to onset of the psychosis depends on the frequency of dosing, the amount of drug in each dose, and individual sensitivity. Griffith et al. (1972) gave small, frequent oral doses of d-amphetamine to normal volunteer subjects. Within five days, eight of the nine subjects manifested symptoms of paranoid psychosis. The symptoms abated, usually within 24 to 36 hrs, after the drug was discontinued. As is generally true in paranoid schizophrenia, the hallucinations occurring during the amphetamine-induced state are predominantly auditory. In addition to the presence of auditory hallucinations, the amphetamine psychosis is characterized by the presence of unreasonable and excessive fearfulness and suspiciousness. Specific ideas of reference develop.

Another characteristic of chronic amphetamine abuse is the appearance of compulsive stereotyped behavior, often preceding the onset of the psychotic episode. The apparently purposeless behavior may consist of, for example, repetitive examination of contents of a handbag, continual counting and rearrangement of objects, and so on. Accompanying the stereotyped behavior may be grinding of the teeth (bruxism), licking of the lips, and shifting of the eyes from side to side. Also characteristic of chronic stimulant overdose is a delusion of formication (ants crawling over one's body). The habitual abuser may show specific physical evidence of the drug-induced phenomena. For example, the teeth may be flattened from chronic bruxism, or the skin may show scarring as a result of continual attempts to pick out the perceived subcutaneous parasites.

During the active paranoid stage, the individual often does not maintain insight into the cause of his condition. The chronic user at this time may be quite hostile and aggressive, a danger to self and others. If the concept of a "drug-crazed dope fiend" has any applicability, it is probably here.

It is of interest that Janowsky, El-Yousef, and Davis (1972) and Davis and Janowsky (1973) found that small amounts of intravenous amphetamine or methylphenidate (a CNS stimulant with actions similar to those of amphetamine) will cause an exacerbation of the schizophrenic symptoms in acute schizophrenic patients.

This exacerbation of symptoms after d-amphetamine was given to schizophrenic patients was not found in a study by Kornetsky, reported in Kornetsky and Mirsky (1966), nor in a study by Modell and Hussar (1963). In the Kornetsky study the patients showed marked resistance to the insomnia-producing effects, and in the Modell and Hussar study there was resistance to the anorectic as well as the insomnia-producing effects of d-amphetamine. In both of these studies the dose of d-amphetamine was significant. Kornetsky used a single 20-mg dose given at 8:00 p.m. for each of seven days, whereas Modell gave a total daily dose of 20 mg in the form of four doses per day, 5 mg each, for 16 weeks.

The most likely explanation for the differences in results between the studies in which d-amphetamine caused exacerbation of schizophrenic symptoms and those in which it did not was that in the former, patients were *acute* schizophrenics, whereas in the latter they were *chronic* schizophrenics.

In an early paper on abuse of amphetamines, Knapp (1952) gives seven detailed case histories of their abuse. He pointed out in 1952 that in spite of the availability of amphetamine for the preceding 15 years, cases of unequivocal abuse were rare. Certainly something in our culture has changed, for there are many cases of marked abuse reported in recent years. The relatively mild effects reported by Knapp are in sharp opposition to the picture today.

In a report of amphetamine use in the San Francisco Bay area, Kramer (1967) indicated that there was a characteristic pattern of behavior in amphetamine abuse. When oral doses reached 150 to 250 mg per day, there was usually a switch to intravenous use. The early intravenous dose levels were usually 20 to 40 mg per dose taken three or four times per day. Doses would then be gradually increased, even in the face of marked toxic symptoms: confusion, paranoid ideas, and hallucinations.

Tolerance and Physical Dependence

Tolerance to the central stimulating effects of amphetamine develops. Chronic users often increase their dosage levels to obtain the marked stimulating and mood-elevating effects, although tolerance to all of the toxic effects does not develop, and the manifestations of chronic use can be quite severe. Tolerance to anorectic effects develops fairly rapidly. Whether the amphetamines produce real physical dependence is not clear. Upon abrupt termination after chronic use, depression is often seen accompanied by fatigue and lassitude, and there is evidence of EEG changes. Despite these signs, discontinuation does not cause the type of major physiologic and biochemical disruption that would warrant a gradual reduction of the drug in withdrawing a patient (Jaffe, 1965).

Therapeutic Use

The amphetamines are used primarily for their central nervous system effects. Other sympathomimetic drugs are usually used for causing the peripheral effects. Since d-amphetamine or methamphetamine have greater central nervous system potency with less peripheral effects than the racemic form, they are generally preferred for producing central nervous system effects. The amphetamines are used in the treatment of obesity, depressive states, fatigue, narcolepsy, and behavior disorders in children. They are used as adjunct therapy in the treatment of epilepsy and have been used in relieving the rigidity seen in parkinsonism (Innes and Nickerson, 1975), although they seem to have little effect on the tremor. The mechanism of action in these latter states has not been elucidated. (See Chapter 13 for further discussion of amphetamine in the treatment of the hyperkinetic child).

SUMMARY

In recent years the amphetamines have acquired a negative image. This has been due to their overuse in the treatment of both obesity, and hyperkinesis in children as well as their popularity as "turn on" drugs by many of the nation's young. There is pressure by some groups to remove the amphetamines from legitimate medical use. Sweden, primarily because of the abuse problem in that country, has removed them from the market. Despite the negative aspects of the amphetamines, it would be unfortunate if we were to follow Sweden's lead. Most of the compounds that would be substituted for the amphetamines cause many of the same problems or even present new problems of toxicity. Illegal users will, as in Sweden, find some other drug to use or will still manage to find available supplies from illegitimate sources. Amphetamines, like all drugs, must be used with care. Amphetamines are not unique in their ability to cause marked toxic effects, and there is evidence that they do have a legitimate place in the therapeutic bag of the physician.

REFERENCES

Alles, G. A. The comparative physiological actions of d,l-beta-phenylisopropylamines. *Journal of Pharmacology and Experimental Therapeutics*, **47**, 1933, 339–354.

Boakes, R. J., Bradley, P. B., and Candy, J. M. A neuronal basis for the alerting action of (+)-amphetamine. *British Journal of Pharmacology*, **45**, 1972, 391–403.

Bradley, P. B., and Elkes, J. The effects of some drugs on the electrical activity of the brain. *Brain*, **80**, 1957, 77–117.

Bradley, P. B. and Key, B. J. The effect of drugs on the arousal responses produced by electrical stimulation of the reticular formation of the brain. *Electroencephalography and Clinical Neurophysiology*, **10**, 1958, 97–110.

Davis, J. M. and Janowsky, D. S. Amphetamine and methylphenidate psychosis. In E. Usdin and S. H. Snyder (Eds.) *Frontiers in Catecholamine Research*. New York, Pergamon, 1973, pp. 977–981.

Griffith, J. D., Cavanaugh, J., Held, J., and Oates, J. A. Dextroamphetamine; Evaluation of psychotomimetic properties in man. *Archives of General Psychiatry*, **26**, 1972, 97–100.

Innes, I. R. and Nickerson, M. Norepinephrine, epinephrine, and the sympathomimetic amines. In L. S. Goodman and A. Gilman (Eds.) *The Pharmacological Basis of Therapeutics*. New York, Macmillan, 1975, pp. 477–520.

Jaffee, J. H. Drug addiction and drug abuse. In L. S. Goodman and A. Gilman (Eds.) *The Pharmacological Basis of Therapeutics*. New York, Macmillan, 1965, pp. 285–311.

Janowsky, D. S., El-Yousef, M. K., and Davis, J. M. The elicitation of psychotic symptomatology by methylphenidate. *Comprehensive Psychiatry*, **13**, 1972, 83.

Killam, E. K. Drug-action on the brain stem reticular formation. *Pharmacological Reviews*, **14**, 1962, 175–223.

Knapp, P. H. Amphetamine and addiction. *Journal of Nervous and Mental Disease*, **115**, 1952, 406–432.

Kornetsky, C. Effects of meprobamate, phenobarbital and dextroamphetamine on reaction time and learning in man. *Journal of Pharmacology and Experimental Therapeutics*, **123**, 1958, 216–219.

Kornetsky, C. and Mirsky, A. F. On certain psychopharmacological and physiological differences between schizophrenic and normal persons. *Psychopharmacologia Berlin*, **8**, 1966, 309–318.

Kornetsky, C., Mirsky, A. F., Kessler, E., and Dorf, J. The effects of dextro-amphetamine on behavioral deficits produced by sleep loss in humans. *Journal of Pharmacology and Experimental Therapeutics*, **127**, 1959, 46–50.

Kramer, J. C., Fishman, V. S., and Littlefield, D. C. Amphetamine abuse: Pattern and effects of high doses taken intravenously. *Journal of the American Medical Association*, **201**, 1967, 305–309.

Laties, V. G. and **Weiss, B.** Performance enhancement by the amphetamines: A new approach. In H. Brill, J. O. Cole, P. Deniker, H. Hippius, and P. B. Bradley (Eds.) *Proceedings Fifth International Congress of Neuropsychopharmacology.* Amsterdam, Excerpta Medica Foundation, 1967, pp. 800-808.

Leake, C. D. *The Amphetamines.* Springfield, Illinois, Charles C Thomas, 1958.

Levy, B. and **Ahlquist, R. P.** Adrenergic drugs. In J. R. DiPalma (Ed.) *Drills Pharmacology in Medicine.* New York, McGraw-Hill, 1965, pp. 463-501.

Marrazzi, A. S. and **Hart, E. R.** Comparison of the effects on evoked cortical synaptic response of mescaline, amphetamine and adrenalin. *Electroencephalography and Clinical Neurophysiology,* **5,** 1953, 317-318.

Modell, W. and **Hussar, A. E.** Failure of dextroamphetamine sulfate to influence eating and sleeping patterns in obese schizophrenic patients. *Journal of the American Medical Association,* **193,** 1963, 95-98.

Nathanson, M. H. The central action of the beta-aminopropyl-benzene (benzedrine): Clinical observations. *Journal of The American Medical Association,* **108,** 1939, 528-531.

Prinzmetal, M. and **Bloomberg, W.** The use of benzedrine for the treatment of narcolepsy. *Journal of the American Medical Association,* **105,** 1935, 265-266.

Smith, G. M. and **Beecher, H. K.** Amphetamine sulfate and athletic performance. I. Objective effects. *Journal of the American Medical Association,* **170,** 1959, 542-557.

Smith, G. M. and **Beecher, H. K.** Amphetamine, secobarbital and athletic performance. II. Subjective evaluation of performance mood and physical states. *Journal of the American Medical Association,* **172,** 1960, 1502-1514.

Snyder, S. H., Banerjee, S. P., Yamamura, H. I., and **Greenberg, D.** Drugs, neurotransmitters and schizophrenia. *Science,* **184,** 1974, 1243-1253.

Stowe, F. R., Jr., and **Miller, A. T., Jr.** The effects of amphetamine on food intake in rats with hypothalamic hyperphagia. *Experentia,* **13,** 1957, 114-115.

Weiss, B. and **Laties, V. G.** Enhancement of human performance by caffeine and the amphetamines. *Pharmacological Reviews,* **14,** 1962, 1-36.

11 ANTIEPILEPTIC DRUGS

Epilepsy is a term used to identify a variety of chronic convulsive disorders that have in common brief episodes of seizures that are associated with loss or alteration of consciousness. These seizures are usually accompanied by abnormal electroencephalographic (EEG) patterns. The seizures are usually, but not always, characterized by rapidly alternating muscular contraction and relaxation (convulsion). The word "epilepsy" is derived from the Greek word for "seizure." Other names have been given to this disease, for example, the "falling disease" or "fits."

The primary function of an antiepileptic drug is to eliminate or reduce seizure or convulsive activity. Not all seizures seen in the various forms of epilepsy are convulsive in nature. Although many drugs can be classified as anticonvulsants, not all anticonvulsants are good antiepileptic drugs. Also, the reverse of this holds true; many good antiepileptic drugs are not good anticonvulsants. Many of the antiepileptic drugs are slow acting and require prolonged use to be effective and thus are not useful in the treatment of acute seizures caused by trauma, elevated body temperature, or toxic materials.

EPILEPSY

Epilepsy and the therapies used to treat the disease have an interesting history. Because of the bizarre manifestations of the disease plus the unpredictability of onset of attacks, epilepsy lent itself to the superstitions and dogma of every historical period. Many famous individuals suffered from epilepsy; these include Julius Caesar, Mohammed, Napoleon, Lord Byron, Guy de Maupassant, and Van Gogh. Vivid descriptions of the disease have appeared frequently in literature. In 95 B.C. the following word picture of a major seizure was given by Lucretius:

> Now rigid, now convulsed, his laboring lungs
> Heave quick, and quivers each exhausted limb,
> Spread through the frame, so deep and dire disease

> Perturbs his spirit; as the briny main
> Foams through each wave beneath the tempest's ire
> But when, at length, the morbid cause declines,
> And the fermenting humors from the heart
> Flow back—with staggering foot the man first treads
> Led gradually on to intellect and strength.

The cause of epilepsy has been ascribed at times to divine visitations and at other times to evil spirits. Along with many theories as to the cause of epilepsy, there have been many "therapeutic" measures tried in the treatment of this malady.

Although the true incidence of this disease is not known, it is believed that there are approximately four million sufferers in the United States (Epilepsy Foundation of America, 1974). During World War II approximately 6 out of every 1000 draftees for the armed forces were diagnosed as epileptic. It is equally prevalent among males and females, and the incidence of the disease is higher among children than among adults.

Hughlings Jackson applied the term "epilepsies" to a variety of different forms of recurring seizures. Stimulated by Jackson, clinicians have classified a dozen or so seizures, each composed of a number of unitary symptoms. Thus such terms as grand mal, petit mal, akinetic, or psychic variant were given to various types of seizure patterns. An attempt at a rational classification based on the anatomy of the brain and the cerebral localization of the cause of the seizure was made by Penfield and Jasper (1954).

Penfield and Jasper divided the epilepsies into three general classes: focal cerebral seizures, centrencephalic seizures, and cerebral seizures. This classification was based on the origin of the epileptic discharge.

TABLE 1. SEIZURE CLASSIFICATION

Type of seizure	Origin of epileptic discharge
1. Focal cerebral seizures (symptomatic seizures)	Hemispherical gray matter, usually cerebral cortex
2. Centrencephalic seizures "highest level" seizures, includes most cases which have been called essential or idiopathic	Central integrating system of higher brain stem
3. Cerebral seizures (unlocalized) not yet classified	Undiscovered or extracerebral cause

After Penfield and Jasper, 1954.

Focal Cerebral Seizures (Focal Epilepsy)

In focal epilepsy the attack begins with abnormal neural discharge at the site of a demonstrable abnormal focus ("lesion") within the CNS. The classic Jacksonian seizure is of this type. Jacksonian seizures are characterized by local movements of some part of the body. In a "Jacksonian March" there is a spread of movement from one part of the body to another.

Psychomotor Epilepsy (Temporal Lobe Epilepsy). This type of epilepsy is characterized by a lapse of consciousness or confused behavior that often begins with head turning, lip smacking, swallowing, and salivation. Often, there will be an automatic continuation, or onset, of apparently purposeful behavior, although the individual may have no recall of the events that transpired. In psychomotor automatism there may be fumbling by the patient with his own person or clothing, and the behavior may continue for a considerable period of time.

Centrencephalic Seizures

Patients classified under this heading are thought to have seizures caused by a neural discharge that originates in the central integrating system of the brain stem. Since this system has connections to both cerebral hemispheres, the EEG abnormalities appear simultaneously over both hemispheres. A number of seizure types (believed by some to be of centrencephalic origin) have been identified.

Petit Mal. This is a minor type of seizure, although its frequency may be quite high. It is characterized by brief periods of loss of consciousness. These periods may be of such a short duration that unless one knows the patient, the "lapses" or "absences" may go unnoticed. If there is no clonic movement such as jerking of the musculature or eyelid blinking, it is called a *pure petit mal absence*. If clonic movements are present, it is sometimes referred to as *myoclonic petit mal*. In petit mal, the EEG during seizure is characterized by a high voltage, bilaterally symmetrical, synchronous, 3-per-second spike-and-wave pattern. Some petit mal seizures are characterized by the continuation, in an automatic fashion, of some ongoing activity. This is referred to as *petit mal automatism*.

Grand Mal. A grand mal seizure is characterized by a major symmetrical convulsion. Usually, there is a maximal tonic spasm (extensor muscles dominating the flexor muscles) followed by synchronous clonic jerking. After the seizure there is a postseizure depression in which the patient is often confused and disoriented. This has been called *postictal automatism* or *postictal twilight state*. The term grand mal has been applied to all types of major seizures; however, Penfield and Jasper believe that the term should be restricted to the major convulsive attacks of centrencephalic origin. However, more than half of all focal seizures are of a grand mal type so that the mere presence of a grand mal seizure should not preclude a search for a focal origin (Ervin, 1967, p. 799). The grand mal seizures of centrencephalic origin differ from seizures of focal origin only in the symmetry of onset.

Cerebral Seizures

This is a catchall classification. All convulsive attacks in which the site of neural discharge cannot be determined are put in this classification. The seizure may be the result of some diffuse abnormality of the brain or it may be the result of some general systemic abnormality, for example, hypoglycemia.

The Penfield and Jasper classification, although tied to the origin of the epileptic discharge in the brain, is not useful as a predictor of response to chemotherapeutic agents. Millichap (1972) states that classification of epilepsies on the basis of the origin of the seizure discharge is misleading from a chemotherapeutic standpoint. Millichap suggests that, considering our present-day knowledge of the mechanism of seizures and response to drugs, it would be better to use a classification of the epilepsies that is based on the clinical pattern of the seizure and the electroencephalographic correlates (see Table 2).

TABLE 2. SPECIFICITY OF ANTIEPILEPTIC DRUGS CORRELATED WITH SEIZURE PATTERNS, ELECTROENCEPHALOGRAPHIC ABNORMALITIES, AND AGE

Age period	Seizure patterns	Electroencephalographic correlates	Most specific therapies
Young children	minor myoclonic and akinetic	polyspike-and-wave 2/sec spike-and-wave	diazepam, primidone
Older children	petit mal	3/sec spike-and-wave	ethosuximide, trimethadione
Adolescents	grand mal and focal motor	spikes, spike-and-wave sharp waves	phenobarbital, diphenylhydantoin, primidone
Adults	psychomotor	temporal lobe spikes sharp waves	primidone, diphenylhydantoin, methsuximide

Abstracted from Millichap, 1972, p. 98.

PHARMACOTHERAPY

The obvious purpose of drug therapy in the epileptic patient is the suppression of seizure activity without causing toxic side effects. To carry out this aim Coatsworth and Penry (1972) suggest the following general principles:

1. A single drug should be used initially and the dosage gradually increased until either drug toxicity or seizure control occurs. If toxicity occurs, the drug is reduced to the previous lower dose. Addition of a second and rarely, a third drug in the same manner may be necessary if one drug fails to give control.
2. Any change in antiepileptic therapy should be done gradually and the effectiveness of the change judged over a long period of time.
3. Medications should not be stopped without medical advice and should be taken regularly, every day, in unvarying dosages.
4. The patient's understanding and acceptance of his disorder often improves previously poor results with medication.
5. Regular visits to the clinic or physician, with an appropriate "seizure calendar," are essential for optimal management.

It is believed that if the above regimen is followed with "patience and persistence," 70 to 80% of all epileptics can have their seizures controlled.

THE DRUGS

Historically, the first successful treatment of epilepsy was with *bromides* in 1857. At the present time bromides are rarely used in the therapy of convulsive disorders. The decrease in their use has been because of their potent sedative and hypnotic actions and other toxic side effects. The next successful drug for the treatment of convulsive disorders was phenobarbital, a long-acting barbiturate.

Barbiturates

The first report of the successful use of phenobarbital in the treatment of epilepsy was in 1912. Today phenobarbital is still considered one of the safest and most effective drugs for the control of grand mal seizures. The most commonly used barbiturates as well as other antiepileptic drugs are listed in Table 3. The most common side effect of phenobarbital in the treatment of seizure disorders is sedation. This effect can be ameliorated by the use of amphetamine or caffeine without any apparent loss of anticonvulsant activity. Slurred speech, nystagmus, and ataxia are rarely seen with the usual therapeutic dose. Doses above the usual therapeutic dose or in the highly sensitive individual may cause the above untoward reactions. Occasionally, a scarlatiniform rash (scarlet

TABLE 3. PRIMARY ANTIEPILEPTIC DRUGS

Class	Indications	Generic name	Trade name
Hydantoinates	Generalized convulsive seizures, all forms of partial seizures	diphenylhydantoin mephenytoin ethotoin	Dilantin Mesantoin Peganone
Barbiturates, Desoxybarbiturate	Generalized convulsive seizures, all forms of partial seizures	phenobarbital mephobarbital metharbital primidone	Luminal Mebaral Gemonil Mysoline
Oxazolidinediones	Generalized nonconvulsive seizures (absences)	trimethadione paramethadione	Tridione Paradione
Succinimides	Generalized nonconvulsive seizures (absences)	phensuximide methsuximide ethosuximide	Milontin Celontin Zarontin

Abstracted from Coatsworth & Penry, 1972, p. 90.

colored rash, similar to that seen with scarlet fever) is observed in some patients, but exfoliative (falling off in scales) dermatitis, a serious complication, is very rare. Patients suffering from acne may have some exacerbation of their skin disorder.

Phenobarbital is most effective in treating grand mal seizures. It is not the drug of choice in other forms of epilepsy and may even increase the frequency of psychomotor automatisms or petit mal seizures.

Patients receiving phenobarbital for long periods of time should not be abruptly withdrawn from this medication because of the possibility that physical dependence may have developed. This by itself could lead to seizure activity and psychotic behavior. The withdrawal syndrome as well as the general pharmacology of the barbiturates is discussed in Chapter 8.

The barbiturates are usually administered by the oral route, although the parenteral route has been used for the immediate relief of *status epilepticus,* a continuous state of convulsive activity.

Two other long-acting barbiturates have been used for the treatment of epilepsy. These are *mephobarbital* and *metharbital.*

Diphenylhydantoin (Phenytoin, DPH)

The first published report of the clinical efficacy of DPH was in 1938 by Merritt and Putnam. DPH is considered the drug of choice in most types of epilepsy with the exception of the petit mal form.

At usual clinical doses DPH has little sedative effect; at doses above the usual clinical dose it may cause central stimulation. Unlike the barbiturates it will not counteract seizures caused by such convulsant drugs as pentylenetetrazol, strychnine, or picrotoxin.

Toxic Effects. Although most patients tolerate the drug very well, an accidental overdose or cumulative overdosing can cause a number of CNS disturbances. These CNS effects will also be seen in the hypersensitive patient. Among the symptoms seen are ataxia, nystagmus, vertigo, blurring of vision, and headache. Overdosing can also cause convulsive seizures. There may be hyperactivity, hallucinations, and confusion. Despite the apparent stimulating effects of overdosage, occasionally one sees drowsiness and slurred speech. There may be loss of appetite, nausea and vomiting, and urinary incontinence.

Hyperplasia (abnormal increase in number of normal cells) of the gums occurs in about 20 percent of patients maintained on DPH. Skin eruption is found in about 5 percent of patients on DPH. Most common is a morbilliform (measleslike) rash. This usually appears about a week after the onset of therapy. Exfoliative (falling off in scales) or hemorrhagic (bleeding) dermatitis is rare. Hirsutism is a common side effect.

Absorption. DPH is readily absorbed from the gastrointestinal tract; however, some of the gastric discomfort reported with the use of DPH is due to its alkalinity. Although it is usually given by the oral route, DPH is available in injectable form for parenteral administration.

Combined with Other Drugs. DPH is often given in combination with phenobarbital in cases where marked side effects to DPH are observed. Since phenobarbital and DPH have different constellations of side effects, this allows a lower dose of each to be used with a concomitant reduction in the severity of side effects.

Ethotoin and Mephenytoin. In addition to DPH, two other hydantoins are used in the clinical control of epilepsy. These are ethotoin and mephenytoin. Ethotoin is usually used as an adjunct to other anticonvulsants. Mephenytoin has been reported to be superior to DPH in the control of grand mal seizures and also to cause fewer minor side effects. There is less gum hypertrophy, ataxia, gastric distress, and hirsutism seen with mephenytoin than with DPH. Also, there is less sedation than is seen with phenobarbital. However, mephenytoin can cause more serious side effects. Death from aplastic anemia has been reported in patients receiving mephenytoin.

Trimethadione

Trimethadione is one of a class of anticonvulsants (*oxazolidinediones*) that has proved to be effective in the treatment of the petit mal patient. It was first used in the mid 1940s. The only other oxazolidinedione in current usage is paramethadione.

Toxicity. A variety of toxic reactions that involve most organ systems have been associated with the use of the oxazolidinediones. Commonly reported by patients is a visual disturbance. This visual disturbance (hemeralopia) is brought on by exposure to bright light and results in a loss of visual acuity. Both black and white as well as color vision is affected. Visual acuity with low illumination is not affected. No external or ophthalmoscopic changes can be detected in patients reporting these effects. The phenomenon is believed to be due to alterations in the retina. Children seem less susceptible than adults to this hemeralopia. Trimethadione will cause sedation in patients, and there have been reports that it can possibly cause an exacerbation of grand mal seizures.

Dermatologic side effects of trimethadione are not uncommon, and they usually occur early in the course of therapy. They are more frequently seen in children under the age of 10. Adverse hematologic effects are considered to be the most troublesome toxic reaction of trimethadione. Moderate neutropenia (decrease in the number of neutrophilic leucocytes in the blood) is not uncommon; however, more severe blood changes have been reported including aplastic anemia. Nephrotic symptoms and hepatitis have been reported. Patients who receive the oxazolidinediones should be carefully followed, especially early in therapy. For further discussion of the toxicity of the oxazolidinediones, the reader is referred to Gallagher (1972).

Ethosuximide

The drug that is most effective in the treatment of petit mal seizures is ethosuximide. At the present time it is considered the drug of choice in the treatment of petit mal seizures by many physicians (Buchanan, 1972).

Toxic Effects. Ethosuximide appears to be a relatively safe antiepileptic drug. Despite the relatively low toxicity compared to the oxazolidinediones, many side effects have been observed. These include gastrointestinal difficulties and CNS symptoms.

The gastrointestinal symptoms include reports of gastric distress, nausea and vomiting, and anorexia. The CNS effects include headache, fatigue, dizziness, and euphoria. These side effects are directly dose related. Other more serious effects have been reported. Among these have been hematological disorders, from relatively minor to severe blood dyscrasias.

Recently, warnings of teratogenicity of the antiepileptic drugs have appeared. Abbott Laboratories, in their package insert for trimethadione (Tridione®) and paramethadione (Paradione®), states:

Warnings: Usage in pregnancy—recent reports strongly suggest an association between the use of anticonvulsant drugs by women with epilepsy and an elevated incidence of birth defects in children born to these women. Data are more extensive with respect to diphenylhydantoin and phenobarbital than with other anticonvulsant drugs, but these are also the most commonly prescribed anticonvulsants. Other reports indicate a possible similar association with the use of other anticonvulsant drugs including Tridione and Paradione. The physician should weigh these considerations in treatment and counseling epileptic women of childbearing potential.

Other Antiepileptic Drugs

In addition to the drugs reviewed, there are a number of additional compounds that are used for the treatment of epilepsy. They are usually used when patients are refractory to the usual drugs used in treatment.

Primidone This drug is a congener of phenobarbital. At onset of therapy with primidone a number of side effects are seen. These are usually not dangerous, but they are unpleasant. They include drowsiness, ataxia, nausea, as well as a number of minor complaints. With continued use these effects tend to recede. Primidone has proven to be effective in cases of grand mal that are refractory to other medications. It is also effective in treating psychomotor epilepsy.

Benzodiazepines Although this class of compounds is usually reserved for the treatment of anxiety (see Chapter 6), they have been used with some success in the treatment of myoclonic spasms in children. With intravenous administration, the benzodiazepines are effective in controlling *status epilecticus*. The drugs of this class that have been useful are *chlordiazepoxide, diazepam, nitrazepam,* and *oxazepam*. For a detailed discussion of the use of the benzodiazepines in the treatment of convulsive disorders, the reader is referred to Mattson (1972).

SUMMARY

The classification of epilepsy proposed by Penfield and Jasper and discussed in the first part of this chapter was an attempt by those workers to provide a rational organization of the seizure disorders that was based on suspected etiology. The difficulty that confronts the clinician is that this classification does not completely correspond to the classification based on the clinical response of the diseases to the various drugs. As an example, the Penfield and Jasper classification groups petit mal and grand mal seizures together as manifestations of centrencephalic epilepsy. Although they both may be of centrencephalic origin, the nature of the neural discharge is different, and the drugs of choice for petit mal are quite different than those for grand mal. Penfield and Jasper as well as others do point out that there are grand mal seizures of focal, cortical origin that are indistinguishable from grand mal seizures of centrencephalic origin, except that the start of the "cortical" seizure is not symmetrical.

Regardless of the assumed site of origin of the seizures, grand mal convulsions do respond to the same antiepileptic drugs.

The fact that different types of seizures respond to different drugs suggests that in some way, no matter the etiology, those drugs that work do so by suppressing abnormal, excessive neural discharge.

There seems to be general agreement concerning which drugs are most beneficial in the treatment of the various types of seizure activity. Millichap (1972, p. 97) believes that the most efficacious treatment can be determined on the basis of the clinical patterns and their EEG correlates, regardless of the proposed etiology. The clinician, using a detailed description of his patient's seizures pattern as his major guideline, will manipulate drug and dose in a manner that will give the best therapeutic response with a minimum of side effects.

The reader is directed to Woodbury and Fingl (1975) for a discussion of the pharmacology and clinical use of the antiepileptic drugs. More detailed discussion will be found in the book, *Antiepileptic Drugs,* edited by Woodbury, Penry, and Schmidt (1972).

REFERENCES

Buchanan, R. A. Ethosuximide: Toxicity. In D. M. Woodbury, J. K. Penry, and R. P. Schmidt (Eds.) *Antiepileptic Drugs.* New York, Raven, 1972, pp. 449–454.

Coatsworth, J. J. and **Penry, J. K.** Clinical efficacy and use. In D. M. Woodbury, J. K. Penry, and R. P. Schmidt (Eds.) *Antiepileptic Drugs.* New York, Raven, 1972, pp. 87–96.

Epilepsy Foundation of America. *Facts and Figures on the Epilepsies,* 1974.

Ervin, R. Brain disorders. IV. Associated with convulsions (epilepsy). In A. M. Freedman and H. I. Kaplan (Eds.) *Comprehensive Textbook of Psychiatry.* Baltimore, Williams and Wilkins, 1967, pp. 795–816.

Gallagher, B. B. Trimethadione and other oxazolidinediones: Toxicity. In D. M. Woodbury, J. K. Penry, and R. P. Schmidt (Eds.) *Antiepileptic Drugs.* New York, Raven, 1972, pp. 409–411.

Mattson, R. H. The benzodiazepines. In D. M. Woodbury, J. K. Penry, and R. P. Schmidt (Eds.) *Antiepileptic Drugs.* New York, Raven, 1972, pp. 497–518.

Merritt, H. H. and **Putnam, T. J.** Sodium diphenylhydantoinate in the treatment of convulsive disorders. *The Journal of the American Medical Association,* 111, 1938, 1068–1073.

Millichap, J. G. Clinical efficacy and use. In D. M. Woodbury, J. K. Penry, and R. P. Schmidt (Eds.) *Antiepileptic Drugs.* New York, Raven, 1972, pp. 97–101.

Penfield, W. and **Jasper, H.** *Epilepsy and the Functional Anatomy of the Human Brain.* Boston, Little, Brown, 1954.

Woodbury, D. M. and **Fingl, E.** Drugs effective in therapy of the epilepsies. In L. S. Goodman and A. Gilman (Eds.) *The Pharmacological Basis of Therapeutics.* (5th ed.). New York, Macmillan, 1975, pp. 201–226.

Woodbury, D. M., Penry, J. K., and **Schmidt, R. P.** *Antiepileptic Drugs.* New York, Raven, 1972.

12 THE NONMEDICAL USE OF DRUGS

The term "nonmedical use of drugs" was used by the Canadian Commission Report (1971) as an alternative to terms such as "illicit drugs," "drug abuse," or "drug addiction." Unfortunately, there is no single term that correctly defines all drug use. Many drugs are taken for legitimate medical reasons, but because of inappropriate prescribing by a physician, many patients become physically and psychologically dependent on the prescribed drugs.

Many of the drugs are taken simply for the pleasure of the effect they produce. These are not necessarily illicit drugs nor do they necessarily cause drug addiction nor do people necessarily abuse these drugs. There are those who state that no drug should be taken for pleasure, yet our society accepts the use of alcohol with all the intrinsic dangers that its use engenders. At the same time our society does not accept the use of the narcotic analgesics for pleasure, despite the fact that the pharmacological actions and the withdrawal syndrome for the narcotic analgesics are much less dangerous to life than the potential pharmacological actions and the withdrawal syndrome of alcohol. I realize that there are those who will disagree with the above statement. It is true that most people who use alcohol never become physically dependent on the drug, whereas this may not be the case with opiates. However, the withdrawal syndrome caused by chronic alcohol use is clearly more dangerous to life than the withdrawal syndrome caused by chronic opiate use.

Most drugs are abused because in some way they produce some pleasurable effect. In a society strongly imbued with the Judeo-Christian ethic, the use of a substance that only gives pleasure is somewhat antithetical to this ethic.

Despite the present attitudes toward drug use, man has indulged in the use of drugs to give him pleasure since at least the time of recorded history. Whether the use of drugs to alter mood is considered abuse depends greatly on the medical and social patterns within a given culture. Certainly, as mentioned, alcohol is an accepted drug in Western society, but in cultures whose ethic is based on the teachings of Mohammed, the use of alcohol is prohibited.

As discussed in previous chapters, all drugs have potential for misuse. There is a marked difference between the occasional marijuana smoker and the compulsive user of marijuana. Jaffe (1970, p. 276) notes that among the hazards in the use of a drug to alter mood and feeling is that for some people ". . . the effects produced by a drug, or the conditions associated with its use, are necessary to maintain an optimal state of well being." Wikler (1973b) points out that the World Health Organization (WHO) has stressed "psychic dependence" as a feature that is common to all types of drug dependence, namely:

". . . a particular state of mind that is termed *psychic dependence*. In this situation, there is a feeling of satisfaction and a psychic drive that require periodic or continuous administration of the drug to produce pleasure or avoid discomfort. Indeed, this mental state is the most powerful of all of the factors involved in chronic intoxication with psychotopic drugs, and with certain types of drugs it may be the only factor involved, even in the most intense craving and perpetuation of compulsive abuse . . . physical dependence is a powerful factor in reinforcing the influence of psychic dependence upon continuing drug use or relapse to drug use after attempted withdrawal."

The compulsive drug user's behavior shows a consistent preoccupation with the seeking and using of the drug. The form that this preoccupation with procurement and use of the drug takes depends very much on the particular drug and the attitude that society has concerning the drug. Some drugs are considered more illegal than other drugs. In addition, some drugs will cause marked physical dependence, whereas other drugs, of which there may be compulsive use, do not.

In the present chapter I discuss each of the drugs separately. However, in some cases I discuss more than one drug at a time since polypharmacy is often practiced by the user of illicit drugs.

OPIATES (NARCOTIC ANALGESICS)

When one thinks of the term "addiction," one conjures up the image of the opiate addict. At the present time this usually means addiction to heroin. The problem of addiction is often seen quite differently by different professional and lay groups. The following, although stressing stereotypes, has a rough ring of truth: To the pharmacologist it is looked at in terms of tolerance and physical dependence; to the psychiatrist it is looked at as a problem of personality maladjustment; to the sociologist it is looked at as a problem of social disorganization; to the law enforcement officer it is looked at as a problem of criminal behavior; to the lay press it is a continual inspiration for stories of human depravity; for the parent it is hopefully something that happens to others' children; to the drug user it runs the gambit from "what is all the fuss about" to a series of physical, personality, and social assaults; and to some members of minority groups it is seen as an attempt by the majority to enslave them.

Brecher (1972, p. 64) points out that earlier use of the term addiction was to describe bondage of one man to another, "... a serf addicted to a master." Shakespeare as well as others of the same period noted the similarity between the bondage of man to man and the bondage of man to alcoholic beverages, and thus they spoke of being addicted to alcohol. Brecher points out that "poets also spoke of men 'addicted to vice' and of young women 'addicted to virginity.'" (Clearly times have changed.) The original use of the term "addicted to," whether it meant to a drug or to virginity, meant to be "enslaved to." This original meaning of addiction was changed in the twentieth century when it was believed that any addict could simply stop taking the drug if he so wished. Society, in helping the addict and believing that it only took willingness to stop the use of drugs, added the incentive of imprisonment for those who did not stop their addiction.

History of Opiate Use

(For a most readable brief history of opiate use, the reader is referred to Brecher, 1972, pp. 3–63; for a more detailed history see *The American Disease* by Musto, 1973.)

Current attitudes toward opiate use are quite different from those held prior to the first part of the present century. Not only were there differences in attitudes but there were differences in the patterns of opiate use in the nineteenth century. As Brecher (1972, p. 3) points out, the United States could be described as a paradise for the opiate user during the nineteenth century. Many of the patent medicines of the period contained opium or morphine. These medicines were administered to infants to assuage the discomfort of teething and given to children and adults for the treatment of cough, diarrhea, or dysentery. Many were sold for the amelioration of pains associated with various "women's complaints." Opiates could be bought over-the-counter without prescriptions, and physicians were not adverse to the dispensing of opiates. Most of this use could be considered for medical purposes. Although the use was extensive, the opiates were probably the most effective remedy that the nineteenth-century physician had for the symptomatic relief of most diseases that afflicted man.

Nineteenth-century society did not consider the use of opiates a problem. Although opiates were used for pleasure, they were only used by relatively few or by people who were not part of the mainstream of Western culture—the Oriental opium smoker. The most well-known portrayal of opiate use of this period is found in Thomas DeQuincey's *Confessions of an English Opium-*

Eater. The "opium eaters" were drinkers of laudanum or other liquids made from opium. Although the nonmedical use of opiates was not illegal in either the United States or England, it was frowned upon. What is important is that despite the fact that it was not completely respectable to use opiates for pleasure, there were not the legal sanctions against its use. These sanctions were not imposed until the twentieth century.

Prior to the Civil War in the United States, the method of taking the opiate drugs, except for the opium smokers, was by means of various liquid preparations. The Civil War introduced the widespread use of the hypodermic syringe. This led a large number of men, who were given morphine by injection, to continue its use after the War. Although this postwar opiate use was frowned on, there was not the stigma attached that appeared later. Opiate use for nonmedical purposes was a vice, but the sanctions against it were no more stringent than for such behavior as dancing, smoking, gambling, or sexual promiscuity. As Brecher (p. 6) points out, "Wives did not divorce their addicted husbands, or husbands their addicted wives . . . addicts continued to participate fully in the life of the community." Thus in the nineteenth century there was not the rise of a deviant subculture that was seen after the laws against opiate use appeared in the twentieth century.

The acceptance of the opiate user in the nineteenth century did not carry over to the opium smoker. Legal sanctions against opium smoking appeared in the last half of the 1800s in the United States. San Francisco passed a city ordinance in 1875 that prohibited the smoking of opium.

Opium smoking was introduced in the United States by the Chinese who were brought to the Western hemisphere as laborers for the building of the railroads in western United States. Many of the Chinese moved to the cities, accepting low-paying jobs. In these cities they established opium smoking houses ("dens"). Just as many other immigrant groups who compete for jobs and who have social customs quite different from the majority, they became the objects of hostility and prejudice. The Chinese had the additional burden of racial differences as well as customs that were certainly more foreign to the people of the United States of that period than those of the European immigrant. They were additionally deprived, for only males were brought to the United States, and thus unlike most other immigrant groups, they were completely shut off from normal family life. Because of their race, they could not easily assimilate and develop a family life. Thus it is not surprising that they continued to use opium in this country. It is highly possible that the Chinese smoked opium not only to assuage the burden of their toil, but for the decrease in sexual drive caused by opium. The pharmacological actions of opium helped to make life more bearable.

Opium smoking did not take root in China until the last part of the eighteenth century. First Portugal, and later Britain, encouraged and participated in the highly profitable importing of opium to China. The Chinese government's attempt to enforce its edicts prohibiting the opium trade led to the Anglo-Chinese (Opium) War of 1839–1842 that was easily won by the British. One might even speculate that our present-day problem of opiate use would never have reached its present scale if the Chinese had won the Opium War.

Prior to the passage of the Harrison Narcotic Act in 1914, the majority of opiate users were women. Also, the average age of users was about 40 years. This is contrary to the present picture where only 13.6 percent of opiate users are over the age of 40 (Brecher, p. 18). Also of interest is the effect that these narcotic laws had on the socioeconomic status of users. The pre-narcotic law users were quite frequently from the upper and middle classes, whereas today narcotic use is more characteristic of lower socioeconomic levels, although during the 1960s there was an increase in the frequency of heroin use among the young middle class.

The Harrison Narcotic Act of 1914 resulted in interpretations that probably were not intended by framers of the law. The Harrison Act was passed as part of the United States' desire to carry out the intent and purpose of the Hague Convention of 1912. The Hague Convention was an attempt to call a halt to the unrestrained international traffic in narcotics. The passage of the Harrison Act was originally looked on as a ". . . simple routine slap at a moral evil, something like the Mann Act or the Antilottery Acts." (Musto, 1973, p. 65). The act was a tax law that on the surface was written to allow for the orderly marketing of opium, morphine, heroin, cocaine, as well as other drugs, in small quantities and only by a physician's prescription. The interpretation of the law that led to it becoming a prohibition law was found in the phrase "in the course of his professional practice." (Brecher, 1972, p. 49). This seemingly innocent clause was interpreted by law enforcement officers to mean that a physician could not prescribe narcotic drugs to a patient to maintain the patient's addiction. Addiction was not considered a disease; therefore, the addict is not sick and cannot be given narcotics by the physician. Many physicians were arrested under this prohibitory interpretation of the law. The net result was to prevent physicians from supplying opiates to the addict and to contribute to illegal trade of opiate drugs.

The original Harrison Act provided for penalties not to exceed 5-years imprisonment. Over the years the penalties have increased, both state and federal, to the extent that present laws include life imprisonment; the death penalty was added in some states during the 1950s. Despite this increase of the penalties, there is little evidence that they have had any impact on the illicit trade and use of the narcotic analgesics. Brecher (1972, p. 56) points out that "The chief effect of such penalties appeared to be as a kind of tranquilizer or opiate on public opinion, persuading the public that severe measures were at last being taken against addiction."

It is unlikely that any punitive state or federal law enacted to control the illicit use of narcotics will succeed in decreasing the use of these drugs. A recent law enacted in the state of New York that provides for mandatory long sentences for the sale of illicit drugs has, in the first nine months of its enforcement, had little effect on the use of drugs or the number of drug addicts. Chayet, writing in 1968 (p. 1), stated

It has become increasingly apparent that the law has failed to offer a constructive means of dealing with the many problems of drug abuse. Rather, the law seems only to have succeeded in alienating thousands of young people and in making a mockery out of an entire segment of our system of criminal justice. Arbitrary enforcement of harsh and often senseless legislation has resulted in the branding of thousands of young people as felons . . .

Chayet was writing not only about the laws to control narcotic use but the laws designed to control such drugs as amphetamines, LSD, and marihuana. Although the above quotation was written in 1968, Chayet's comment on the law holds true today, with the possible exception of some recent relaxation concerning marihuana laws.

Despite the fact that most authorities in the field of drug abuse are convinced that legal sanctions against drug use lead us nowhere (Freedman, 1973), public policy has generally taken the road toward stronger laws. Ward and Hutt (1972) concluded that our national policy has "bred" an illegal market that is sustained only by criminal activity.

Causes of Addiction

Why people take opiates and continue to take them in the presence of strong social and legal sanctions against their use, is not known. A number of theories have been proposed. For the most part these theories have stressed the psychological and/or the social factors leading to drug use.

Psychological Factors. There have been many studies that have suggested that there are basic personality characteristics of the addict that make him especially vulnerable to narcotics. The addicts (at least those who were patients at the U.S. Public Health Service Hospital in Lexington, Kentucky) answered the items in the Minnesota Multiphasic Personality Inventory (MMPI) in a unique way. Hill, Haertzen, and Glaser (1960) made use of those items in the MMPI that identified an addict population as the basis for an "Addiction Scale." Beckett, reporting in 1974, stated "that heroin addiction in some is symptomatic of an underlying chronic depression in a wounded personality and in others of a failure of personality development." Despite such diagnoses as character disorder, inadequate personality, and so on, tagged to the addict, there is little evidence suggesting that there is a unique vulnerable personality.

All of the personality studies have been retrospective. The profound effects of the opiates plus the marked change in life-style caused by opiate use makes these personality studies most difficult to interpret.

Wikler (1952), in a unique study of a patient who was allowed to self-regulate his morphine intake, suggested that addicts have difficulty in obtaining satisfaction of their "primary needs." The pharmacologic dependence that develops leads to a continuous cycle of a drug-induced "need." The gratification of this need will motivate behavior in a manner similar to the recurrent cycles of such primary motivations as hunger and thirst.

Wikler also states that ex-addicts have reported the presence of withdrawal symptoms long after they have been withdrawn from opiates, when they are in environments in which narcotics are readily available. The similarity of these reports to a conditioning model has led Wikler to propose and to experimentally model a conditioning theory of drug addiction (Wikler and Pescor, 1967; Wikler, 1973a, 1973b). It should be noted that Wikler is not implying that physical dependence to opiates is conditioned but that the repeated cycling of mild to severe withdrawal symptoms and their relief by the self-administration of opiates are instrumental in opiate dependence. Wikler (1973b) has defined drug dependence as ". . . habitual, non-medically indicated drug-seeking and drug-using behavior which is contingent for its maintenance upon pharmacological and usually, but not necessarily, upon social reinforcement." By defining drug dependence in this way, Wikler points out that the strength of drug dependence can then be measured by its resistance to extinction.

The continual drug seeking and repeated use of opiates by the physically dependent individual can be explained by this definition. Also, the former addict, who relapses long after he is "cured" of his "habit" is explained by such a model. Further, the model allows for the experimental study of drug dependence in animals. The conditioning of the opiate abstinence syndrome has been done by two methods. The technique that Wikler uses (Wikler and Pescor, 1967) is the pairing of the abstinence phenomenon with a specific physical environment. A second technique is to pair an opiate antagonist-precipitated abstinence with a specific stimulus (Goldberg and Schuster, 1967). The importance of the conditioning model at its simplest level of interpretation is that it suggests a method for treating the drug user and thus will allow clinical testing of the theory.

It is clear that simple detoxification along with long detention in a drug-free environment does not lead to the extinction of the drug-seeking behavior. The magnitude of the relapse rate in patients treated at the U.S. Public Health Service Hospital in Lexington, Kentucky attests to the failure of simple forced abstinence, even when accompanied by psychotherapy. If we are dealing with a conditioning model, then the appropriate technique of producing extinction of the behavior would be to allow drug-seeking behavior along with the self-administration of heroin. If the effect of heroin could be blocked so that it ceased to be reinforcing, then extinction of the behavior should result. Since we now have means of completely blocking the effects of opiates by the use of narcotic antagonists, this model is now being tested in a number of research-treatment centers in the United States. However, as Wikler points out, there may be other reinforcers of narcotic use. One such reinforcer that has been identified is peer-group pressure.

Some support for Wikler's hypothesis can be found in the drug-use histories of returning Viet Nam veterans (Robins, 1974, p. 84). Robins found that the incidence of illicit drug use within the population under study was 7 percent prior to duty in Viet Nam, 33 percent during the stay in Viet Nam, and 5 percent after return from Viet Nam. Clearly, these data indicate that use alone of illicit drugs is neither a primary determinant nor predictor of continued abuse. When the soldiers returned to an environment in which they had not experienced drug effects or withdrawal, drug use was discontinued. Wikler's hypothesis would suggest that those soldiers who had used illicit drugs while in Viet Nam but did not continue to do so on their return to the United States would relapse if they returned to Viet Nam (not an unreasonable prediction).

Although there are many studies that indicate that there may be personality factors that account for the use of opiates, as previously pointed out, all of these studies have been retrospective. The search for an "addictive personality" is probably doomed to failure, for what might look like a personality that is addiction-prone may be conditioned by the addiction process or will describe only a particular subgroup of those who use illicit drugs.

Unfortunately, most studies of the "addictive personality" have failed to use an adequate control group in their studies. Ideally, the proper control group should be matched with the experimental group for a number of variables including social class, and in addition, the control group should be equally exposed to drug use in that they live in an area of extensive use. Thus the question can be asked: Why did they not become users despite the high risk for use? A study that attempted to have such a control group was done a number of years ago by Gerard and Kornetsky (1955).

In the study by Gerard and Kornetsky 32 consecutive patient admissions at the U.S. Public Health Service Hospital in Lexington, Kentucky were studied. They were all under 21 years of age and all were males. What makes this study unique is the method of selecting the control subjects. The control subjects were selected from a pool of subjects who were friends of addict patients being treated at the Riverside Hospital in New York. Ideally, it would have been better to have obtained the control subjects from a pool of names obtained from the experimental group; however, this was not possible. In addition to being a friend of an addict (or at least known by an addict), the criteria for selection of the control group were: residence in a high-drug-use census-tract area in New

York City, 16 to 21 years of age, not attending college, no history of opiate addiction, no current drug use, no known record of delinquency, and roughly matched to the experimental group for ethnic composition. The nonaddictive use of drugs terminating at least six months prior to the study did not preclude the inclusion of a person as a control subject. The results of this study, which made use of the Rorschach Test, Draw-a-Person, and the Bender Gestalt, clearly yielded differences between the groups. In each of the tests only those aspects in which objective scoring could be applied were used. Also, the Rorschach Test was immediately readministered to the subjects using a method of Jernigan (1951). In this method subjects are instructed to produce only responses that were not given the first time the test was given.

Specifically, the results of this study were that the addict group's Rorschach as compared to the control group's was characterized by few responses, lack of use of shading and color, and responses that were more typical of the standard responses given to the cards. Also, in the repeat testing, responses appeared to be more pathological in nature in the addict group. In this study none of the addict subjects were diagnosed as normal adolescents, whereas almost half of the control subjects were considered such. Although these results are strongly suggestive, the psychiatric evaluation was done with full knowledge of which subjects had been previously physically dependent on heroin and which subjects were the controls. Supporting the psychiatric diagnoses were the results obtained on the various psychological tests. These were not scored until all the data were collected and the scoring was done "blind."

Whether the significant amount of personality maladjustment postdated or antedated drug use can only be inferred from other information obtained in this study. The life-history data shown in Table 1 indicates that prior to addiction, the addict group had been significantly more involved in adjustment difficulties than the control group.

Chein, Gerard, Lee, and Rosenfeld (1964, p. 194), in writing about the young addict, state two major propositions:

I. The addiction of the adolescents we have studied was an extension of, or a development out of, long lasting, severe, personality disturbance and maladjustment.
II. The addiction of the adolescents we have studied was adaptive, functional and dynamic.

The first proposition very boldly states that any personality deviation seen in the addicts studied was not conditioned by the addiction but was present long before these youths started to use drugs. Among the evidence supporting this proposition is that given by Chein et al. (1964, pp. 109–148), which shows a history of the drug user's interests and life-style preceding the onset of drug use that is considered less "constructive" than that seen in their control group (see pages 196–197, this chapter).

TABLE 1. A COMPARISON OF FREQUENCY OF ADJUSTMENT DIFFICULTIES IN PREDRUG USE PERIOD OF ADOLESCENT ADDICTS AND CONTROL SUBJECTS

Problem	Addicts	Controls
School adjustment (truancy, authority problems, etc.)	10	5
Behavior that led to psychiatric study	4	0
Behavior that led to correctional institutions	2	0
Probation	0	1
Alcoholism	5	2
Gambling as *modus vivendi*	2	0
Runaway from home	2	0
Theft	5	0
Club fighting	10	2
(a) Subjects with none of these features	9	15
(b) Subjects with any of these features	23 (72%)	8 (34.8%)

Abstracted from Gerard and Kornetsky, 1955.

The argument in the Chein et al. study that there is a longlasting severe personality disturbance seems well documented and is congruent with the earlier findings of Gerard and Kornetsky (1955). However, these findings must be looked at in the context of the group studied. The pathology observed may not be present in other groups of addicts, for example, those coming from different backgrounds. Other addict groups may show different types of preaddiction pathology. Also, the Chein study was conducted in the 1950s, and it is possible that the epidemiology of use has changed sufficiently so that even a sample gathered in the same manner as in the Chein study's sample might show a different picture today. However, the Chein et al. study is a landmark investigation of addiction in New York City, and it is this author's belief that much that was written then would hold true today. Further, in this chapter I will discuss some of the sociological aspects of their study.

Chein et al.'s second formulation that addiction is "adaptive and functional" is not as clearly documented as their first formulation which concerns personality and drug use. Khantzian (1974) apparently agrees that this formulation is not well documented; however, surprisingly, he then mentions a report by himself and one by Wurmser (1972) given at the Fourth National Methadone Conference that support the Chein et al. formulation. Both Khantzian and Wurmser argued that narcotics are used ". . . as a means to counteract the disorganizing influences of rage and aggression, affects with which addicts have particular difficulty." (Khantzian, 1974).

The concept of addiction as "adaptive and functional" is a compelling hypothesis. It is, however, a difficult hypothesis to prove. Khantzian (1974) states that the "craving" for narcotics can be ". . . viewed as a desire for relief from threatening and dysphoric feelings associated with unmitigated aggression." How can we know that the addict takes drugs to decrease dysphoric feelings? Even though there is sufficient evidence that narcotic drugs reduce overt aggression, we do not know that this is the action desired by the opiate user. I feel that only if we concisely describe and document the behavior of the drug user before and after the start of regular opiate use can we come to any conclusions regarding a possible "adaptive and functional" theory of drug use. Both Khantzian's (1974) argument that opiate use protects the user from feelings associated with "unmitigated aggression" and the earlier hypothesis of Wikler (1952) that the pharmacological action of opiates reduces aggressive and sexual drive support the notion that opiate use is adaptive.

In the studies by Gerard and Kornetsky (1954a, 1954b, and 1955) there is the suggestion that the adolescent addict's use of drugs provides a means of warding off more severe psychopathology. Thus the addiction of many of the subjects in the Gerard and Kornetsky studies as well as in the more detailed studies of Chein et al. (1964) might have masked an underlying pathology that would have become fully manifest only had the subject not turned to narcotics. This hypothesis cannot be proven, for it would be impossible to do the critical experiment that would demonstrate that the potential addict who did not become addicted developed severe psychopathology. Also, it is possible that the adolescent addicts that Kornetsky and Gerard and Chein studied in the 1950s were very different from adolescent addicts of today; however, recent descriptions of today's users suggest that many are, in fact, quite similar to those studied in the 1950s.

Bourne (1974) states that a significant number of individuals who become addicted to the opiates suffer from severe psychopathology and that there is a higher incidence in this group of schizophrenia and depression that clearly antedates the use of the opiates. He further states that some schizoid individuals do seem to function much more adequately as addicts than they did prior to their addiction. Wurmser (1972) states that the opiates keep many addicts from becoming completely dysfunctional by keeping their affective reactions under control. He further argues that the narcotics perform a unique therapeutic function for such individuals.

Social Factors. Despite recent accumulation of a myriad of data on the opiate user, the most systematic studies of drug use in an urban area were done in the middle to late 1950s and early 1960s; these are described in a book by Chein, Gerard, Lee, and Rosenfeld, *The Road to H* (1964). "'H' is for heaven; 'H' is for hell; 'H' is for heroin" (Chein, et al., 1964, p. 3). Although this book was written over 10 years ago, the addict today would probably agree with these three meanings of 'H.' The authors of this book asked the questions: "How and why does addiction happen? What, if anything, should be done about it?" With these questions in mind, the book is a model of a social and psychological study of the problem of addiction, and despite its apparent obsolescence, most of what was written then probably is true for similar users today.

What is clear from the Chein et al. book and reports of other writers in the field, is that there is no single social factor that accounts for drug abuse. Certainly poverty, social disorganization, and racial prejudice do not alone create drug addicts. However, all of these factors contribute to a milieu in which drug addiction is more likely to flourish. In the Chein et al. report the variables that consistently distinguished the "epidemic" areas from the "nonepidemic" areas of drug abuse in New York City, based on the 1950 U.S. census, were the following:

Percentage of population that was Negro.
Percentage of population that was of Puerto Rican origin.
Percentage of wives separated from husbands.
Average number of male adolescents per city block.
Percentage of husbands separated from wives.
Percentage of excess adult females over males.
Percentage of married couples not living in their own homes.
Percentage of income units earning less than $2000 in 1949.
Percentage of dwelling units that were highly crowded.
Percentage of men employed in "lower" occupations.
Percentage of adults with fewer than 8 years of schooling.
Percentage of unemployed men.
Percentage of working women.
Percentage of dwelling units without television.

With a few exceptions the above items would probably still distinguish today between high and low drug-use areas of our large urban centers. Chein et al. make a point that is often ignored in this type of social-epidemiological study. They state that it cannot be concluded that the differences found between the epidemic and nonepidemic areas are, either individually or collectively, directly responsible for the use of opiate drugs. All that can be concluded is that areas that are relatively high in these characteristics are fertile ground for opiate use.

When Chein et al. looked at the characteristics of their opiate-user population compared to those of nonusers from the same epidemic areas, they were surprised to find evidence of differences that antedated the use of drugs. Table 2 is an example of the types of differences that were found between a sample of users and nonusers. The table clearly shows that prior to drug use, the drug users made significantly less use of opportunities in the community than did the nonusers.

TABLE 2. USE OF COMMUNITY AND SCHOOL RESOURCES BY ADOLESCENT OPIATE USERS AND CONTROL SUBJECTS

Use	Controls (%)	Users (%)
Used library or book club	63	28
Liked to read books on "how to improve yourself" (explicit mention in answer to open-ended question)	17	4
Was interested in extracurricular activities	50	21
Was active in extracurricular activities	40	6
Went on camping trips, and so on	22	5
Stayed in school at least until age sixteen	88	27
Total cases	(50)	(50)

From Chein et al., 1964, p. 146.

One somewhat surprising finding was that the Puerto Rican and white drug users came from homes of less socioeconomic deprivation than did the nondrug users living in the same epidemic areas. The opposite was found for the black subjects. The picture for the black subjects was in agreement with the findings of others with respect to juvenile delinquency, regardless of race: delinquents have more socioeconomic deprivation than nondelinquents coming from the same urban areas. Gerard and Kornetsky (1955) found that their addict subjects came from homes of less socio-economic deprivation than did their controls, although both groups were living in high incidence areas. The data of the Gerard and Kornetsky study differed from that of the Chein et al. study in that subjects in the former were predominantly black. Thus from these two studies it is difficult to draw any final conclusion except to state that poverty, per se, is not a primary predictor of addiction vulnerability. Having said that, I would like to emphasize the fact that the total environment of a community in which there is socioeconomic deprivation provides a multitude of opportunities for opiate use to flourish.

A recent report by Robins (1974) supports the previously described findings that the opiate user's behavior and life style prior to opiate use was different from that of the nonuser. The study by Robins was precipitated by the extensive use of drugs by United States soldiers in Viet Nam. The extent of drug use in Viet Nam was significant. Of the approximately 13,760 Army enlisted men who had returned from Viet Nam in September 1971, approximately 1400 were found to have urine tests that were positive for narcotics, amphetamines, or barbiturates. Obviously, those found to have urines positive for drugs were not the only soldiers who used drugs. Robins points out that about half of all of the United States soldiers in Viet Nam used drugs. She further states that the use of drugs was not randomly distributed. Table 3 summarizes some of her findings regarding predictors of drug use in Viet Nam.

I would like to conclude this section on causes of addiction with some speculation concerning the continual use of opiates by the physically dependent individual. One of the fascinating aspects of opiate use in some individuals is its compulsive nature. Part of this can be explained by the relatively rapid development of tolerance with the concomitant development of physical dependence. The dose used is increased because of tolerance, and this increases the degree of physical dependence. It is believed that because of tolerance, the user is obtaining very little of the pleasurable effects of the drug so that it is usually concluded that the continued driving force is the need to avoid the manifestations of withdrawal. I would like to suggest an alternate hypothesis which is that only part of the reason for the continued use is to avoid the unpleasantness of abstinence. The other factor contributing to this continued desire for the drug is that a "high" is still obtainable. It is known that

TABLE 3. PREDICTORS OF DRUG USE IN VIET NAM

Factor	Users of narcotics, barbiturates, or amphetamines (Interviewed: $N = 205$)	No drugs or marijuana only (Interviewed: $N = 246$)
Drugs and Alcohol		
Used marijuana	69%	7%
Used narcotics, barbiturates, or amphetamines before Viet Nam	54	0
Heavy drinking	58	31
Civilian arrest	44	20
Large city[a]	38	28
Service Status		
Enlisted	62	29
Draftee	34	53
Career	4	18
Education		
Did not complete high school	39	23
Age in 1970		
Under 20	25	8

[a] $p < .05$. All others: $p < .001$.
Abstracted from Robins, 1974, p. 38.

tolerance to opiates does not develop to the same degree in all physiological systems. Some work previously mentioned in Chapter 7 indicates that morphine lowers the threshold for electrical stimulation to reward systems in the brain and at the same time, raises the threshold for electrical stimulation to aversive areas of the brain. Preliminary experiments suggest that tolerance to morphine may not develop to the same degree in the reward areas as in the aversive areas of the brain. If this is the case and the effect in the reward system is related to the opiate "high," then the physically dependent individual who is tolerant to the depressant effects of morphine is still obtaining the "high" associated with opiate administration.

Treatment Methods

The causes of opiate abuse are certainly varied. Various theories concerning the etiology have had impact in terms of public policy and treatment programs. If you believe that personality abnormalities are the primary cause of addiction, then the obvious treatment method is psychotherapy. If you believe that the problem is fundamentally similar to an infectious disease model, then you could isolate those diseased from those uninfected. If you believe that a conditioning model explains the continued use of the narcotics, then the proper treatment technique would be to use a blocking agent as a tool in extinguishing the opiate-seeking behavior. If you believe that the problem is primarily caused by the availability of drugs, then you would attempt to eliminate the drugs. Our attempts to limit the growing of opium in Turkey is an example of this approach.

The above are just examples of the manner in which theory has had an impact on public policy and the selection of therapeutic approaches. The field of drug addiction research is not lacking in theories or in treatment methods based on each of the theories. I can state gratuitously and without fear of contradiction that the problem of addiction is very complex and that no single theory adequately explains opiate abuse. I can further state that our image of the opiate user as some kind of "fiend," or criminal, has led to laws that make little sense and have had little impact on the problem except perhaps to make the problem worse.

Jaffe (1973), former Director of the U.S. Special Action Office for Drug Abuse Prevention, states that there are at least eight conceptually and operationally distinct treatment methods used in the treatment of compulsive narcotic use:

1. Medical-distributive
2. Supervisory-deterrent
3. Self-regulating community (character restructuring)
4. Psychotherapeutic

5. Benign maintenance/specific deficit correction
6. Conditioning—narcotic antagonists
7. Faith and dedication
8. Multimodality

The *medical-distributive* treatment model is the one currently used in Great Britain. Its use is based on the assumption that addiction is almost impossible to "cure," and thus it is preferable to provide drugs under medical supervision rather than to force the addict to obtain his drugs illegally. The British make the assumption that compulsive opiate use is an illness and, if all curative methods dealing with the disorder are equally unsuccessful, then making the drugs available under the aegis of the medical profession is probably the most humane treatment (Bewley, 1973). Bewley goes on to say that we must learn to live with the casualties of our society and that the compulsive drug user is one of the casualties. One of the values of the medical model is that sickness is socially more acceptable than sin.

The *supervisory-deterrent* model is based on the premise that regardless of the primary cause of the addiction, the individual who is no longer physically dependent can be kept drug free. The model employs detoxification in an institutional setting followed by a controlled drug-free period in the institution. After this period the individual is returned, under supervision, to the community. If there is a relapse to the use of drugs, the individual is returned to the institution. This method, at its best, allows for counselling or psychotherapy in the institution, followed by a great deal of support when the person returns to the community. At its worst it involves incarceration in a correctional institution with no support when the individual returns to the community.

The *self-regulating communities* are self-contained, voluntary residential therapeutic communities. The first organization of this type was Synanon, which started in the late 1950s in California. It received a great deal of notoriety and became the model for many of the subsequently appearing groups (see Meyer, 1972, pp. 63–75). The program in the therapeutic community is based on the premise that the drug addict is someone whose way of life has been incorrectly styled. The therapeutic community will restructure the life style of the individual by changing his goals, values, and expectations. Each of these treatment communities maintains a rigid social hierarchy. On being admitted into the program the novitiate is given few privileges and is required to carry out the menial tasks that are necessary for the functioning of the center. As the program progresses he moves up in the social heirarchy of the center. These programs are usually organized around a charismatic leader who is most authoritarian in his leadership. Different approaches to group living are used. Courses in psychopathology may be given, and various forms of group therapy are used with the emphasis on the encounter group. These confrontation-model therapeutic communities have been successful in producing a cadre of ex-addicts who are well trained in this mode of treatment. The advocates of this method are convinced that it is the only successful way to treat the addict. The question of how successful the method is for the majority of drug addicts has not been answered. Meyer (1972, p. 72) states that a problem in assessing the confrontation model of a therapeutic community arises from the "passionate commitment of its followers and their belief in the absolute efficacy of the treatment." This "myopia" leads members of the group to respond to outside evaluation as an unwanted intrusion. From available data it appears that this type of treatment modality is acceptable to only a small minority of the narcotic users. Those who do complete a program seem to do very well; however, according to Meyer's review of the available data, these communities are able to keep in the program no more than 7 to 20 percent of persons entering. Thus the actual number of addicts who successfully complete the program and reenter society is small.

The *psychotherapeutic model* is based on the hypothesis that there is a severe psychological maladjustment that antedates drug use. This model assumes that after withdrawal from the drug, a change can be effected in the individual by use of one form of psychotherapy or another. Psychotherapy is often combined with other treatment modalities. As previously mentioned in this chapter, even if there were a personality maladjustment that antedated the drug use, there is no evidence that psychotherapy is particularly successful in changing the lifestyle of the narcotic addict.

The model that Jaffe (1973) refers to as the *benign maintenance/specific deficit correction* method is similar to the British method in that subjects are maintained on an opiate for long periods of time. This treatment method, known as *methadone maintenance,* was pioneered by Vincent Dole and Marie Nyswander (1965, 1968). This treatment method was based on their theory that chronic exposure to opiates causes cellular changes that remain long after detoxification has occurred and that these changes account for the high rate of relapse seen in the heroin addict. Evidence that there are long-term cellular changes is seen in animal studies in which, long after even a single dose of morphine, there is an altered response to a subsequent dose of the drug (Cochin and Kornetsky, 1964; Kornetsky and Bain, 1968; Friedler, 1974). Dole draws the analogy between the heroin addict who seems to require continual narcotic administration and the diabetic who requires an external source of insulin for the duration of his life (Dole and Nyswander, 1968). Whether or not Dole and Nyswander are correct, it is clear that methadone will substitute for heroin, and if the dose of methadone is adequate, it will preclude heroin seeking in most addicts.

When Dole and Nyswander, over ten years ago, introduced methadone maintenance as a treatment method, there was a great deal of resistance, both from the established "addictionologist" and from the U.S. Bureau of Narcotics. Dole and Nyswander literally started a crusade for the use of the method, and without their persistent efforts, a significant treatment method would never have been accepted.

Even if the theories supporting the use of methadone as a treatment are incorrect, methadone has clear advantages as a maintenance drug. It is a longer-acting opiate than heroin; it is well absorbed orally; it does not seem to produce a "high" in the addict. The latter may be a function of oral administration and/or the degree of tolerance. The method allows addicts the opportunity to lead relatively normal lives. They can hold jobs, as they are not spending all their time "hustling" for drugs. Some proponents of this treatment method feel that eventually the addict will be able to withdraw from methadone. The method seems to work best in those programs that give additional psychological support to the subject. Methadone maintenance is often criticized because the method is simply the substitution of one addiction for another. Pharmacologically and psychologically, this is true. However, if addicts receiving methadone can function, whereas they could not before, if they are not hustling for drugs, whereas they were before, if they are not in and out of jail, whereas they were before, and if they are not at risk for hepatitis or a heroin overdose, whereas they were before, then we can say that methadone maintenance is an effective way of treating the problem. What is also clear is that if the addict's behavior prior to his addiction was maladaptive and asocial, the use of methadone alone will not change his way of life.

The basis for the *conditioning-narcotic antagonist* model has already been discussed in this chapter under the section on theories of opiate drug use. The basic method is to give adequate doses of naloxone or some other narcotic blocking agent to the detoxified opiate addict so that any time he takes heroin, he will experience no drug effect. In this way the heroin-seeking behavior will be extinguished. Although there is sufficient experimental evidence to support this approach, the problem is to keep the subject taking the naloxone. It would seem that this method will work only on those addicts who have already made a strong commitment to stop their heroin use. At the present time there is a great deal of effort being expended toward the development of a long-acting narcotic blocking agent. The search is for an agent in which the duration of action would be longer than one week.

The method of *faith and dedication* is not a treatment method that is useful for most addicts. It has its roots in religious conversions and Addicts Anonymous, an organization similar to Alcoholics Anonymous. The Black Muslims and various fundamentalist Protestant sects have made use of this technique that requires complete abstinence from the "sinful" ways of drug use if one wishes to be a member of the group. Group pressure and group support are integral parts of such programs. Some groups have substituted political and revolutionary goals for moral and religious goals (Meyer, 1972, p. 63). The number of people who can be successfully treated by means of this type of "religious" conversion is probably small, and although there are no statistics concerning the usefulness of the methods, there are enough anecdotal reports to suggest that the method is probably helpful for some.

Jaffe (1973) defines the *multimodality* approach as an eclectic approach that defines the treatment method in terms of the needs of the particular patient. The theoretical basis for this approach, by now probably obvious to the reader, is that the reasons for drug addiction are varied and that no single procedure is appropriate for all subjects. Also, different approaches may be appropriate for the same subject at different times in the course of the treatment.

A few final points on opiate use. Not all users are compulsive addicts. Probably a large number of users never reach a level of daily consumption. And as Jaffe (1973) points out, most users of opiates probably use other psychoactive drugs such as the barbiturates, alcohol, and amphetamine. Addiction to opiates per se does not preclude maintenance of a relatively normal lifestyle. Although rare, there are many examples of individuals who held jobs and performed in a professional capacity for decades while they were physically dependent on opiates. Opiates do not produce violence or aggression in men. Violent men may even behave less violently when they are taking opiates. However, the desire for opiates in the physically dependent individual may lead him into situations in which the potential for violent crime is present.

THE HALLUCINOGENS

Many drugs and chemical compounds can cause hallucinations; most of them, however, do not belong to the drug class usually described by the term hallucinogen (psychotomimetics, psychedelics, psychodysleptics, fantastica). A substantial proportion of all pharmacologically active substances, either in unusually high doses or in the presence of idiosyncratic sensitivity, cause toxic metabolic disturbances. Among the consequences of these metabolic disturbances may be organic brain syndromes that are accompanied by hallucinations (Brawley and Duffield, 1972). These toxic psychoses have been caused by sulfonamides; hormones such as adrenocorticotrophin (ACTH), prednisolone, and thyroxine; cardiac glycosides; phenacetin; disulphiram; methyl and ethyl alcohol; and the industrial chemicals. A second group of substances that Brawley and Duffield refer to as *deliriants* causes a delirious state usually accompanied by hallucinations without concomitant metabolic disturbances. Most of these drugs are anticholinergic compounds, for example, scopolamine and atropine.

Although in some cases the separation of the hallucinogens from the deliriants may be difficult, the primary characteristic of the true hallucinogenic drug is that it will produce, in the presence of a clear sensorium, a psychotic-like state in which the subject is oriented to time, place, and person. The deliriants characteristically cause memory loss, confusion, and often slurring of speech and ataxia.

The hallucinogens are of intrinsic interest because of the love affair that man has had since early times with the mystical and religious implications of altered states of consciousness. The compounds are of interest to the biologist because of their possible relevance to the understanding of the psychoses. The hallucinogens are among the oldest-known psychoactive substances. Although their pharmacology has been extensively studied since the discovery of the hallucinogenic properties of lysergic acid diethylamide thirty years ago, it is said of these drugs (Brawley and Duffield, 1972) that "the pharmacological and physiological bases of their hallucinogenic potency are not yet understood."

Although the hope that the study of the hallucinogens would provide the key to the understanding of schizophrenia reached almost hysterical proportions in the 1950s, we find today that the key has only opened the door to an anteroom, and it may turn out that there are a series of rooms that we must go through before we enter the house. Some investigators believe that the key will not, in fact, be provided by studying classical hallucinogens but by the study of the chronic use of amphetamines.

Mescaline

Mescaline (3,4,5-trimethoxyphenethylamine) is one of the many alkaloids found in the peyote cactus, a plant indigenous to northern Mexico and the southwestern United States. The term "peyote" is derived from the Aztec word "peyotl" ("devine messenger") (del Pozo, 1967). Peyote has different names among the various southwest Indians who use it in their religious rituals.

Mescal buttons or mescal beans are the dried tops cut from several species of peyote cactus. These buttons have the appearance of mushroom-like discs. Mescal buttons are not to be confused with mescal, a distilled liquor that is a common intoxicant in Mexico.

In addition to the hallucinogenic effects of mescaline, the most common pharmacological effect is mydriasis, and many users also experience nausea and vomiting. Scientific study of the hallucinogenic effects of mescaline was carried out in the 1920s. In 1926 Heinrich Klüver published a paper in the *American Journal of Psychology* entitled "Mescal visions and eidetic visions," and in 1928 he published a monograph on the subject that has recently been reissued with the addition of a paper on the "Mechanisms of hallucinations" (Klüver, 1966). The reports published in this book on the visual hallucinations caused by mescaline are as descriptive as any that I have read. The following is Klüver's report of his own personal experience with the drug (Klüver, 1966, p. 17–18):

"We refer now to our personal observation to demonstrate some other aspects of mescal visions. 23 g. of the powdered buttons were taken in doses of 13 and 10 g. Half an hour after taking the second dose vomiting occurred. Soon hereafter phenomena of the following kind could be observed with closed eyes: 'Clouds from left to right through optical field. Tail of a pheasant (in center of field) turns into bright yellow star; star into

THE HALLUCINOGENS

sparks. Moving scintillating screw; 'hundreds' of screws. A sequence of rapidly changing objects in agreeable colors. A rotating wheel (diameter about 1 cm.) in the center of a silvery ground. Suddenly in the wheel a picture of God as represented in old Christian paintings.—Intention to see a homogeneous dark field of vision: red and green shoes appear. Most phenomena much nearer than reading distance. —The upper part of the body of a man, with a pale face but red cheeks, rising slowly from below. The face is unknown to me. —While I am thinking of a friend (visual memory-image) the head of an Indian appears. —Beads in different colors. Colors always changing: red to violet, green to bright gray, etc. Colors so bright that I doubt that the eyes are closed. —Yellow mass like saltwater taffy pierced by two teeth (about 6 cm. in length). —Silvery water pouring downward, suddenly flowing upward. —Landscape as on Japanese pictures: a picture rather than a real landscape. —Sparks having the appearance of exploding shells turn into strange flowers which remind me of poppies in California. —(Eyes open): streaks of green and violet on the wall. Then a drawing of a head changing into a mushroom (both of natural size). Then a skeleton (natural size) in lateral view turned about 30° to the left. Head and legs are lacking. Try to convince myself that there are only shadows on the wall, but still see the skeleton (as in X-ray). —(Eyes closed). Soft deep darkness with moving wheels and stars in extremely pleasant colors. —Nuns in silver dresses (about 3 cm. height) quickly disappearing. —Collection of bluish ink-bottles with labels. —Red, brownish and violet threads running together in center. —Autumn leaves turning into mescal buttons. —Different forms emitting intense greenish light. —Forms in different colors; contours often dark. —Strange animal (length perhaps 10 cm.) rapidly turns into arabesques. —Gold rain falling vertically. On stationary background rotating jewels revolving around a center. Then, with a certain jerk, absence of all motion. —Regular and irregular forms in irridescent colors reminding me of radiolaria, sea urchins and shells, etc., in symmetrical or asymmetrical arrangement. —Shells illuminated from within radiating in different colors, moving towards the right, turned about 45° towards the right and somewhat towards me. A little piece in every shell is broken out. —Slow majestic movements along differently shaped curves simultaneously with 'mad' movements. —Feeling there is 'motion *per se*'. —Man in greenish velvet (height about 7-8 cm.) jumping into deep chasm. —Strange animal turns into a piece of wood in horizontal position.'''

Lysergic Acid Diethylamide (LSD)

LSD was synthesized by Hofmann in 1938 at Sandoz Laboratories in Basel, Switzerland, but it was not until 1943 that he discovered its hallucinogenic properties. The report of his discovery is of some interest (Hofmann, 1959).

"In the afternoon of 16 April 1943, when I was working on this problem, I was seized by a peculiar sensation of vertigo and restlessness. Objects, as well as the shape of my associates in the laboratory, appeared to undergo optical changes. I was unable to concentrate on my work. In a dreamlike state I left for home, where an irresistible urge to lie down overcame me. I drew the curtains and immediately fell into a peculiar state similar to drunkenness, characterized by an exaggerated imagination. With my eyes closed, fantastic pictures of extraordinary plasticity and intensive colour seemed to surge towards me. After two hours this state gradually wore off.

The nature and course of this extraordinary disturbance immediately raised my suspicions that some exogenic intoxication may have been involved, and that the lysergic acid diethylamide, with which I had been working that afternoon, was responsible. However, I could not imagine in which way I could have absorbed a sufficient quantity of this compound to produce such phenomena. Moreover, the nature of the symptoms did not coincide with those previously associated with ergot poisoning. However, I decided to get to the root of the matter by taking a definite quantity of the compound in question. Being a cautious man, I started my experiment by taking 0.25 mg of d-lysergic acid diethylamide tartrate, thinking that such an extremely small dose would surely be harmless, and bearing in mind that the natural ergot alkaloids produce toxic symptoms in man only with doses exceeding several milligrams.

After 40 minutes, I noted the following symptoms in my laboratory journal: slight giddiness, restlessness, difficulty in concentration, visual disturbances, laughing.

At this point the laboratory protocol ends. The last words are hardly legible and were written only with the greatest difficulty. It was now obvious that LSD was responsible for the earlier intoxication. I requested my laboratory technician to accompany me home. Since it was war time and no car available, we went by bicycle. This journey is about 4 miles and I had the feeling of not getting ahead, whereas my escort stated that we were rolling along at a good speed. I lost all count of time. I noticed with dismay that my environment was undergoing progressive changes. My visual field wavered and everything appeared deformed as in a faulty mirror. Space and time became more and more disorganized and I was overcome by a fear that I was going out of my mind. The worst part of it being that I was clearly aware of my condition. My power of observation was unimpaired. I was not, however, capable by any act of will, of preventing the breakdown of the world around me. At home the physician was called.

At the height of the experience, the following symptoms were most marked:

Visual disturbances, everything appearing in impossible colours, objects out of proportion. At times the floor seemed to bend and the walls to undulate. The faces of the persons present changed into colourful grimaces.

Marked motor restlessness alternating with paralysis. Limbs and head felt heavy as if filled with lead and were without sensation. My throat felt dry and constricted.

Occasionally I felt as if I were out of my body. I thought I had died. My ego seemed suspended somewhere in space, from where I saw my dead body lying on the sofa."

Chemistry. LSD is an ergot alkaloid that chemically resembles ergonovine. Since ergot derivatives are produced by a fungus that grows on rye, it is very possible that many of the mass psychoses reported in Europe during the Middle Ages were due to the ingestion of fungus infected flour.

Physiological Effects. Recognition of the tremendous potency of LSD (doses as low as 20 to 25 micrograms can cause effects in man) was instrumental in fostering the scientific quest for an endogenous substance in schizophrenic patients that was similar to LSD. Unfortunately, no such easy solution to the etiology of schizophrenia was found.

LSD has marked effects on the autonomic nervous system with some predominance of sympathetic actions. It causes marked mydriasis with little pupillary responsiveness to light. Pupillary dilatation is not seen when the drug is directly applied to the eye. Tachycardia, nausea, tremor, gooseflesh, numbness, muscular weakness, and hyperthermia are among the actions of LSD. Tolerance develops rapidly to LSD in that after three to four daily doses, there is little physiological or psychological response.

Behavioral Effects. For the most part, animals are quite resistant to the effects of LSD; however, as already mentioned, the drug is quite potent in man. In man the effects of LSD are a good example of the interaction between direct pharmacological effects and nonspecific factors. The personality of the subject and the setting in which the drug is taken are important determinants of the response to LSD (Jarvik, 1968). In a comprehensive study of the effects of LSD, Barr et al. (1972, p. 164) stated that one of their major findings was "that reactions to LSD are patterned and meaningfully related to the preexisting personalities of the subjects. . . ."

The hallucinations caused by LSD are primarily visual. Colorful displays and strange geometric patterns are commonly seen. Colors seem more saturated, objects seem to move and are often mistaken for faces. Although auditory hallucinations are rare, some subjects report an amplification of background noises. Some subjects experience synesthesias, for example, sounds "have" color, or colors "have" texture. Time seems to pass slowly. Although subjects will report an enhancement of perception after LSD, almost all experimental studies on visual perception, as well as on cognitive and motor performance, report impairment.

Emotional responses to LSD will vary greatly between individuals as well as within the same individual during a single LSD exposure. Apprehension may be present and in some cases will culminate in panic. Subjects will move from feelings of marked euphoria to depression and back again. (For further discussion and review of the pharmacologic and behavioral effects of LSD, the reader is referred to Brawley and Duffield, 1972; Jarvik, 1968, 1970; Cohen, 1970; and Barr et al., 1972. Also, for an interesting report of one psychologist's personal experience with an overdose of LSD, I would suggest the paper by Bennett, 1960.)

One of the common reports of the user of LSD is that perception is enhanced, as I mentioned previously. Despite this subjective feeling, the objective evidence clearly shows that LSD impairs perception. This lack of agreement between scientific evidence and subjective reports is not a new phenomenon in science. Usually we completely accept the scientific evidence when there is disparity between subjective and objective observations.

However, subjects receiving LSD may not be telling us that visual acuity is enhanced by LSD. When one perceives the environment outside of the laboratory setting, there are many factors that contribute to the "world" that is seen. Previous experience with the objects viewed and the setting in which the objects viewed reside are important determinants of perception. There is certainly adequate experimental evidence to support the role of personality and environment in perception. If one listens to the reports of LSD users, one hears statements to the effect that the walls of a room (painted with one color) are of different colors, that the walls seem to be sloping in, that people look bigger or smaller than they actually are. One possible explanation for these apparent distortions of the environment is that the drug is breaking down perceptual constancies. When one stands in a cubical room, one knows that it is cubical in shape from past experience, but what is impinging on the retina is really a trapezoidal design. Certainly, even in a room painted one color, what is actually seen are various intensities of color depending on the amount of light reflecting on each of the surfaces. Thus what the LSD user sees is perhaps the actual world as it impinges on the retina. This breakdown of constancies can be quite disturbing to the subject for without these constancies, he would not be able to determine such obvious things as whether someone is small but relatively near in the visual field or large but relatively far away in the visual field. This interpretation of some of the visual phenomena suggests that LSD extinguishes a type of behavior that is learned very early in life and that in a strange but nonadaptive way, it enhances perception.

Some Other Common and Not-so-common Psychotomimetics. There are a variety of compounds that have been used for their hallucinogenic effect. The effects of these are similar to the effects of LSD or mescaline; however, there may be differences in potency and in the magnitude of side effects.

1. *Bufotenine* (n,n-dimethyl-5-hydroxytryptamine). This is found in Cohoba Snuff, the skin and parotid gland of the toad (Bufo marinus) and in small amounts in the fly agaric mushroom (Amanita muscaria). At doses of this drug that will cause the hallucinogenic effects, there are severe and uncomfortable autonomic effects.

2. *Psilocybin* (n,n-dimethyl-4-phosphoryltryptamine) and *Psilocin* (n,n-dimethyl-4-hydroxytryptamine). These are found in Psilocybe mexicana and related mushrooms. They are active alkaloids that, except for a relative lack of potency and shorter duration of action, have effects that are comparable to those of LSD.

3. *Harmine* (A Harmala alkaloid from Banisteriopsis caapi). The South American vine that harmine comes from is also called caapi, yage, and

ayahuasca. The Amazon natives use portions of this vine to make snuff and an intoxicating beverage. It causes vivid imagery but also marked somatic effects. These include nausea and vomiting and numbness.

4. *STP* (2,5-dimethoxy-4-methylamphetamine, DOM). STP, at least among some of the street users, stands for Serendipity, Tranquility, and Peace. DOM are initials for the chemical name. Cohen (1970) states that STP is probably the first synthetic hallucinogen that has gone directly from the animal pharmacology laboratory to the street user. It is claimed that STP causes prolonged hallucinogenic effects lasting as long as 24 to 48 hours. Among the somatic effects are systolic hypertension and mydriasis. STP's reputed duration of action is most likely an exaggeration that evolved when street doses of the drug became available in quantities that were contaminated with other compounds, most likely belladonna alkaloids.

5. *DMT* (*n,n*-dimethyltryptamine). DMT is found in Cohoba snuff made from the seeds of Piptadenia peregrina. DMT is not a very effective hallucinogen when taken orally; however, taken intravenously, smoked, or snuffed, it causes an LSD-like syndrome of short duration but with more severe sympathomimetic actions. *DET* (diethyltryptamine) is the synthetic form of DMT.

6. *American Tropical Morning Glory Seeds* (Ipomoea violacea, Rivea corymbosa, *Ololiuhqui*). The active ingredients in these seeds are lysergic acid amide and isolysergic acid amide. The morning glory seeds have definite sedative properties. The hallucinogenic properties are only seen when large amounts of the seeds are ingested. Nausea and vomiting are common side effects.

7. *Nutmeg* (Myristicin). Nutmeg can cause psychotomimetic effects when large amounts are eaten. There are marked unpleasant effects that include agitation, anxiety, dry mouth, tachycardia, marked flushing of the face, and a heavy feeling in the extremities. As a flavoring agent nutmeg is quite popular and pleasant. As an hallucinogen nutmeg is neither popular nor very effective.

It should be noted that many of the drugs sold on the street may not be what they are labeled. Many are manufactured in private underground laboratories that make no attempt to make certain that chemicals are pure. Many of the severe side effects seen with street drugs may be due to chemicals that contaminate the drug during synthesis or that are subsequently added. Also, a particular name may be used for several substances that have similar effects. (For further information concerning these natural products, the reader is referred to Efron, Holmstedt, and Kline, 1967.)

MARIHUANA

Marihuana (marijuana, marywana, maraguana, Indian hemp—*Cannabis sativa*) has been described in the following terms by P. O. Wolff (cited by Lasagna, 1965):

"At the price of a few fleeting minutes of pseudocelestial miracles for a few, a hell of moral catastrophes arises for the community, for public health, and for the sane and laborious people. The individual himself is subjugated by this weed, messenger of a false happiness, panderer to a treacherous love, which can provide a superhuman enjoyment and misery, likewise superhuman, which makes him sick—morally more than physically—and changes thousands of persons into nothing more than human scum. It is this weed which sunders the bonds of inhibition that make it possible for men to live together in a society; weed of the brutal crime and of the burning hell; this weed which splits the personality, which invades the prison and the asylum, the hovel and the palace, which subjugates the savage and the cultured; this weed which attempts to convert paupers into kings, weaklings into champions, minutes into years, and evil into good; this weed which brings dreams, which sets free the spiritual and the bestial, and, with the ease that Baudelaire and Gautier pen famous pages, makes the rabble bespatter pages with blood. There you have the picture of this diabolical resin which approaches under the mask of pleasant friendship."

It is likely that there are still many who would agree with the above description. For the most part, however, societal attitudes toward marihuana have evolved to the point where the question of whether marihuana should be legalized is being debated in some state legislatures. Still, a recent book by Nahas (1973) stresses the negative aspects of cannabis.

Marihuana is the crude preparation of the flowering tops, leaves, seeds, and stems of female plants of Indian hemp. The intoxicating constituents are found in the sticky resin that is exuded from the tops of the plants. At one time it was believed that only the resin taken from the female plant was high in concentration of the psychotropic ingredient. However, Valle, Lapa, and Barros reported in 1968 that the psychotropic ingredient was, in fact, present in equal concentrations in both male and female plants. It is believed that the primary active ingredient in cannabis is delta-9-tetrahydrocannabinol (THC). THC can be made synthetically. Marihuana can be grown in almost any climate, although the hemp grown in warmer climates is higher in THC content.

Indian hemp is prepared and used in a number of ways. Marihuana is usually smoked. In Africa a preparation of marihuana that is to be smoked is called *dagga* or *kif*. *Bhang* is an Indian name for a drink made only from the leaves of the plant. *Ganja,* used only in India, is made from the dried flowering tops of cultivated plants. Although ganja is usually smoked, it is also made into a tea. It is higher in THC content than European or American marihuana. The most potent form of cannabis is *charas* (India) or hashish. Hashish is the resin of the plant that has been pressed into blocks. Since most of the THC is found in the resin, hashish has the highest concentration of THC of any of the cannabis preparations.

In the latter part of the nineteenth century cannabis was extensively used in medicinals. Medical journals of this period extolled its application for a variety of conditions including such things as migraine headaches, insomnia, coughs, menstrual cramps, and asthma (Snyder, 1971, pp. 8–9. Bonnie and Whitebread, II, 1974, p. 4). It is of interest that recent work by Vachon et al. (1973, 1976) and Tashkin et al. (1973, 1974) indicates that marihuana, when smoked, has marked bronchodilator effects in normal subjects and in asthmatics. Harris et al. (1974) have reported that THC retarded tumor growth in mice.

History of Nonmedical Use. The American use of marihuana as an intoxicant started in South America and the West Indies. Marihuana use was quite common by the end of the nineteenth century in Mexico. It is reported that soldiers in Pancho Villa's army used cannabis freely. Bonnie and Whitebread, II (1974, p. 5) point out that the use was memorialized by a familiar Mexican folk song describing the inability of the cockroach to march without marihuana to smoke:

> La cucaracha, la cucaracha
> Ya no puede caminar
> Porque no tiene, porque no tiene
> Marihuana que fumar

The history of marihuana use as an intoxicant in the United States makes an interesting story of public morality, hysteria, legal contradictions, and the abdication by the medical profession of its responsibility not to succumb to the hysteria.

Although there was extensive cultivation of marihuana almost from the time of the founding of the first colonies, its extensive use as an intoxicant in the United States probably did not appear until early in the twentieth century. Hemp was a primary source of fiber for rope and consequently was a cash crop until the decline of the sailing ship in the last half of the last century. United States entrepreneurs then discovered other uses for the hemp. It was used in the manufacture of paper. Birdseed manufacturers used the cannabis seeds in their mixtures. It was used as a medicinal, and tincture of cannabis could be prescribed by physicians until 1937. It is of interest that George Washington was cultivating hemp in 1765. It has been suggested that Washington may have attempted to cultivate the plant for medicinal purposes as well as for the fiber (see Brecher, 1972, p. 403).

Although itinerant Mexican farmers are often blamed for the introduction of the use of marihuana as an intoxicant in the 1920s, it is clear that there was much earlier use in the United States. In 1856 an account of marihuana-eating experiences by Fritz Hugh Ludlow of Poughkeepsie, New York was published. This was followed by an expanded account by Ludlow in a book, *The Hashish Eater,* that was published the following year (Brecher, 1972, p. 406). Throughout the latter half of the nineteenth century and into the twentieth century the lay press carried articles on the recreational use of marihuana.

According to Brecher (p. 410), it was the legal prohibition of alcohol (the Eighteenth Amendment) in 1920 that resulted in the large-scale marketing of marihuana for recreational use. Alcohol beverages during this period rose in price and/or were inferior to those prior to Prohibition. By the 1930s every major American city had at least a few marihuana smokers. Many of the users during this period were the mexican workers, blacks, and Jazz musicians. Grinspoon (1971, p. 16) states that much of the hostility toward marihuana as well as the user could probably be attributed to ". . . fear of that which is alien and unAmerican. . . ."

The Federal Bureau of Narcotics was founded in 1930. At that time only 16 states had laws prohibiting the use of marihuana. By 1937 nearly every state had laws outlawing marihuana. A campaign was undertaken by the Federal Bureau of Narcotics to educate the public as to the "dangers" of marihuana. It was portrayed as a drug that released aggression and incited normal people to lead a life of violent crime. The Federal Bureau of Investigation (FBI) joined the crusade. With reference to the marihuana user, they issued the following warning:

"He becomes a fiend with savage or 'cave man' tendencies. His sex drives are aroused and some of the most horrible crimes result. He hears light and sees sound. To get away from it, he suddenly becomes violent and may kill."

(Grinspoon, 1971, p. 17).

The campaign of the Bureau of Narcotics had help from many other groups including the press; this culminated in 1937 with the passage of the Tax Act. This Act provided that individuals who used the plant for defined industrial or medical use pay a tax of $1.00 per ounce. However, individuals using the plant for purposes undefined by the Act would have to pay a tax of $100.00 per ounce. The penalties for failure to comply called for a fine of $2000.00 and/or a prison sentence not to exceed five years. Although on the surface the bill seemed to be a simple means of raising revenue, the real motivation was the control of marihuana use. The individual who wished to smoke marihuana was forced to pay $100.00 per ounce. The effect of this was to force him underground, exposing him to the risk of tax evasion.

From 1937 on, the state laws concerning the use of marihuana became more punitive. Many of the laws punished offenses related to marihuana in the same manner as offenses related to the opiates. Although in some states the mere possession for private use was a misdemeanor, in others simple possession was a felony, and conviction could result in sentences of life imprisonment. In the state of Massachusetts, until recently, one could be arrested without a warrant and be imprisoned for not more than five years if found where marihuana was kept.

For a number of decades there was a tacit social consensus supporting the marihuana laws. Bonnie and Whitebread, II (1974, p. 222) point out that this marihuana consensus was ". . . buttressed by a number of ideological and disruptive propositions." These included: the belief that marihuana was a "narcotic," the fact that people who used it were members of racial and ethnic minorities (at least until the upsurge of use by middle class youths in the 1960s), and the fact that failure of the medical and scientific communities to study the drug gave tacit approval to the consensus. The complicity of organized medicine was exemplified by a denouncement in an editorial in the *Journal of the American Medical Association* in April 1945 of a study initiated by New York's Mayor Fiorello La Guardia (Mayor's Committee on Marihuana, 1944). The Committee reported that marihuana smoking does not alter the personality structure of the smoker nor does it cause sexual overstimulation.

Beginning in the middle 1960s the marihuana consensus began to dissolve. Drug use, especially marihuana use, increased on the college campuses to what some people believed were epidemic proportions. The absurdity of the laws only became evident to white America when children of the middle class were directly confronted with these laws. There is a remark that was made by Bill Russell, a well-known former professional basketball player, that characterizes some of the change in attitude. Although not an exact quotation, he said something to the effect that "When marihuana was used by poor Blacks and Mexicans it was called a weed. When marihuana use increased by the white middle class it was called grass." The reader is directed to Bonnie and Whitebread, II (1974), Grinspoon (1971), and Brecher (1972) for detailed reviews of the history of marihuana use.

Pharmacology of Cannabis

Physiological Effects. The immediate physiological effects of cannabis are relatively slight, especially when marihuana is smoked. There is an increase in heart rate and swelling of the small conjunctival blood vessels. This gives the "red eye" look to the smoker. Although it was believed that cannabis caused dilation of the pupil, careful studies indicate that there are no pupillary changes. Some individuals report initially increased salivation followed by dryness of the mouth. Throat irritation and coughing are commonly reported by marihuana smokers. There is also an increase in the frequency of urination. Occasionally, nausea may occur when cannabis is taken orally. Although it has been believed that marihuana alters blood sugar levels, studies have been inconclusive. Appetite, however, is increased. Blood pressure changes have been inconsistently reported, although a recent experimental study by Vachon, Sulkowski, and Rich (1974) demonstrated a small but significant increase in systolic blood pressure. The maximum rise in blood pressure was seen one hour after smoking. The mean increase was 7 mm of mercury. As already mentioned, after brief exposure to marihuana there is a bronchodilator effect in normals and asthmatics (Vachon et al. 1973, 1976 and Tashkin et al. 1973, 1974). However, Tashkin et al. (1976) report that "very heavy marihuana smoking for six to eight weeks causes mild but statistically significant airway obstruction." (See Vachon's critique of Tashkin et al. in the New England Journal of Medicine, 1976).

Long-term effects of cannabis have only been studied retrospectively. There are many reports from Eastern countries of chronic poor health among heavy long-term users of hashish. Unfortunately, these studies did not include adequate control groups. Campbell et al. (1971) report evidence of cerebral atrophy in 10 young men who smoked marihuana daily for 3 to 11 years. This study, like many attempting to show long-term toxicity, is confounded by the possibility of concomitant use of other drugs and by the lack of adequate controls. For a selective review of acute and chronic toxicity of cannabis, the reader is directed to Nahas (1973, pp. 104–114). It should be noted that most scientists in the field do not share Dr. Nahas' negative attitude toward cannabis. (The reader is referred to *The Interim Report of the Canadian Government Commission of Inquiry,* 1971, and *First Report of the National Commission on Marihuana and Drug Abuse,* 1972.)

Despite the conclusion of the majority of members in the research community that the acute effects of marihuana are minimal and that there is little evidence of chronic toxicity, there have been some recent disquieting reports. In a special two-part article, *Science* published a review of the negative aspects of marihuana (Maugh, II, 1974) under the titles "Marihuana: The Grass May No Longer Be Greener" and "Marihuana II: Does It Damage the Brain?" Maugh, II lists six possible potential hazards associated with prolonged heavy use of cannabis: (1) chromosome damage, (2) interference with functioning of the immune system, (3) hormonal changes that may lead to impotence and temporary sterility and to the development of enlarged breasts in males, (4) injury to the bronchial tract and lungs, (5) severe personality changes, and (6) irreversible brain damage. In these *Science* articles Maugh, II reported on a number of different studies; however, he made no attempt to evaluate the validity of these studies.

There have been a number of papers in recent years reporting the effects of marihuana on perceptual, motor, and cognitive functioning. As might be expected, the effects are dose related in that effects vary with the THC content of the marihuana and with the amount inhaled. One of the first of these papers is by Weil, Zinberg, and Nelsen (1968). Among the more recent are papers by DeLong and Levy (1973), Roth et al. (1973), Vachon, Sulkowski, and Rich (1974), and Vachon and Sulkowski (1976). All of these studies show only slight impairment in performance of subjects under the influence of marihuana. Speed of response and cognitive ability seem most vulnerable to marihuana-induced impairments. A question that is often asked concerns the effects of marihuana on the ability to drive. Crancer et al. (1969) compared the effects of marihuana to those of alcohol on the performance of volunteers on a simulated driving test. All subjects were marihuana users, and they were allowed to titrate their marihuana intake to a level of a "social marihuana high." Although marihuana impaired performance, the impairment was not as great as that seen after alcohol. This study might be criticized on the grounds that when subjects were tested under the influence of marihuana, they were allowed to regulate the amount of drug taken, as described above; however, subjects tested under the influence of alcohol were given a predetermined dose. This dose was equivalent to 6 ounces of 86-proof whiskey for a 120-pound individual, and although for most people this would induce only a mild "social high," for some it might induce a much stronger intoxication.

The marihuana "high" varies greatly between individuals. For some there seems to be a stimulating effect and for others a depressant effect. Euphoria is often present. There is no evidence that cannabis has any direct sexual stimulating effect although increased enjoyment of sex while under the influence of the drug has been reported. It should be observed that in studies by Isbell et al. (1967) with THC, there were dose-related effects, and at the higher dosages used the effects were similar to those of LSD.

The question of whether marihuana smoking is dangerous has to be answered in relative terms. The use of any drug has potential for producing dangerous effects. Certainly the available evidence suggests that casual use of marihuana carries with it little risk to the user or to society. In fact, one could argue that under present laws, the major risks that the user incurs may be from the law. However, the use of any substance in high doses and for long periods of time increases the potential for pharmacological and physiological risks. It is believed by some investigators that chronic use of marihuana leads to a condition referred to as the "amotivational syndrome" (Allen and West, 1968; McGlothlin and West, 1968). Among the characteristics of the syndrome are apathy, retarded physical movements, lack of goals except for marihuana acquisition and use, and lack of interest in personal appearance. There is also mental confusion and difficulty with recent memory, and speech lacks logical cohesiveness. It is believed that this is directly the result of cannabis use since retrospective information suggests that life-style and behavior prior to use were quite different. However, whether this is a direct effect of chronic use has not been determined. Recent work by Rossi, Mendelson, and Meyer (1974) gave a somewhat contrary picture to that described above. They found that chronic marihuana users did not show any indications of a lack of motivation in an experimental situation that allowed subjects to earn some money. However, if a subject's life revolves entirely around marihuana, its acquisition and use, it is clear that he will no longer share the goals and aspirations of the majority of the people.

COCAINE

The natives of the South American Andes have been using the leaves of a shrub (*Erythroxylon coca*) since before the time of the Spanish conquests. The leaves are chewed causing mild euphoria and stimulation. The Andean coca leaf chewers seem to be able to survive the rigors of a very harsh life at very high altitudes. It is believed that the use of coca facilitates their ability to survive the rigors.

In the nineteenth century coca became an ingredient in patent medicines and in the soft drink Coca-Cola. By 1906 coca leaves were no longer used in the manufacture of Coca-Cola. Brecher (1972, p. 271) notes that a search of the medical literature has revealed little data that would suggest that the chewing of coca leaves or the drinking of beverages containing small amounts of coca is any more harmful than drinking coffee or tea.

The active ingredient in coca leaves, cocaine, was isolated in 1844. In 1883 a German Army physician reported that soldiers on maneuvers were more able to overcome fatigue when they took cocaine. A young Viennese neurologist read the report and obtained the drug to try it for cases of "heart disease and nervous exhaustion." This neurologist, Sigmund Freud, tried cocaine himself and became ecstatic about the effects. A detailed account of Freud's "love affair" with cocaine is given in Ernest Jones' (1953) biography of Freud.

Freud not only used cocaine himself, he urged members of his family as well as friends to use this wonderful drug. Freud used cocaine to treat his own depression. He also attempted to use cocaine as a local anesthetic but was not successful, although later the usefulness of cocaine as a local anesthetic was well documented.

Pharmacology

Cocaine has marked stimulating effects on the central and sympathetic nervous systems. Acute cocaine poisoning is not rare. Fatal doses are estimated to be 1.2 grams; however, severe toxic effects have been reported at doses as low as 20 mg (see Ritchie, Cohen, and Dripps, 1970). In acute cocaine poisoning the patient becomes excited, anxious, and confused. Pulse is rapid, respiration irregular, and the pupils are dilated. Sensations of crawling objects are felt on the skin. Nausea and vomiting are not uncommon. Death is the result of convulsions and respiratory arrest. The specific recommended treatment for acute cocaine poisoning is the intravenous administration of short-acting barbiturates.

Although cocaine abuse has been confused with narcotic abuse, the actions of the drugs are quite different not only in terms of acute effects but because cocaine does not cause physical dependence. Jaffe (1970) describes the effects of cocaine abuse as similar to the effects observed with amphetamine. A common method of self-administration of cocaine is by means of a snuff ("sniffing" or "snorting"). Since cocaine causes marked vasoconstriction when topically applied, it results in a decrease in blood flow to the mucosa of the nose resulting in lesions and often perforations of the septum. Cocaine is taken intravenously, either alone, or mixed with heroin. This latter preparation is called a "speedball" and results in some reduction of the stimulating effect of the cocaine. Devotees of cocaine liken the experience of an intravenous shot of cocaine to that of an orgasm. They also feel that intravenous cocaine is the ultimate drug experience. In addition to these fleeting effects, intravenous cocaine causes euphoric excitement and exaggerated feelings of increased strength and mental capacity. Cocaine is rapidly metabolized, and to maintain the "high," some users will repeatedly inject large doses at frequent intervals. When this abuse pattern is maintained, feelings of anxiety and suspiciousness often supervene the original euphoria, and a condition similar to that described as the amphetamine paranoid psychosis may ensue (Jaffe, 1965). (See Chapter 10.)

SUMMARY

In this chapter I have tried not only to describe the above drugs and their actions but to give something of the flavor of their use. I have not been all inclusive and obviously have omitted some important aspects of the drug-abuse problem. What should be clear to the reader, however, is that the nonmedical use of drugs is a very complex issue.

Among the factors that have complicated a rational approach to the problem of nonmedical use of drugs is the Calvinistic ethic prevalent in our society. There is a remark that is attributed to Margaret Mead commenting on the drug scene, "Virtue can be defined as pain followed by pleasure; sin can be defined as pleasure followed by pain." This Calvinistic tradition is ". . . said to prohibit us from even exploring whether the use of hallucinogens could improve the healthy, or possibly transform Western society into Zen elysium." (Freedman, 1967). It has been suggested that the "tradition-bound" scientist will usually conclude that the only proper use of the hallucinogens is for research and medical application and that illicit abuse is only for kicks and cults (McGlothlin, 1965).

Although drugs used in a nonmedical setting have predictable pharmacological actions, these actions are more susceptible to "nonspecific factors" than when the drugs are used in the usual medical context. Whether the hallucinations are auditory or visual is determined by properties of the drug itself, but the content of the aberrations is determined more by individual characteristics. The specific hallucinations and fears that a drug will cause do not reside in the drug molecules but are the contribution of the individual, his experience, and the environment in which he finds himself.

There have been debates in recent years concerning the legalization of marihuana and the removal of penalties for the use of other drugs. Among the arguments given is that the social use of marihuana is less dangerous than the social use of alcohol and that it is less likely to cause the social and personal catastrophes that are associated with alcohol use. Freedman (1969) directly confronts this issue. He points out the relative lesser dangers of marihuana as compared to alcohol but does correctly state that we do not know what the impact would be to society if marihuana were legalized. Before we can legalize a drug like marihuana, we must know such things as: what would be the epidemiology of use; for example, what percent of users would be expected to become the equivalent of the alcoholic? In other words, what would be the social costs to society? I believe that we cannot seriously consider legalization of any drug until we have answered questions like these. Before a new product is introduced for sale, extensive marketing research is done by the manufacturer. Similarly, extensive research should be done on marihuana before allowing it to become a legal product for sale. Until this research is done I agree with Freedman (1969) that we must not treat marihuana "... as an opiate, narcotic, nor equate personal possession with a major crime or disease...," although I would not even wish to equate possession with a minor crime. Further, I believe that we cannot continue to treat possession and use of the opiates as a crime. As Freedman (1969) points out, "The population of drug users constantly changes; there are different problems of use in different subpopulations; group patterns and ideologies play a crucial role in induction of drug experimentation and use." Thus there can be no single philosophy, no single treatment modality, no single law that can apply to all drugs and all people.

REFERENCES

Allen, J. R. and West, L. J. Flight from violence; Hippies and the green rebellion. *American Journal of Psychiatry*, **125,** 1968, 365–370.

Barr, H. L., Langs, R. J., Holt, R. R., Goldberger, L., and Klein, G. S. *LSD: Personality and Experience.* Wiley-Interscience, New York, 1972.

REFERENCES

Beckett, H. D. Hypotheses concerning the etiology of heroin addiction. In P. G. Bourne (Eds.) *Addiction*. New York, Academic, 1974, pp. 38–54.

Bennett, C. C. The drugs and I. In L. Uhr and J. G. Miller (Eds.) *Drugs and Behavior*, New York, Wiley 1960, pp. 596–609.

Bewley, T. H. Treatment of opiate addiction in Great Britain. In S. Fisher and A. M. Freedman (Eds.) *Opiate Addiction: Origins and Treatment*, Washington, D.C., Winston 1973, pp. 141–161.

Bonnie, R. J. and Whitebread, C. H., II. *The Marihuana Conviction—A History of Marihuana Prohibition in the United States*. Charlottesville, University Press of Virginia, 1974.

Bourne, P. G. Issues in addiction. In P. G. Bourne (Ed.) *Addiction*. New York, Academic, 1974, pp. 1–19.

Brawley, P. and Duffield, J. C. The pharmacology of hallucinogens. *Pharmacological Reviews*, 24, 1972, 31–66.

Brecher, E. M and the Editors of Consumer Reports. *Licit and Illicit Drugs*. Boston, Little, Brown, 1972.

Campbell, A. M. G., Evans, M., Thompson, J. L. G., and Williams, M. J. Cerebral atrophy in young cannabis smokers, *Lancet*, 7736, 1971, 1219–1224.

Canadian Commission Report. *The Non-Medical Use of Drugs, Interim Report of the Canadian Government's Commission of Inquiry*. Harmondworth, Middlesex, England, Penguin, 1971.

Chayet, N. L. Legal aspects of drug abuse. *Suffolk University Law Review*, 3, 1968, 1–22.

Chein, I., Gerard, D. L., Lee, R. S., and Rosenfeld, E. *The Road to H*. New York, Basic Books, 1964.

Cochin, J. and Kornetsky, C. Development and loss of tolerance to morphine in the rat after single and multiple injections. *Journal of Pharmacology and Experimental Therapeutics*, 145, 1964, 1–10.

Cohen, S. The hallucinogens. In W. G. Clark and J. del Giudice (Eds.) *Principles of Psychopharmacology*. New York, Academic, 1970, pp. 489–503.

Crancer, H., Dille, J. M., Delay, J. C., Wallace, J. E., and Haykin, M. D. The effects of marihuana and alcohol on simulated driving performance. *Report of the State of Washington Department of Motor Vehicles*, No. 021, April 1969.

DeLong, F. L. and Levy, B. I. Cognitive effects of marihuana, described in terms of a model of attention. *Psychological Reports*, 33, 1973, 907–916.

del Pozo, E. C. Empericism and magic in Aztec pharmacology. In D. H. Efron, B. Holmstedt, and N. S. Kline (Eds.) *Ethnopharmacologic Search for Psychoactive Drugs*. U. S. Government Printing Office. Public Health Service Publication, No. 1645, Washington, D.C., 1967, pp. 59–76.

Dole, V. P. and Nyswander, M. E. A medical treatment for diacetylmorphine (heroin) addiction. *Journal of the American Medical Association*, 193, 1965, 646–650.

Dole, V. P. and Nyswander, M. E. Methadone maintenance and its implications for theories of narcotic addiction. In *The Addictive States*, Research Publications Association for Research in Nervous and Mental Disease, 46, 1968, 359–366.

Efron, D. H., Holmstedt, B., and Kline, N. S. *Ethnopharmacologic Search for Psychoactive Drugs*. U. S. Government Printing Office, Public Health Service Publication, No. 1645, Washington, D.C., 1967.

Freedman A. M. Narcotic Addiction: The middle-range outlook. In S. Fisher and A. M.

Freedman (Eds.) *Opiate Addiction: Origins and Treatment.* Washington, D.C., Winston, 1973, pp. 225–233.

Freedman, D. X. Perspectives on the use and abuse of psychedelic drugs. In D. H. Efron, B. Holmstedt, and N. S. Kline (Eds.) *Ethnopharmacologic Search for Psychoactive Drugs.* U. S. Government Printing Office. Public Health Service Publication, No. 1645, Washington, D.C., 1967, pp. 77–102.

Freedman, D. X. Drug abuse-comments on the current scene. In J. R. Wittenborn, H. Brill, and J. P. Smith (Eds.) *Drugs and Youth.* Springfield, Charles C Thomas, 1969, pp. 345–361.

Friedler, G. Long-term effects of opiates. In J. Dancis and J. C. Hwang (Eds.) *Perinatal Pharmacology; Problems and Priorities.* New York, Raven 1974, pp. 207–220.

Gerard, D. L. and **Kornetsky, C.** A social and psychiatric study of adolescent opiate addicts. *Psychiatric Quarterly,* **28,** 1954a, 113–125.

Gerard, D. L. and **Kornetsky, C.** Adolescent opiate addiction; A case study. *Psychiatric Quarterly,* **28,** 1954b, 367–380.

Gerard, D. L. and **Kornetsky, C.** Adolescent opiate addiction: A study of control and addict subjects. *Psychiatric Quarterly,* **29,** 1955, 457–486.

Goldberg, S. R. and **Schuster, C. R.** Conditioned suppression by a stimulus associated with nalorphine in morphine-dependent monkeys. *Journal of the Experimental Analysis of Behavior,* **10,** 1967, 235–242.

Grinspoon, L. *Marihuana Reconsidered.* Cambridge, Harvard University Press, 1971.

Harris, L. S., Munson, A. E., Friedman, M. A., and **Dewey, W. L.** Retardation of tumor growth by Δ^9-tetrahydrocannabinol (Δ^9-THC). *Pharmacologist,* **16,** 1974, 259.

Hill, H. E., Haertzen, C. A., and **Glaser, R.** Personality characteristics of narcotic addicts as indicated by the MMPI. *Journal of General Psychology,* **62,** 1960, 127–139.

Hofmann, A. Psychotomimetic drugs chemical and pharmacological aspects. *Acta Physiologica et Pharmacologica Neerlandica,* **8,** 1959, 240–258.

Isbell, H., Gorodetsky, G. W., Jasinksi, D., Claussen, U., Spulak, F., and **Korte, F.** Effects of (−) delta-9-trans-tetrahydrocannabinol in man. *Psychopharmacologia (Berlin),* **11,** 1967, 184–188.

Jaffe, J. H. Drug addiction and drug abuse. In L. S. Goodman and A. Gilman (Eds.) *The Pharmacological Basis of Therapeutics.* (3rd ed.). New York, Macmillan, 1965, pp. 285–311.

Jaffe, J. H. Drug addiction and drug abuse. In L. S. Goodman and A. Gilman (Eds.) *The Pharmacological Basis of Therapeutics.* (4th ed.). New York, Macmillan, 1970, pp. 276–313.

Jaffe, J. H. Multimodality approaches to the treatment and prevention of opiate addiction. In S. Fisher and A. M. Freedman (Eds.) *Opiate Addiction: Origins and Treatment.* Washington, D.C., Winston 1973, pp. 127–140.

Jarvik, M. E. The behavioral effects of psychotogens. In R. C. DeBold and R. C. Leaf (Eds.) *LSD, Man and Society.* Middletown, Connecticut Wesleyan, 1968.

Jarvik, M. E. Drugs used in the treatment of psychiatric disorders. In L. S. Goodman and A. Gilman (Eds.) *The Pharmacological Basis of Therapeutics.* (4th ed.). New York, Macmillan, 1970, pp. 151–203.

Jernigan, A. J. A Rorschach study of normal and psychotic subjects in a situation of stress. Ph.D. dissertation, University of Kentucky, 1951.

Jones, E. *The Life and Work of Sigmund Freud,* Vol. *I* (1856–1900). New York, Basic Books, 1953.

Khantzian, E. J. Opiate Addiction: A critique of theory and some implications for treatment. *American Journal of Psychotherapy,* **28,** 1974, 59–70.

REFERENCES

Klüver, H. *Mescal and Mechanisms of Hallucinations.* Chicago, University of Chicago Press, 1966.

Kornetsky, C. and Bain, G. Morphine: Single-dose tolerance. *Science,* 162, 1968, 1011–1012.

Lasagna, L. Addicting drugs and medical practice; Toward the elaboration of realistic goals and the eradication of myths, mirages and half-truths. In D. M. Wilner and G. K. Kassenbaum (Eds.) *Narcotics.* New York, McGraw-Hill 1965, pp. 53–66.

Maugh, T. H., II. Marihuana: The grass may no longer be greener. *Science,* 185, 1974, 683–685.

Maugh, T. H., II. Marihuana (II): Does it damage the brain? *Science,* 185, 1974, 775–776.

Mayor's Committee on Marihuana. *The Marihuana Problem in the City of New York.* Lancaster, Pennsylvania, 1944, pp. 65–132.

McGlothlin, W. H. Hallucinogenic drugs: A perspective with special reference to peyote and cannabis. *Psychedelic Review,* 6, 1965, 16–57.

McGlothlin, W. H. and West, L. J. The marihuana problem; An overview. *American Journal of Psychiatry,* 125, 1968, 370–378.

Meyer, R. E. *A Guide to Drug Rehabilitation—A Public Health Response.* Boston, Beacon, 1972.

Musto, D. F. *The American Disease—Origins of Narcotic Control.* New Haven, Yale University Press, 1973.

Nahas, G. G. *Marihuana—Deceptive Weed.* New York, Raven, 1973.

National Commission. *Marihuana: A Single of Misunderstanding.* First Report of the National Commission on Marihuana and Drug Abuse, U. S. Government Printing Office. Washington, D.C., 1972.

Ritchie, J. M., Cohen, P. J., and Dripps, R. D. Cocaine; Procaine and other synthetic local anesthetics. In L. S. Goodman and A. Gilman (Eds.) *The Pharmacological Basis of Therapeutics.* (4th ed.). New York, Macmillan, 1970, pp. 371–401.

Robins, L. N. *The Vietnam Drug User Returns.* Special Action Office Monograph Executive Office of the President, Special Office for Drug Abuse Prevention. U. S. Government Printing Office. Series A, No. 2, Washington, D.C., May 1974.

Rossi, A. M., Mendelson, J. H., and Meyer, R. Experimental analysis of marihuana acquisition and use. In J. H. Mendelson, A. M. Rossi, and R. Meyer (Eds.) *The Use of Marihuana—A Psychological and Physiological Inquiry.* New York, Plenum, 1974, pp. 25–43.

Roth, W. T., Tinklenberg, J. R., Whitaker, C. A., Darley, C. F., Kopell, B. S., and Hollister, L. E. The effect of marihuana on tracking task performance. *Psychopharmacologia,* 33, 1973, 259–265.

Snyder, S. *Use of Marijuana.* New York, Oxford University Press, 1971.

Tashkin, D. P., Shapiro, B. J., and Frank, I. M. Acute pulmonary physiologic effects of smoked marihuana and oral Δ9-tetrahydrocannabinol in healthy young men. *New England Journal of Medicine,* 289, 1973, 336–341.

Tashkin, D. P., Shapiro, B. J., and Frank, I. M. Acute effects of smoked marihuana and oral Δ9-tetrahydrocannabinol on specific airway conductance in asthmatic subjects. *American Review of Respiratory Disease,* 109, 1974, 420–428.

Tashkin, D. P., Shapiro, B. J., Lee, Y. E., and Harper, C. E. Subacute effects of heavy marihuana smoking on pulmonary function. *New England Journal of Medicine,* 294, 1976, 125–129.

Vachon, L. The smoke in marihuana smoking. *New England Journal of Medicine,* 294, 1976, 160–161.

Vachon, L., FitzGerald, M. X., Solliday, N. H., Gould, I. A., and Gaensler, E. A. Single-dose effect of marihuana smoke—bronchial dynamics and respiratory—center sensitivity in normal subjects. *New England Journal of Medicine,* **288,** 1973, 985–989.

Vachon, L., Mikus, P., Morrissey, W., FitzGerald, M., and **Gaensler, E.** Bronchial effects of marihuana smoke in asthma. In S. Szara and M. Braude (Eds.) *Proceedings of the International Conference on the Pharmacology of Marihuana.* New York, Raven, 1976, in press.

Vachon, L. and **Sulkowski, A.** Attention, learning, and speed in psychomotor performance. In S. Szara and M. Braude (Eds.) *Proceedings of the International Conference on the Pharmacology of Marihuana.* New York, Raven, 1976, in press.

Vachon, L., Sulkowski, A., and **Rich, E.** Marihuana effects on learning, attention, and time estimation. *Psychopharmacologia (Berlin),* **39,** 1974, 1–11.

Valle, J. R., Lapa, A. J., and **Barros, G. G.** Pharmacological activity of cannabis according to the sex of the plant. *Journal of Pharmacy and Pharmacology,* **20,** 1968, 798–799.

Ward, P. M. and **Hutt, P. P.** *Dealing With Drug Abuse, A Report to the Ford Foundation.* New York, Praeger, 1972.

Weil, A. T., Zinberg, N. E., and **Nelsen, J. M.** Clinical and psychological effects of marihuana in man. *Science,* **162,** 1968, 1234–1242.

Wikler, A. A psychodynamic study of patients during experimental self-regulated readdiction to morphine. *Psychiatric Quarterly,* **26,** 1952, 270–293.

Wikler, A. Dynamics of drug dependence: Implications of a conditioning theory for research and treatment. *Archives of General Psychiatry,* **28,** 1973a, 611–616.

Wikler, A. Dynamics of drug dependence: Implications of a conditioning theory for research and treatment. In S. Fisher, and A. M. Freedman (Eds.) *Opiate Addiction: Origins and Treatment.* Washington, D.C., Winston 1973b, pp. 7–21.

Wikler, A. and **Pescor, F. T.** Classical conditioning of a morphine abstinence phenomenon, reinforcement of opioid-drinking behavior and "relapse" in morphine-addicted rats. *Psychopharmacologia (Berlin),* **10,** 1967, 255–284.

Wurmser, L. Methadone and the craving for narcotics: Observations of patients on methadone maintenance in psychotherapy. *Proceedings of the National Conference on Methadone Treatment, 4th,* 1972, 525.

13 MINIMAL BRAIN DYSFUNCTION (THE HYPERKINETIC SYNDROME) AND DRUGS

Most teachers find a certain joy and satisfaction in teaching most students. However, since the time of the first classroom there probably have always been a few children who seem to be unable to learn or do not seem to want to learn. This has been the special problem of the educator, and in recent years society has been turning to the use of various pharmacological agents as adjuncts to the educational process in some children. The use of drugs has not been without its problems. Its detractors have pointed out that drugs are being used as substitutes for good teaching practices and for keeping the difficult child "doped up"; they say that it leads to drug abuse, and that it is part of a plan of the majority to enslave the minority.

The physician who is asked by parents to treat their child because of a behavior disorder is faced with a difficult problem. The putative pathological condition may not be pathological in the manner that physicians define pathology. The condition is not as easily defined as when the presenting symptoms are fever and an inflamed throat. He is confronted with a pattern of behavior in which the degree of abnormality is relative to the total behavioral manifestations of a child who comes from a particular background and social class.

For many children in our society the first recognition of a behavior problem is by the teacher. As our social and educational programs improve, the physician will be asked, if not compelled, to attend to children who have rarely been seen by a physician. These are children whose mothers did not seek out a physician from the moment of conception, whose prenatal care was not instituted until the mother was in labor, whose contact with physicians may have only been in a hospital emergency room, whose mothers are not aware of the

---

Some material in this chapter originally appeared in my chapter "Minimal Brain Dysfunction and Drugs," in *Perceptual and Learning Disabilities in Children,* edited by William M. Cruickshank and Daniel P. Hallahan (Syracuse: Syracuse University Press, 1975), Vol. 2, *Research and Theory,* pp. 447–81.

latest (not necessarily the best) child-rearing practices. The fact that a child is hyperactive or withdrawn in the classroom or does not learn may, in many instances, be more of a social problem than one of psychopathology or pathology or organic disease.

Despite the difficulties in diagnosis, the point of view that I will present in this chapter is that drugs are useful in some children with certain types of learning disabilities. They are not a panacea and they can never substitute for good teaching practices.

For the most part, the drugs that have been employed in the treatment of the condition called minimal brain dysfunction (MBD) have been the drugs that are classified as central nervous system stimulants. The two most common CNS stimulants used are the amphetamines and methylphenidate (Ritalin). There have been clinical reports of the usefulness of some of the phenothiazine drugs, drugs used in the treatment of schizophrenia, as well as some of the drugs used in the treatment of depression. The latter two classes of drugs are not classified as CNS stimulants, although the antidepressant drugs do have some similarity in mechanism of action with the amphetamines.

The present chapter discusses the syndrome called minimal brain dysfunction, the pharmacology of the drugs used in treating MBD, effects of the drugs on the MBD child, and finally the socio-political implications of drug therapy. No attempt is made to be all-inclusive. The reader is referred to the following reviews for further reading on the use of drugs in children: Grant (1962), Eisenberg (1966), Millichap and Fowler (1967), Millichap (1968), Werry (1968), Fish (1968), Cole (1969), Conners (1971), and Millichap (1973), and to a recent book by Wender (1971) and a report of the New York Academy of Sciences (De La Cruz, Fox, and Roberts, 1973) for detailed reviews of the various aspects of MBD.

DRUGS

Amphetamines

The amphetamines belong to the general class of compounds called sympathomimetic amines. Drugs of this group have actions in the peripheral nervous system that are, more or less, similar to those seen when the sympathetic branch of the autonomic nervous system is stimulated (see Chapter 10).

Methylphenidate Hydrochloride (Ritalin)

Methylphenidate is considered the drug of choice in the treatment of the minimal brain dysfunction (MBD) child by many clinicians (Millichap, 1973) because of its putative lesser tendency than amphetamines to cause anorexia. Methylphenidate is a mild CNS stimulant. It has many of the same sympathomi-

DRUGS

metic actions as the amphetamines. However, respiration and blood pressure seem to be affected less than with amphetamine at doses that cause central stimulation.

Magnesium Pemoline (Cylert)

Pemoline is a CNS stimulant that is structurally distinguishable from amphetamine and methylphenidate. Despite this difference, it does cause many of the same side effects seen with the other CNS stimulants used in the treatment of MBD. The most common side effects are anorexia and insomnia. As of this writing, it has only been approved for investigational use for the treatment of hyperkinetic syndrome in the United States. It is very likely that it will soon receive approval by the FDA for clinical use. It has already received approval for clinical use in the United Kingdom in the treatment of the MBD child.

Phenothiazines

The phenothiazines are a class of compounds used mostly in the treatment of schizophrenic patients. Although some success has been reported with these compounds in the treatment of the MBD child, they have proved to be significantly poorer as therapeutic agents in the treatment of the hyperkinetic child.

The two most commonly used drugs of this class have been chlorpromazine (Thorazine) and thioridazine (Mellaril). These drugs are not CNS stimulants and seem to make use of their central-depressant effects in decreasing hyperkinesis. The most common side effect seen in the MBD child treated with phenothazines is drowsiness; however, these drugs are capable of causing a number of other side effects, some of which are only bothersome, such as dry mouth and nasal stuffiness; however, others, such as skin rash, jaundice, extrapyramidal effects, and blood dyscrasias, may be dangerous to life. As far as this writer is aware, these more severe effects have not been reported in the MBD child treated with phenothiazines. The lack of serious side effects may be due to the relatively low doses of phenothiazines used as compared to doses used in the treatment of the schizophrenic patient and/or the fact that relatively few MBD children have been treated with these drugs (see Chapter 5).

Chlordiazepoxide (Librium)

Chlordiazepoxide is a minor tranquilizer used primarily for the treatment of anxiety. It is a member of a class of drugs called benzodiazepines. Two other drugs of this class are extensively used in the treatment of the anxious patient. These are diazepam (Valium) and oxazepam (Serax). In addition to their putative antianxiety properties, the benzodiazepines have skeletal muscle-relaxing properties. The major side effects are drowsiness and ataxia. More severe but less frequent side effects are nausea and skin rash (see Chapter 6).

Antidepressants

The antidepressant that has been most commonly used in the treatment of MBD is imipramine (Tofranil). Among the side effects of imipramine are dry mouth, nasal stuffiness, hypotension, constipation, and urine retention. The latter effect led to its use in the treatment of enuretic children. The incidence of side effects is relatively high with this drug. In one study reviewed by Millichap (1973) side effects were observed in nineteen of 52 children given the drug (see Chapter 6).

Summary

In a number of studies reviewed by Millichap (1973) it was clear that either methylphenidate or amphetamine was superior, both in therapeutic outcome and, in many cases, in terms of fewer side effects, to the other drugs used. It must be remembered that drug effects are dose related, that is, the larger the dose the greater the effect. This is true for the therapeutic action of the drug as well as the unwanted side effects. The ideal medication will produce the wanted therapeutic action with no or minimal side effects. Some side effects are not dose related but are due to idiosyncratic responses of an individual to a drug. Also, it must be remembered that not all individuals show the same sensitivity to drugs. Some patients will respond therapeutically at relatively low doses, whereas others require larger doses. This holds true not only for the therapeutic action but also for the side effects of a drug. Often, a patient will not respond to one drug or will have excessive side effects but will respond very favorably to another drug that is quite similar in action.

MINIMAL BRAIN DYSFUNCTION (MBD)

Behavior

The MBD syndrome has come to be used synonymously with the constellation of symptoms and signs that has been called hyperkinesis. The term hyperkinesis (also hyperkinesia) literally means pathological excessive motion. Clinically, MBD refers to children who are characterized by restlessness and hyperactivity, distractability and poor attention span, low frustration tolerance and emotional lability, as well as aggressive behavior. MBD is not associated with low intelligence; however, there are learning or behavioral impairments. These deviations will manifest themselves by various combinations of perceptual, conceptual, language, or memory impairment.

The difficulty with the above description of the MBD syndrome is that the terms used to define the characteristics are terms used to describe, to a lesser or greater degree, the behavior of all children at some time. That is, the normal child will not manifest all of these characteristics at the same time, but the normal child shows some hyperactivity or distractibility, exhibits emotional lability, or may have had difficulty with learning. This use of terms that describe most children at some time, probably has led to a great deal of confusion, the overdiagnosing of MBD, as well as the failure to recognize it in many cases.

The syndrome may be organized as dysfunction in the following areas of behavior: motor activity and coordination, attention and cognitive function, impulse control, interpersonal relations, and emotionality. The child may not show equal dysfunction in all of these areas of behavior, but the extent of dysfunctioning will be consistent and severe so that parents usually report a long history of disturbed behavior. Parents report that the child was active and restless during infancy, stood and walked early, "... and then, like an infant King Kong, burst the bars of his crib asunder and sallied forth to destroy his parents' house." (Wender, 1971, p. 12). He would often break his toys, and it was often a struggle for the parents to preserve the physical integrity of the household from the inadvertent assault of the child. Colic during infancy as well as sleep disturbances and feeding problems have been reported (Stewart et al., 1966). Increase in motor activity is often accompanied by increase in verbal activity that lacks a focus. Many of the children exhibit significant incoordination, the two left hands and two left feet syndrome. However, there are many reported histories of MBD children with good athletic ability. Although many walk at an early age, they have a history of being described as clumsy. The child is slow to learn to tie his shoelaces or ride a two-wheeled bicycle, and buttons are a challenge. The child's handwriting is usually poor.

The MBD child seems unable to concentrate and maintain attention. The child does not engage in the same activity for any length of time and quickly moves from one thing to another. Failure to attend in the classroom situation is often labeled "daydreaming" by teachers. The "daydreaming" is not characterized by a richness of fantasy but is more often the anticipation of activities once released from the confines of the school. Poor performance in school may be a function of this seeming inability to focus attention or concentrate; however, there may be learning difficulties associated with dyslexia among the MBD children.

Although learning difficulties are one of the most common difficulties of the MBD children, poor performance in school is not diagnostic of MBD. Unfortunately, there are many reasons "why Johnny won't learn" besides the possibility of MBD. Wender (1971, p. 16) states, without documentation, that one-half to two-thirds of MBD children manifest learning difficulties in school and "... that among children with normal intelligence and with good school experience MBD is a very frequent source of academic difficulty." Among children diagnosed as dyslexic, a heterogeneous group, the single most common subgroup consists of children with MBD. Unfortunately, the specific data to confirm this statement of Wender is not available, except that repeated studies have shown that poor school performance is one of the most characteristic behaviors of the MBD child.

MBD children often show marked differences in emotionality and impulse control as compared to normal children. They are often reckless and seem to show no concern for their own safety. This leads to frequent injuries and reports that the child is accident prone. They show a low level of tolerance to frustration, often responding violently to small frustrations. They often show evidence of emotional problems as manifested in irritability, acute anxiety, aggressiveness, depression, and a lack of responsiveness to external controls. Whether these symptoms are primary is unknown. However, it is more likely that the lack of impulse control may be primary, and this, plus many of the other factors, certainly could lead to some of the emotional symptoms seen.

Neurological Signs

Benton (1973) has characterized MBD as "... a behavioral concept with neurological implications." Benton notes that a patient can have clear evidence of a disease of the brain without any observable evidence of functional abnormality. However, a child cannot have MBD without behavioral manifestations. Furthermore, the term MBD implies that there is a cerebral abnormality that is the primary basis for the behavior. In this section some of the evidence of central nervous system bases is discussed for at least some of the children who are called hyperkinetic or MBD.

Many investigators have investigated the possibility of central nervous system pathology. It is generally agreed that there is an increased prevalence of soft neurological signs in the MBD child. One or more of the following soft signs will be revealed in neurological examination of the MBD child: abnormalities of resting muscle tone, some clumsiness of either gross or fine motor movements, hyperactive deep-tendon reflexes, extensor plantar responses, abnormal extraocular movement, frequent tics and grimaces, disturbed position sense, choreiform movements, dyskinesias, mild ataxia, minimal gait abnormalities with asymmetries of associated movement, left-right confusion, poor visual motor skills, dyslexia. There does not seem to be any relationship between hard neurological signs and the MBD syndrome. Soft neurological signs are slight and often inconsistently present. They are not associated with specific neural pathology. (For a more detailed listing of neurological signs see Clements, 1966, p. 12.)

Soft neurological signs are not diagnostic of MBD. They occur in a relatively high percentage of normal children; however, it is believed that 50 percent of MBD children show such soft signs (Wender, 1971, p. 27). Wikler, Dixon,

TABLE 1. TOTAL NEUROLOGICAL SOFT SIGNS

Subjects	Total soft signs	
All patients ($N = 24$)	92	$p < .01$
All controls (($N = 24$)	39	
Hyperactive patients ($N = 11$)	43	$p < .01$
Matched controls ($N = 11$)	21	
Nonhyperactive patients ($N = 9$)	33	$p < .01$
Matched controls ($N = 9$)	14	
Hyperactive patients ($N = 11$)	43	N.S.
Nonhyperactive patients ($N = 9$)	33	

Abstracted from Wikler, Dixon, and Parker, 1970.

and Parker (1970), in a study of 24 patient children with 24 matched controls, found that 20 of their control children had one or more soft neurological signs. In the patient group soft neurological signs were found in 22 of the 24 subjects. However, there was a total of 92 soft signs in the patients as compared to 30 in the normal group. In the Wikler, Dixon, and Parker study 24 children who had no evidence of classical neurological disease and who were referred to a psychiatric outpatient clinic because of a variety of scholastic and behavioral problems were compared to 24 matched control children. The age range of the children was 5 to 15 years. The control children were matched with the experimental children for age, race, sex, I.Q., and socioeconomic class. Of the 24 experimental children 11 were definitely considered hyperactive and 9 definitely hypoactive. Table 1 summarizes the total neurological soft signs reported by this group of investigators. It is of interest that even those children who were nonhyperactive showed a greater incidence of soft neurological signs than the appropriate matched controls.

EEG Findings

Stevens, Sachdev, and Milstein (1968) and Wikler, Dixon, and Parker (1970), in reviewing the literature going back to 1938, report that there is a repeated finding of EEG abnormality in children with behavior disorders. Most of the children sampled in these studies would meet the criteria of the MBD syndrome. In the studies reported by Stevens et al. the range of the mean percent of control children with abnormalities in the EEG was from 5 to 27 percent, whereas in the experimental series the range of mean percent of behavior-disordered children was from 35 to 73 percent. In the actual experimental study of Stevens et al. a total of 97 children, ages 6 to 16 years, had behavioral abnormalities that were, for the most part, compatible with the diagnosis of MBD. The control group consisted of 88 children matched to the experimental group with respect to age and sex, and they were matched for socioeconomic background as closely as possible. Control subjects were obtained from pediatric, medical, and orthopedic outpatient clinics of the hospital as well as from the schools. As in previously reported studies there was a significantly higher incidence of EEG abnormality in the experimental group than in the control group.

The study by Stevens et al. (1968) is of interest because of the detailed analysis of the EEG that was made as well as the investigators' search for EEG correlates of specific behavioral patterns. The authors comment that the presence or absence of abnormality in the EEG by itself is of little value in predicting clinical or etiological factors. However, their results suggest that there are relationships between specific behavioral traits, predisposing factors, and specific abnormalities in the EEG. For example, they found slowing of EEG frequencies was associated with hyperactivity, whereas EEG spike activity was associated with disturbances in attention, time sense, ideation, and finger agnosia.

The Wikler et al. (1970) study is somewhat unique, for not only did it compare behavior-problem children with matched controls but it compared hyperactive-behavior-problem children with nonhyperactive-behavior-problem children. In addition, this study compared these groups to matched controls. Also unique in the Wikler et al. study was that their analyses of the EEG took into account the age differences between the subjects. The primary finding of the study was the emergence of two relatively distinct syndromes. The first is characterized by hyperactive behavior, perceptual motor deficits, high incidence of soft neurological signs, and an EEG with excessive slow activity and abnormal transient discharges. The EEG changes were not age dependent. The second syndrome was similar in terms of soft neurological signs and excessive slow activity in the EEG; however, the latter was age dependent; that is, the amount of slow activity decreased with age. The group was different from the hyperactive group in their lack of hyperactivity and lack of perceptual motor deficits.

Satterfield, Cantwell, Lesser, and Podosin (1972) studied a group of 31 children diagnosed as hyperkinetic with a control group of 21 children matched for age. The mean age for both groups was 7.75 years with a range of 6 to 9 years. However, the groups differed significantly in I.Q. with a mean WISC score of 104 for the hyperkinetic children and 118 for the control children. They did not match each patient subject with a paired control subject as in the Wikler et al. study, and unfortunately, they do not describe the method used for obtaining the control group, though they go into a great deal of detail describing the criteria of selection of the hyperkinetic children. Although the method of EEG analysis was different than in the Wikler et al. study, the results were similar in that there was more slow-wave activity in the hyperkinetic children than in the control group.

From the results of various neurological studies of behavior-problem children, it would seem that it is difficult to accept the view that these children are not suffering from some central nervous system abnormality. In general, most EEG studies report slowing of the EEG as one of the most common characteristics, and in the study by Stevens et al. (1968) there is strong evidence that specific behavior patterns are correlated with specific abnormalities of the EEG.

One of the clearest experimental demonstrations that the MBD child has a CNS that is abnormally sensitive to stimulation is an experiment by Laufer, Denhoff, and Solomons (1957). As far as this writer knows, no one, including the original investigators, ever replicated this experiment. Considering the procedure used, the failure to replicate this study is understandable. The thesis was that a dysfunction of the diencephalon is related to the hyperkinetic syndrome. The procedure that was used was the photo-Metrazol technique of Gastant (1950) and Gastant and Hunter (1950). The procedure consists of determining the threshold dose of pentylenetetrazol (Metrazol) in mg/kg of body weight necessary to cause EEG spike-wave bursts and myoclonic jerking of the forearms when the patient was subjected to stroboscopic stimulation. In human and animal subjects the threshold was lower in those subjects in which there was some dysfunction of subcortical areas.

Laufer and his co-workers studied 32 children who were diagnosed as hyperkinetic impulse disordered, with 11 of the 32 having an unequivocal history of brain organicity. The remaining 18 children had a diagnosis of behavior disorders other than the hyperkinetic syndrome. The results of this study are of considerable interest, for it is the only study that has come to my attention where there was direct experimental manipulation of the CNS. These investigators found a significant separation between the hyperkinetic and nonhyperkinetic groups (see Table 2). Although it was possible to identify the hyperkinetic children with a history of organic brain damage from those without such a his-

TABLE 2. COMPARISON OF THE NUMBER OF HYPERKINETIC AND NONHYPERKINETIC CHILDREN WHO WERE ABOVE AND BELOW THE MEDIAN OF THE PHOTO-METRAZOL THRESHOLD DOSE

Number	Above Median	Below Median	Total
Hyperkinetic children	9	23	32
Nonhyperkinetic children	16	2	18

Abstracted from Laufer, Denhoff, and Solomons, 1957.

tory, both groups together differed from the nonhyperkinetic group. Of further interest is that these investigators selected 13 of the hyperkinetic children who had a low pentylenetetrazol threshold to the photic stimulation and repeated the procedure with and without d-amphetamine. The control threshold value in this group was 4.8 mg/kg of pentylenetetrazol, whereas after d-amphetamine the threshold mean was 6.7 mg/kg. This difference was statistically significant. It is unfortunate that these investigators did not do the same d-amphetamine experiment with some of their nonhyperkinetic subjects. This additional experiment would have allowed them to determine whether a real paradoxical effect exists, at least as far as the excitability of the central nervous system is concerned.

Etiology

Wender (1971, pp. 37–43; and 1972) reviewed the evidence, suggesting that the MBD syndrome was due to organic brain damage and/or a genetic factor. He concluded that there was a well-documented association between complications in pregnancy and during birth and the later manifestation of MBD syndrome. Wender points out that despite this association of the MBD syndrome (as well as other behavior pathology) with complications of pregnancy, most children who could be described as at risk escape such pathology and do not become symptomatic. Why some children seem to escape possible consequences of this early insult is not presently known. The failure of many children who are at risk, due to complicated pregnancy or birth, to manifest subsequent behavioral disorders speaks well for the resiliency of the biological system. However, there may be sequelae of this early assault that are either subtle enough that they are not noticed, or it may be that our instruments for measuring human behavior are not sensitive enough to measure these slight impairments. Another possibility is that the early prenatal and perinatal assault may cause specific organic alteration in the CNS, but as a result of the tremendous redundancy of the biological system, these "lesions" of the CNS are of no significant consequence.

There is reason to believe that specific toxic substances ingested during pregnancy or during early infancy could be responsible for some of the later behavioral manifestations. Two recent reports of studies in rats and mice in which varying concentrations of lead were given to nursing mothers yielded significant changes in the chemistry of the brains (Sauerhoff and Michaelson, 1973) and alteration in the behavior (Silbergeld and Goldberg, 1973) of the offspring. In the Silbergeld and Goldberg study there was an increase in the motor behavior of the mice that had a high lead content in the diet which could be reversed by the administration to the animal of appropriate doses of d-amphetamine, l-amphetamine, or methylphenidate (Silbergeld and Goldberg,

1974). Phenobarbital not only did not attenuate this hyperactivity of the mice but caused a further increase in their activity.

Wender (1971, pp. 40–43) suggests a possible genetic etiology in some instances of MBD. However, he bases this possibility on three clinical observations not documented by published studies. He has observed: (1) a "pronounced clustering" of MBD within the same family, (2) an apparent higher incidence of severe psychopathology in the parents of MBD children, and (3) a few instances of the syndrome in adopted children whose biological parents had severe psychopathological disturbances. Wender does point out that there seems to be a familial clustering of dyslexia, a specific reading disorder that is often associated with MBD. There are two studies demonstrating such a familial relationship of dyslexia, the most recent published in 1967 (Hallgren, 1950; Frisk et al., 1967). Considering the recent increase in the identification and interest in the dyslexic child, it is somewhat surprising that there would not have been additional studies on the familial aspects of dyslexia. Dyslexia is a specific reading disability that indicates some failure in cerebral organization, so that if there are familial factors, it might be relatively easy to identify them. However, MBD is a constellation of symptoms, and what we call MBD may be a number of diseases, each with its own etiology. Also, some of those children diagnosed as MBD may not be suffering from anything more than misdiagnosis.

The fact that many MBD children respond favorably to stimulant drugs has led some to cite this as qualified support for the concept that the disease is due to some biochemical abnormality that is reversed by the drug (Wender, 1972). Wender does point out that response to treatment is not proof of etiology, since the treatment may reverse abnormalities anywhere ". . . from the primary abnormality through its causal chain." However, despite that qualification, he does state, ". . . the drug responsiveness of MBD children does suggest a fairly specific biochemical lesion." Thus if we knew how amphetamines or other stimulants work in the MBD child, we might know the cause of the disorder. However, the specific mechanism of action of amphetamine or other central nervous system stimulants in decreasing hyperkinetic behavior is not known. Common sense would suggest that a central nervous system stimulant, if anything, would make the hyperkinetic child worse, and the drug of choice would be one of the central nervous system depressants such as a barbiturate. Laufer and Denhoff (1957), in reviewing the literature on drug treatment of the MBD child, reported that not only are barbiturates ineffective but they often result in an increase of the behavior problems of the child; the ". . . reaction is so marked as almost to provide a specific diagnostic test itself." Eisenberg (1966), in reviewing the pharmacotherapy of the MBD child, states that barbiturates are contraindicated because of the frequency of paradoxical excitement they may cause in these children.

Hyper- versus Hypoarousal

Until recently, it was generally accepted that the MBD child is both behaviorally and centrally hyperaroused and that the therapeutic response to CNS stimulants is a paradoxical effect. However, recent research has begun to question the central hyperarousal model. Stevens, Sachdev, and Milstein (1968) found a relationship between hyperactivity and inattentiveness and the slowing of cortical EEG frequencies recorded from the occipital area. Wikler, Dixon, and Parker (1970) reported that the MBD child showed an increase in low-frequency waves when compared to a control group. Slow waves in the EEG are usually associated with hypoarousal. The impairment on various psychological tests, especially those that putatively measure attention (Conners and Rothschild, 1968; Sprague, Barnes, and Werry, 1970) could be interpreted as either hypo- or hyperarousal, thus the psychological test data by itself gives us no clue as to the central arousal state of the child. Further evidence supporting the hypoarousal theory can be found in the results of experiments by Satterfield and Dawson (1971). These investigators studied the galvanic skin response (GSR) in 24 hyperkinetic children. The GSR gives two resistance measures, the basal resistance level and the change in resistance to a specific stimulus (this is the actual GSR). Satterfield and Dawson found that basal resistance levels were higher than those in a normal control group. Higher basal levels are considered a measure of low arousal. They also found that the response to specific stimuli was less than the controls and that there were fewer spontaneous GSRs than in the normal child.

These studies suggesting hypoarousal are in conflict with the previously mentioned experimental results of Laufer et al. (1957). By means of the photo-Metrazol test, Laufer and collaborators directly tested the responsivity of the central nervous system of the hyperkinetic child and found a lower threshold for sensory stimulation that was reversed by amphetamine (see page 231). The apparent paradoxical effect of amphetamines in the centrally aroused subject may be more apparent than real. Connors (1966) and Conners and Rothschild (1968) also suggested that the action of the CNS stimulants in the hyperkinetic child is not a true paradoxical effect but merely one of the characteristics of this class of compounds. The CNS stimulants, in addition to their general exciting action, also cause an increase in focused attention. If the drug does have as its major action the ability to focus attention, then responses to interfering stimuli would be decreased, and this could result in the child being more amenable to positive reinforcement by both parents and teachers.

DRUG TREATMENT

In this section studies in which drugs have been used in the treatment of the MBD child are briefly reviewed.

DRUG TREATMENT

Although there are probably reports in the literature prior to 1937 in which children with behavior disorders were treated with drugs, most reviews of the field take as their starting point a report by Charles Bradley (1937) on the effects of amphetamine. It is of some historical interest that Matthew Molitch and August Eccles (1937) published a report on the effects of amphetamine on intelligence test scores in behavior-problem children in the same month and in the same journal in which Bradley's paper appeared. Molitch published another paper on the same subject the same year (Molitch and Sullivan, 1937). Despite the apparently simultaneous reports of Bradley and Molitch and his co-workers, Bradley is usually given credit for the discovery of the use of amphetamines in the treatment of behavior problems in children.

Bradley reported in his 1937 paper that Benzedrine (amphetamine) caused a "spectacular" improvement in school performance in 15 out of 30 children studied. He stated that ". . . a large proportion became subdued without losing interest in their surroundings." This paper was followed a few years later by a report by Bradley and Bowen (1940) on the effects of amphetamine on schoolroom performance. They reported that the drug improved performance in arithmetic, but the drug only had variable effects on spelling performance. The 1940 paper was quickly followed by a report by Bradley and Bowen (1941) of the use of amphetamine in the treatment of 100 hospitalized problem children. The drug caused a subdued type of behavior in 54 of the children, failed to have any effect in 21 of the children, caused behavioral stimulation in 19 of the children, and improved school performance in 6 of the children with no evidence of side effects. Bradley and Bowen suggested that the drug altered the child's emotional reaction to irritating situations rather than causing any direct effect on the specific behavior problem.

In the two 1937 studies by Molitch and collaborators one of the reports dealt with 93 males, age 11 to 17, whereas the other reported results in which 96 males of the same age range were studied. It is not clear from the reports whether the subjects used in the first study were included in the second. In these studies a placebo was used as a control for the medication. Molitch and his co-workers found that more of the subjects showed an improvement in their performance on an intelligence test after receiving amphetamine than after receiving a placebo. No statistical analyses of the data were done in these early studies. This could be considered fortunate or unfortunate depending on whether the reader believes that amphetamines are useful in treating behavior problems.

Among the early workers with amphetamine in children was Lauretta Bender (Bender and Collington, 1942). Although she used no objective measures in her studies, she was impressed with the results achieved with amphetamine and wrote, ". . . Benzedrine is a useful adjunct to the treatment of the neurotic child in that it gives him a feeling of well being and temporarily allows him to feel secure and loved."

Lindsley and Henry (1942) reported the effects of amphetamine, diphenylhydantoin (Dilantin), and phenobarbital on the behavior and EEG in 13 subjects, 8 to 12 years of age, with behavior problems. The behavior problems included negativism, hyperactivity, impulsiveness, destructiveness, aggression, and distractibility (all symptoms used to describe the MBD child). Only amphetamine and diphenylhydantoin were effective in ameliorating the symptoms, with amphetamine the more effective drug of the two. The EEGs of the children who were considered abnormal prior to treatment did not reflect the improvement in behavior. These early studies did not have all the appropriate controls that are considered a necessary part of a modern clinical study of a drug. Statistical analyses yielding an unacceptable probability level could have precluded work with amphetamines as a pharmacotherapy of behavior problems for many years.

Fisher (1959) and Fish (1968), in reviewing research in child psychopharmacology published in English up to 1959, reported that out of 159 studies only 33 contained ". . . some aspect of experimental design." Among these 33 reports, 13 were primarily studies of adults or of neurological disorders. Of the remaining studies all were flawed to some degree except for 3 that could be considered acceptable by present standards. Freeman (1966), in reviewing drug studies on learning in children, concluded that ". . . it remains difficult to draw firm conclusions about the influence of drugs on learning behavior."

Millichap and Fowler (1967) took a more sanguine attitude. They felt that despite the lack of scientific acceptability in many of the studies, some drugs consistently proved to be useful. During the past ten years there have been a number of studies that have met the criteria of the more rigorous clinical pharmacologists and that have demonstrated effectiveness of these drugs in improving performance on a variety of cognitive, perceptual, and psychomotor tests.

Problems in Research

Conners (1971), reviewing some of the problems inherent in research with drugs in children, states that there are special problems that are not found in research with adults, plus all the difficulties that are found in drug experimentation in man. Since the research is always within a clinical treatment context, it may not be feasible to meet all the criteria needed for good experimental design. The heterogeneity of the diagnostic characteristics of the children under study may be impossible to control. This leads to a large diagnostic variability, or the experimenter is forced to study very small samples. Conners goes on to state that treatment studies of children are influenced to a greater degree by the immediate family as well as the school environment than are such studies of adults.

Organicity as a Prediction of Response to Drugs

Many of the studies of the MBD child, including some of the earlier ones, looked for organic etiology as well as for the presence of some signs of organicity. As already mentioned, the incidence of soft neurological signs is higher in the MBD child than in comparable control groups. The later studies attempted, in a systematic manner, to look for specific behavioral deficits in this group of children as well as specific deficits that would most likely respond to pharmacotherapy. The MBD syndrome is seen in children with a history of possible organic etiology including birth trauma, encephalitis, and head injury. However, the syndrome is also seen in children who present no clear-cut history of organic factors. It was suggested as early as 1942 that only the more "organic" group responds to pharmacotherapy (Lindsley and Henry, 1942) and later by Lytton and Knobel (1959). Subsequent studies have indicated that MBD children with and without organic signs respond to drug treatment; however, there does seem to be a better response to drug therapy in the "organic" than the "nonorganic" MBD children (Epstein et al., 1968).

Attention

Psychopharmacological studies that have attempted to delineate the action of drugs in the hyperkinetic child or the child with learning disabilities have focused on those actions usually associated with learning skills. For anyone to learn or perform any task, the first factor that is necessary, but certainly not sufficient, is the ability to attend to the task. Unless the attention is maintained in the task at hand, no learning or successful performance can take place. Sprague and Sleator (1973), summarizing their own work as well as the work of others, observe that sustained attention is a particular impairment of the hyperkinetic child and that the central stimulants either reverse or ameliorate this deficit. Conners and Rothschild (1968) and Conners (1970) used a modified form of the Continuous Performance Test (CPT) (Rosvold et al., 1956) to study the effects of d-amphetamine or methylphenidate on attention or vigilance. They found that both d-amphetamine and methylphenidate decreased errors of omission and commission on these tasks.

Two more recent studies have made use of the Continuous Performance Test (Sykes, Douglas, and Weiss, 1971; and Sykes, Douglas, and Morgenstern, 1972). In these studies the performances of hyperactive and control children on the CPT were compared. These investigators found significant relative impairment in the hyperkinetic children that was reversed by methylphenidate. In one of the studies the researchers compared the performance of the children on an experimenter-paced task, the CPT, with a similar task in which the subject had control of the presentation of stimuli. On the experimenter-paced task the hyperkinetic children showed greater impairment, relative to the control subjects, than on the subject-paced task. This finding further supports the notion that there is a specific attentional dysfunction in the hyperkinetic child that is reversed by the central stimulants. Sprague, Barnes, and Werry (1970) studied the effects of methylphenidate or thioridazine on a vigilance task in 12 boys with a history of poor school performance. In this study classroom observation was made and performance data on the attention task was obtained. The investigators were interested in whether the objective performance data was predictive of what happens in the classroom. The child's task was to look at a number of pictures presented simultaneously for a brief exposure and then, after a lapse of a few seconds, indicate whether a particular picture was among those presented. This is a modification of the Continuous Performance Test. Methylphenidate significantly increased correct responding as well as speed of responding in the hyperkinetic children. In this study methylphenidate was compared to thioridazine (a phenothiazine drug). The latter drug caused the opposite effect, greater number of errors and slower response time. In these same children methylphenidate increased the hyperkinetic child's attention in the school situation, as measured by a standard observational scale, and, in addition, increased appropriate social behavior in the classroom.

Motor Activity

One of the most commonly reported behaviors of the MBD child is hyperactivity. A study reported by Millichap (1973) in which motor activity was measured before and after treatment with methylphenidate showed a marked reduction in activity following drug administration. However, this reduction in motor activity was most pronounced in those children who, prior to treatment, had the highest level of motor activity, and some of the children with the lowest activity level even showed an increase in activity when treated with methylphenidate.

Impulsive Behavior

Conners (1971) states that impulsive behavior is characteristic of many poor learners and that the drugs may enhance the child's ability to "... delay, plan, and respond in a more controlled, integrated manner." He goes on to state that this general "inhibitory" quality of medication "... is perhaps the single most important effect on behavior in children." This only slightly qualified unequivocal statement is based on the results that Conners and his colleagues obtained in studies in which the performance of children on the Porteus Maze was enhanced by amphetamine or methylphenidate (Conners, Eisenberg, and Barcai, 1967; Conners, Eisenberg, and Sharpe, 1964; Conners and Eisenberg, 1963; Conners et al., 1969; and Conners and Rothschild, 1968).

The Porteus Maze requires the subject to find his or her way with a pencil through a maze. Successful performance on the task seems to require some ability to plan ahead, and performance is correlated with other types of intelligence tests. Although the results of these studies are clear, what is not clear is the interpretation. Failure on the test could certainly be attributed to lack of attention, and improvement caused by drug could be attributed to the drug's ability to focus attention. This seems like a more parsimonious explanation than evoking some "inhibitory" action of the drug.

Motor Skills

The CNS stimulants also enhance performance on a variety of motor skill tests. These studies have measured hand steadiness and tapping speed (Conners, 1971). Conners suggests that the drugs may allow the child to exert greater control of his motor behavior or possibly increase the motivation of the child to perform well. The best evidence that Conners (1971) gives for the disinhibitory-inhibitory action of stimulants is in the study in which the CPT was used (Conners and Rothschild, 1968). The latency of responses to the critical stimulus was longer in the stimulant-treated children than in the placebo-treated children, whereas errors were greater in the latter group. Thus it was believed that the stimulant drugs reduced impulsive behavior that seems to be one of the characteristics of the MBD child.

Intelligence

There have been a few studies, starting with the one by Molitch and Eccles (1937), demonstrating that intelligence test scores of behavior- or learning-problem children are improved by treatment with CNS stimulants. Zimmerman and Burgermeister (1958) and Knights and Hinton (1968) reported improvement on the WISC performance I.Q. in children treated with methylphenidate, and Epstein, Lasagna, Conners, and Rodriguez (1968) obtained similar results with d-amphetamine. Since an intelligence test taps many functions, it is not clear what exactly is being improved with stimulant drugs. In the studies cited above improvement was found only on the performance scale of the WISC. Bradley and Green (1940) stated that in their results there were no striking I.Q. changes that could be attributed to stimulant drugs. This apparent contradiction in findings could be accounted for by a number of variables that include the sample of subjects used, the I.Q. test employed, and what is meant by "striking" or "significant" improvement.

School Performance

One of the major problems concerning the use of drugs is the heterogeneity of children with learning disabilities. Many children not specifically diagnosed as

MBD children but who seem to have learning disabilities and/or school behavior problems seem to respond to the CNS stimulants. Conners, Eisenberg, and Barcai (1967) conducted a systematic study specifically designed to determine whether a sample of children with learning problems who were not specifically selected because of psychiatric and neurological diagnoses would show improvement in school behavior (as determined by the teachers) when given *d*-amphetamine. The study was conducted in two elementary schools in the Baltimore area. The schools were in low-income areas of Baltimore, and all of the 52 children studied were black. The authors state that many of the problems reported by the teachers could be related to the ". . . condition of economic and cultural deprivation."

Table 3 lists the teachers' referral complaints of the children. Also many of the behaviors listed have been used to describe the MBD child. The authors used two dependent measures in their study of these children: teacher ratings and a number of objective situational tests. The teachers used a checklist

TABLE 3. EXAMPLES OF TEACHER REFERRAL COMPLAINTS

1. Poor study habits and always fails written tests. Is shy and slow when called on for oral recitation, but does not seem embarrassed when he cannot respond. Very defiant.
2. Very slow child. Does not respond to stimulation. Not an active member in the class.
3. Very restless and inattentive. Disturbs others most of the time.
4. Very inattentive. Has difficulty concentrating. Is failing in all subjects.
5. Sullen and sulky. Frequent behavior problem. Not emotionally or physically adjusted to his class.
6. Has outbursts of temper and laughter. Below-average skills in reading and language arts.
7. Very nervous and fidgety. Below average in reading. Frequently does not participate orally. Stutters a little.
8. Aggressive and bullying. Fights constantly. Seeks attention.
9. Inattentive, compulsive, talkative, aggressive, and stubborn.
10. Appears nervous but can keep still long. Very fidgety, very talkative. Likes to play with small objects.
11. Very arrogant and defiant. Has little respect for authority. Shows little effort. Exhibits very little self-control.
12. Very shy, withdrawn, does not socialize. Is very submissive. Does not engage in classroom activities.
13. Frequently daydreams. Very short attention span.
14. Poor reader. Restless. Playful. Often uncooperative. Has very poor work and social habits. Is a disturbing element in classroom. A poor achiever.

Abstracted from Conners, Eisenberg, and Barcai, 1967.

divided into three areas: classroom behavior, group participation, and attitude toward authority.

The experimental design called for a crossover treatment of 10-mg d-amphetamine or placebo. The study made use of a double-blind procedure. The duration of the study was two months, with active medication for one month and a placebo for one month. This study was most carefully designed to rule out teachers' expectations of benefits to be derived from drug treatment. The children who were selected exhibited behavior that teachers could not help but respond to negatively so that the mere presence of a research project in the school, in which the teachers were active participants, could lead to improvement independent of the drug. This is reflected in the significant order effect. That is, subjects were rated as improved even when receiving a placebo. However, the degree of improvement under placebo conditions was significantly less than that seen under drug treatment. Unfortunately, the authors did not directly compare the behavior scores prior to treatment to those scores after treatment. In addition, there were mean differences in the pretreatment scores between those subjects who received the drug first and those receiving the placebo first. No statistical results are presented to enable the reader to determine if these pretest differences were significant. The authors did make use of a covariance analysis using the pretest scores as the covariate so that their statistical analysis did control for pretest behavior scores.

The crossover design controlled for the possible teacher bias. Conners et al. (1967) added one additional important control that is often lacking in crossover-design experiments. They did not inform the teachers that such a crossover of treatments would take place. There are various levels of double blindness in drug studies, and if the observers know exactly when critical periods of the experiment occur, they cannot be considered blind, unbiased observers.

The authors confront another possible area of influence on the teacher ratings. There is the possibility that side effects caused by d-amphetamine would let the teacher know that a child was receiving the active medication and not the placebo. They point out that this type of bias is controlled by the unannounced drug crossover. Further, they indicate that the dosage of d-amphetamine used leads to few observable side effects and that teachers did not report any clues that might have influenced their ratings. This latter point could be disputed because 10 mg of d-amphetamine can cause side effects that could be observed by the teachers. The failure of teachers to report side effects or cues may not necessarily be because cues were not observed but could be because the teachers were not specifically asked to report such changes.

Despite some of the minor points of difficulty that could preclude an unequivocal interpretation of the results, this study is a very good example of a well-controlled study of the action of stimulants on school behavior, and it clearly indicates that a student's behavior problems in school can be ameliorated to some degree by a central nervous system stimulant.

As mentioned previously, many of the referral complaints of the teachers are characteristic of the MBD child. These children, at least in the Conners study, were not diagnosed as MBD children. The sample used consisted of 51 out of 61 children originally referred by the principals and faculty of two schools. All the children were in the fifth and sixth grades of these two schools. It would have been of interest to know the total number of children in the fifth and sixth grades of these schools. If 51 children is a large percentage of the children suffering from MBD in these grades, the issue of whether society wishes to treat with drugs such a percent of children in a school must be considered.

The prevalence of behavior problems in the schools as defined by the Conners et al. study is probably not as high in our suburban communities as it is in our core cities. Eisenberg, (1966) in a study of the epidemiology of reading retardation in the entire sixth grade of a large urban area, found that 29 percent of the children were two or more grades below expected levels and that there was a decrease in the amount of retardation in reading the further away the child lived from the central city. If reading disabilities and behavior problems decrease the further one lives from the core city and if we can correctly assume that socioeconomic level correlates with the distance one lives from the core city, then it would strongly indicate a relationship between behavior, learning problems, and socioeconomic level of the family. This by itself does not explain the behavioral problems. Although it is not the scope of this chapter to analyze the manner in which social class, disorganization of the community, and so on, contribute to the problem, it is important that we confront the fact that, at least for the children who come from the same social class as in the Conners et al. study, drugs will produce effects that we might prefer to see produced by social change. However, as previously mentioned, the hyperkinetic child is not simply a manifestation of the disorganization of community or family.

Although the treatment of the MBD child with central stimulant drugs decreases attentional and motor disorders that interfere with the child's school performance, drugs do not directly improve learning. They allow the child to function more adequately in the school situation and thus he is more likely to learn. Eisenberg (1972) strongly states that the central stimulants are far superior to other drugs in the treatment of the MBD child. Millichap (1973), in reviewing drug therapy, states that methylphenidate is the treatment of choice. Although the central actions of these two drugs are similar, methylphenidate seems to cause less anorexia. Eisenberg (1972) does note that a given child will sometimes respond to one and not the other.

Eisenberg, who was instrumental in stimulating as well as doing research on the effects of drugs in the MBD child during the 1960s, believes that too many clinicians abandon treatment after only a brief and inadequate trial of medication. He states that the strategy is to begin with a small dose of 5 mg of d-amphetamine or 10 mg of methylphenidate. The drug should be given once each morning with breakfast at 2- to 3-day intervals. If improvement in behavior does not result, the dosage should be increased in like increments. The suggested maximum daily dose is 40 mg for d-amphetamine or 80 mg for methylphenidate.

Long-Term Effects of Drug Treatment

One of the major concerns of drug treatment of the MBD child is what are the effects of long-term therapy. Before we can intelligently answer that question, we must first ask the question—what happens to the MBD child who is not treated or at least is not treated by means of pharmacotherapy?

Menkes, Rowe, and Menkes (1967) evaluated 14 of 18 cases that were previously seen on one or more occasions during the years 1937 to 1946 at The Johns Hopkins Hospital Child Psychiatry Out-Patient Clinic. All were originally seen because of hyperactivity and learning difficulties. The selected subjects had exhibited the following behavior that is characteristic of the MBD child: distractibility, short attention span, emotional lability, impulsivity, and a low frustration threshold. In addition, the subjects selected presented with hyperactivity, learning difficulties, and they had one or more of the following neurological signs: poor coordination of fine motor movements, visual-motor deficits, and impaired or delayed development of speech.

At the time of follow-up, the patients ranged in age from 22 to 40 years of age. Table 4 summarizes some of the presenting factors and status of the patients at the time of follow-up. Most of the patients reported that "restlessness" had disappeared about the time of adolescence. However, three subjects reported that they still felt "restlessness." They said that they found it difficult to settle down to anything, including watching television; they changed jobs frequently. Four subjects were institutionalized with a reported diagnosis of

TABLE 4. SUMMARY OF THE FOLLOW-UP DATA ON 14 PATIENTS PREVIOUSLY DIAGNOSED AS HYPERKINETIC CHILDREN

$\bar{x}$ age	\multicolumn{4}{c}{Neurological abnormalities}	Institutionalized	Past history of Institutionalization
	Definite	Probable	None	Not seen		
30.9	8	1	2	3	4	4

Abstracted from Menkes, Rowe, and Menkes, 1967.

psychosis at the time of the follow-up; two others were diagnosed as retarded and were supported by their families. Although 8 subjects were self-supporting, 4 of these had spent time in institutions.

There is much wrong with this follow-up study. It would have been a much better study if a matched group of children were also followed up and the follow-up examinations and testings were done in a double-blind fashion. Despite these major shortcomings, the study strongly suggests that the MBD child who is untreated or treated with nondrug therapies has a poor prognosis.

Other follow-up studies of the hyperkinetic child showed that these problems continue and that the prognosis for good outcome without treatment is poor, although not as bad as in the Menkes et al. (1967) study. Weiss, Minde, Werry, Douglas, and Nemeth (1971) did a five-year follow-up study of 64 hyperkinetic children. They found that despite the diminished hyperactivity in adolescents in this group, social, psychological, attentional, and learning disorders persisted. All of the children in the follow-up study had been initially treated with chlorpromazine. At the time of follow-up, only 5 were still taking medication. Most had taken chlorpromazine for one to two years (it should be noted that chlorpromazine is not presently believed to be the drug of choice with the MBD child). Some of the children were treated with other medications, and they report that 20 percent had remained on these for "varying periods." It is of interest that despite a high incidence of academic difficulty at referral, only 15 percent of the children received remedial education. The authors point out that ". . . this small percentage reflects the dearth of, rather than any lack of, need for remedial educational facilities."

The findings of this study are interesting for they certainly suggest long-term persistence of various components of the syndrome, despite a decrease in hyperactivity at adolescence. Unfortunately, the results are not unequivocal for no control group was used, and, although it is unlikely, it could be concluded from this study that treatment for one to two years with chlorpromazine could lead to the long-term poor outcomes. The authors' findings of persistent disability do agree with other observations of the long persistence of sequelae of the syndrome (Mendelson, Johnson, and Stewart, 1971). Further evaluation of the data from this group (Minde, Weiss, and Mendelson, 1972) considered duration of treatment with chlorpromazine as it related to good or poor outcome. No significant relationship was observed. They did comment on a trend that was far from significant, that those who took the drug more than 3 years were the more poorly adjusted. They state that this confirmed their impression that families who relied on medication alone as therapy were "often disappointed." This report, like many in the follow-up area, lacks certain information that would allow at least an approach to unequivocal answers. Some of the subjects received d-amphetamine at some time, but the details concerning the number of subjects and duration of treatment is not given. The study lacks a control group of children matched for significant variables but not diagnosed as hyperkinetic.

The study by Mendelson, Johnson, and Stewart (1971) of 83 children between the ages of 12 and 16 who had been diagnosed as being hyperkinetic 2 to 5 years earlier found that about 50 percent of the children were markedly impaired, 25 percent remained unchanged, and the remaining 25 percent fell somewhere in between. Although the authors state that 92 percent of the children had been treated with either *d*-amphethamine or methylphenidate, they do not relate length of therapy with eventual outcome.

Laufer (1971), by means of a questionnaire sent to 100 former hyperkinetic children treated with amphetamine or methylphenidate, obtained responses from 66 of the subjects. At the onset of drug therapy the children ranged in age from 3 to 13 years, and at the time of the written inquiry they ranged from 15 to 26. Although this study is based only on questionnaire material, the responses received do not suggest any dire outcome from long-term use of the central stimulants in the hyperkinetic child. Out of 37 who were 19 years of age or older, 18 were employed and 14 were attending college or graduate school. Of 57 subjects who responded to the question regarding experimentation with drugs such as marijuana or LSD, only 5 subjects responded that they had tried these drugs. None reported that they were "hooked." None reported habitual use of stimulants to produce a "high," and only 3 subjects reported some ". . . experimentation with Dexedrine, Benzedine, "Speed", etc." Twenty of 56 respondents reported need of psychiatric help, mostly in early adolescence. However, only 5 were in psychiatric treatment at the time of the questionnaire. Overall, the group was much more adjusted than untreated groups. However, unequivocal answers cannot be given because of the lack of an appropriate control group, the failure to receive response from 34 of the subjects, the failure of the subjects to answer all questions, and the failure of the experimenter to interview the subjects for verification of the validity of the responses.

Sleator, von Neumann, and Sprague (1974) followed up 42 hyperkinetic children who had previously been used as subjects in a double-blind study of the effects of methylphenidate on behavior and school performance. Thirteen were followed for two years and 24 for one year. During one month of the school year, with teachers and subjects "blind," placebos were given. Seventeen of the 42 subjects showed deterioration in behavior and school performance during the placebo month. Five of the subjects could not be kept on placebos because of the extreme regression in their behavior. Sleator et al. found that 11 of the subjects showed no deterioration when placed on placebos. These investigators state that their findings indicate that physicians treating the hyperkinetic child with stimulants, ". . . should periodically try drug-free periods during the school year."

Denhoff (1973), in reviewing the available evidence from the few follow-up studies, concluded that there was no evidence to suggest that properly prescribed stimulant drugs have any long-term harmful effects. Despite the lack of real evidence that the drugs are causing any long-term problems in the children as they mature, there is also a paucity of evidence that the drugs cause a real long-term gain in these children. Although there is a wealth of experimental evidence indicating the effectiveness of the medication in some children, we do not know for sure if 10 years after treatment, the child who received pharmacotherapy is any better off than the child who did not.

There is one published paper that strongly suggests a negative effect from long-term use of central stimulants in the treatment of the hyperkinetic child (Safer and Allen, 1973). In this study the effects of two or more years of treatment were evaluated in 49 children (29 received *d*-amphetamine and 20 received methylphenidate) and compared to 14 hyperkinetic children who received no medication. These investigators found a significant reduction in growth, weight and height, in the drug-treated group when compared to the nondrug-treated group. This suppression of growth was most pronounced in the *d*-amphetamine group and the high dose methylphenidate group (> 20 mg/day). This study is a replication of an earlier study by these same investigators in which the differences were less, but a small sample size was used. Considering the number of children currently receiving central stimulants, it would be most important to have this study repeated. Unfortunately, the subjects in the study were not preselected. The controls were hyperkinetic children whose parents refused to permit the use of medication. Data was presented in terms of percentile changes based on age and sex norms for a normal population rather than actual weight and height changes. Another point in the paper that makes evaluation difficult is that the number of years between the first and last weights used in the study was significantly larger for the control group than for the drug groups. Despite these shortcomings, this is an important finding and, as mentioned, the study should be repeated.

SOCIAL-POLITICAL IMPLICATIONS

There has been a great deal of criticism of the use of drugs in the MBD syndrome. Some of the criticism seems well founded in that MBD diagnoses can be abused, and there is a tendency to treat every child who is difficult to manage in school with drugs (Divoky, 1973). An article by Charles Witter (1971) summarized the position of those who are against the use of drugs in the treatment of MBD children. Witter was staff director for Congressman Cornelius E. Gallagher who was chairman of the House Privacy Subcommittee that held hearings in the Fall of 1970 on the use of stimulant drugs in children (see Gallagher, 1970). The fears of those who are against the use of drugs in children is succinctly stated by Witter (1971, p. 31) ". . . it must be recognized that drugs are a cheap alternative to the massive spending so obviously necessary to revitalize the public school system." Many have expressed fear that the drugs will be used to control black children and that the drugs will be a substitute for social change. These fears have led the Black Caucus of the legislative body of the Commonwealth of Massachusetts to sponsor and to have passed a law that makes it illegal to use children in any of the public schools in Massachusetts as research subjects in studies involving the use of drugs. As one worker in the field stated, "The use of drugs in children will not be stopped, the only thing that will be stopped is our finding out how they work" (Cole, personal comment).

The evidence is strong that the CNS drugs do work in many of the children with a diagnosis of MBD. What is needed is not a decrease in research nor an increase in controls that will not allow the researcher access to the subject but safeguards for the subject and more research that will delineate the syndrome. We must know in what way the CNS stimulants modify the behavior of the hyperkinetic child if we are to understand the hyperkinetic child. If all we wish to do is to control all acting-out behavior, we could, for example, give large enough doses of depressant drugs such that we would suppress all behavior. The CNS stimulant drugs do not seem to cause a general depression in behavior but seem to allow the child to take better advantage of those factors in the environment that will allow a fuller and more useful life for the child and for society.

Statements such as the following are attributed to Congressman Gallagher by Witter (1971, p. 34) ". . . the suspicion still exists that these programs will be used to modify the behavior of black children to have them conform to white society's norm." If learning to read, if exploiting available educational resources, if becoming a more adequate person is conforming to "white society's norm," then I would think it would also be the norm of the black community or at least a goal of that community.

Eisenberg (1972) asks the question, ". . . are these drugs mind control agents to suppress rebellion against excessively rigid teachers and school?" Eisenberg answers his own question by indicating that the answer could only be forthcoming if the drugs were administered to normal children. The implication is that only by the study of the effects of these drugs in the normal child could we determine if the drugs are "mind-control agents." If the normal child was stimulated by the drug rather than "controlled," it would certainly indicate that stimulant drugs cannot be used to indiscriminately control classroom behavior. Eisenberg appropriately notes that giving drugs to the normal child would be a breach of ethics. However, the answer that he gives to the question of "mind control" would not answer the question. The problem is that the question is a political one rather than a scientific or medical one. Certainly, large numbers of MBD children improve when given central stimulant drugs. The improvement is not only seen in poor schools in the large urban areas, but the improvement is also seen in what could be considered good schools. The improvement in behavior is not only in the school but in the home. Eisenberg states that there is schoolroom behavior that could be classified as overactivity and distractibility in which drugs would be "grossly inappropriate." The first point that he makes is that it is important to make the proper diagnosis. Many of the behavioral symptoms of MBD could be caused by intense anxiety in the presence of a grossly disorganized family situation. The second condition that he lists is that inability to concentrate can be caused by hypoglycemia in a malnourished child who often does not eat breakfast. As mentioned previously, there is the strong possibility that lead poisoning could lead to many of the symptoms seen in MBD. Malnourishment or physical disabilities, for example, poor hearing or poor eyesight, might cause distractibility and poor performance in school. As mentioned in the introduction of this chapter, there are many children whose only contact with a physician is in the emergency room of a hospital.

The third point that Eisenberg makes is one concerning the state of the environment in which the child is required to do his learning. Is the classroom inadequate and crowded? Is the teacher competent? It is this writer's opinion that the question of the classroom adequacy or inadequacy is not the problem in the case of the MBD child. Certainly, an inadequate school will contribute to the problem, but an adequate school will not solve the problem.

The stimulant drugs, as previously mentioned, do not sedate, and as Eisenberg states, ". . . the myth that stimulants make hyperkinetic children into 'conforming robots' is arrant nonsense." If they do not make "conforming robots" out of the diagnostically confirmed MBD child, there is no reason to assume that the stimulants will make "conforming robots" of the nonMBD child who unfortunately goes to a school in which the environment is not conducive to good learning. If we want to make our classrooms quiet, if we want children to lockstep, I would not recommend a stimulant drug. Even if one used depressant drugs, in other words, barbiturates, there would be a significant number of students in the classroom who would manifest excitement unless the dose was sufficiently large to guarantee complete suppression of all behavior.

The answer to the problem of the nonhyperkinetic child who does not learn in school is not with medicine. Learning problems are for the educators to solve. However, for those children who clearly fit the definition of the MBD child—and this usually includes a history of MBD prior to entering school—the answer may not simply be that the teaching is inadequate. That child may be helped with medication, and the failure to adequately diagnose and treat an MBD child is just as criminal as treating the difficult child with drugs rather than with good teaching. Just because the hyperkinesis of the MBD child seems to disappear in adolescence is no reason to ignore and not treat the syndrome. Maladaptive behavior in the early school years that is not properly handled leads to continued maladaptive behavior in subsequent years. Failure in the second grade, no matter the cause, is much more amenable to remedial help in the second grade than failure in the second grade that is treated in the sixth grade. The teacher, with the parent, and if there is suspicion of MBD, with the physician, must vigorously not allow the second-grade problem to become the third-, fourth-, and fifth-grade problem.

REFERENCES

Bender, L. and Collington, F. The use of amphetamine sulfate (Benzedrine) in child psychiatry. *American Journal of Psychiatry,* **99,** 1942, 116–121.

Benton, A. L. Minimal brain dysfunction from a neuropsychological point of view. In F. F. De La Cruz, B. H. Fox, and R. H. Roberts (Eds.) "Minimal Brain Dysfunction" *Annals of the New York Academy of Sciences,* **205,** 1973, 29–37.

Bradley, C. The behavior of children receiving benzedrine. *American Journal of Psychiatry,* **94,** 1937, 577–585.

Bradley, C. and Bowen, M. School performance of children receiving amphetamine (Benzedrine) sulfate. *American Journal of Orthopsychiatry,* **10,** 1940, 782–788.

Bradley, C. and Bowen, M. Amphetamine (Benzedrine) therapy of children's behavior disorder. *American Journal of Orthopsychiatry,* **11,** 1941, 92–103.

Bradley, C. and Green, E. Psychometric performance of children receiving amphetamine (Benzedrine) sulfate. *American Journal of Psychiatry,* **97,** 1940, 388–394.

Clements, S. D. Minimal brain dysfunction in children: Terminology and identification phase one of a three phase project. NINDB Monograph No. 3, U.S. Department of Health, Education, and Welfare, 1966.

Cole, J. O. The amphetamines in child psychiatry: A review. *Seminars in Psychiatry,* **1,** 1969, 174–178.

Conners, C. K. The effect of Dexedrine on rapid discrimination and motor control of hyperkinetic children under mild stress. *Journal of Nervous and Mental Disease,* **142,** 1966, 429–433.

Conners, C. K. Symptom patterns in hyperkinetic, neurotic and normal children. *Child Development,* **41,** 1970, 667–682.

Conners, C. K. Drugs in the management of children with learning disabilities. In L. Tarnopol (Ed.) *Learning Disorders in Children: Diagnosis, Medication, Education.* Boston, Little, Brown, 1971, pp. 253–301.

Conners, C. K. and Eisenberg, L. The effects of methylphenidate on symptomatology and learning in disturbed children. *American Journal of Psychiatry,* **120,** 1963, 458–464.

Conners, C. K., Eisenberg, L., and Barcai, A. Effect of dextroamphetamine on children: Studies on subjects with learning disabilities and school behavior problems. *Archives of General Psychiatry,* **17,** 1967, 478–485.

Conners, C. K., Eisenberg, L., and Sharpe, L. Effects of methylphenidate (Ritalin) on paired-associate learning and Porteus Maze performance in emotionally disturbed children. *Journal of Consulting Psychology,* **28,** 1964, 14–22.

Conners, C. K. and Rothschild, G. H. Drugs and learning in children. *Learning Disorders,* **3,** 1968, 195–223.

Conners, C. K., Rothschild, G. H. Eisenberg, L., Shwartz, L., and Robinson, E. Dextroamphetamine sulfate in children with learning disorders: Effects on perception, learning and achievement. *Archives of General Psychiatry,* **21,** 1969 182–190.

De La Cruz, F. F., Fox, B. H., and Roberts, R. H. (Eds.) Minimal brain dysfunction. *Annals of the New York Academy of Sciences,* **205,** 1973.

Denhoff, E. The natural life history of children with minimal brain dysfunction. In F. F. De La Cruz, B. H. Fox, and R. H. Roberts (Eds.) Minimal brain dysfunction. *Annals of the New York Academy of Sciences,* **205,** 1973, 188-205.

Divoky, D. Toward a nation of sedated children. *Learning,* **1,** 1973, 6-12.

Eisenberg, L. The management of the hyperkinetic child. *Developmental Medicine and Child Neurology,* **8,** 1966, 593-598.

Eisenberg, L. Symposium: Behavior modification by drugs. III. The clinical use of stimulant drugs in children. *Pediatrics,* **49,** 1972, 709-715.

Epstein, L. C., Lasagna, L., Conners, C. K., and Rodriguez, A. Correlation of dextroamphetamine excretion and drug response in hyperkinetic children. *Journal of Nervous and Mental Disease,* **146,** 1968, 136-146.

Fish, B. Methodology in child psychopharmacology. In D. H. Efron (Ed.) *Psychopharmacology. A Review of Progress 1957-1967.* U. S. Government Printing Office. Public Health Service Publication, No. 1836, Washington, D.C., 1968, pp. 989-1001.

Fisher, S. (Ed.) *Child Research in Psychopharmacology.* Springfield, Charles C Thomas, 1959.

Freeman, R. D. Drug effects on learning in children: A selective review of the past thirty years. *Journal of Special Education,* **1,** 1966, 17-44.

Frisk, M., Wegelius, B., Tenhunen, T., Windholm, O., and Hortling, H. The problem of dyslexia in teenage. *Acta Paediatrica Scandinavica,* **56,** 1967, 333-343.

Gallagher, C. E. (Presiding) Federal involvement in the use of behavior modification drugs on grammar school children of the right to privacy inquiry. Hearing before a *Subcommittee of the Committee on Government Operations House of Representatives.* 91 Congress, Second Session, September 29, 1970, U. S. Government Printing Office, pp. 1-175.

Gastant, H. Combined photic and Metrazol activation of the brain. *Electroencephalography and Clinical Neurophysiology,* **2,** 1950, 249-261.

Gastant, H. and Hunter, J. An experimental study of the mechanism of photic activation in ideopathic epilepsy. *Electroencephalography and Clinical Neurophysiology,* **2,** 1950, 263-287.

Grant, G. R. Psychopharmacology in childhood emotional and mental disorders. *Journal of Pediatrics,* **51,** 1962, 626-637.

Hallgren, B. Specific dyslexia ("congenital word blindness"): A clinical and genetic study. *Acta Psychiatrica Scandinavica Supplement,* **64,** 1950, 1-287.

Knights, R. M. and Hinton, G. The effects of methylphenidate (Ritalin) on the motor skills and behavior of children with learning problems. *Research Bulletin,* No. 102, University of Western Ontario, 1968 (as reviewed in Conners, 1971).

Laufer, M. W. Long-term management and some follow-up findings on the use of drugs with minimal cerebral syndromes. *Journal of Learning Disabilities,* **4,** 1971, 518-522.

Laufer, M. W. and Denhoff, E. Hyperkinetic behavior syndrome in children. *Journal of Pediatrics,* **50,** 1957, 463-474.

Laufer, M. W., Denhoff, E., and Solomons, G. Hyperkinetic impulse disorder in children's behavior problems. *Psychosomatic Medicine,* **19,** 1957, 38-49.

Lindsley, D. B. and Henry, C. E. Effects of drugs on behavior and the electroencephalograms of children with behavior disorders. *Psychosomatic Medicine,* **4,** 1942, 140-149.

Lytton, G. V. and Knobel, M. Diagnosis and treatment of behavior disorders in children. *Diseases of the Nervous System,* **20,** 1959, 334-340.

REFERENCES

Mendelson, W., Johnson, N., and Stewart, M. A. Hyperactive children as teenagers: A follow-up study. *Journal of Nervous and Mental Disease,* **153,** 1971, 273–279.

Menkes, M. M., Rowe, J. S., and Menkes, J. H. A twenty-five year follow-up study of the hyperkinetic child with minimal brain dysfunction. *Pediatrics,* **39,** 1967, 393–399.

Millichap, J. G. Drugs in management of hyperkinetic and perceptually handicapped children. *Journal of the American Medical Association,* **206,** 1968, 1527–1530.

Millichap, J. G. Drugs in management of minimal brain dysfunction. In F. F. De La Cruz, B. H. Fox, and R. H. Roberts (Eds.) Minimal brain dysfunction. *Annals of the New York Academy of Sciences,* **205,** 1973, 321–334.

Millichap, J. G. and Fowler, G. Treatment of "minimal brain dysfunction" syndromes: Selection of drugs for children with hyperactivity and learning disabilities. *Pediatric Clinics of North America,* **14,** 1967, 767–777.

Minde, K., Weiss, G., and Mendelson, N. A 5-year follow-up study of 91 hyperactive school children. *Journal of the American Academy of Child Psychiatry,* **11,** 1972, 595–610.

Molitch, M. and Eccles, A. K. Effect of benzedrine sulfate on intelligence scores of children. *American Journal of Psychiatry,* **94,** 1937, 587–590.

Molitch, M. and Sullivan, J. P. Effects of benzedrine sulfate on children taking the new Stanford Achievement Test. *American Journal of Orthopsychiatry,* **7,** 1937, 519–522.

Rosvold, H. E., Mirsky, A. F., Sarason, I., Bransome, E. D., and Beck, L. H. A continuous performance test of brain damage. *Journal of Consulting Psychology,* **20,** 1956, 343–350.

Safer, D. V. and Allen, R. P. Factors influencing the suppressant effects of two stimulant drugs on the growth of hyperactive children. *Pediatrics* **51,** 1973, 660–667.

Satterfield, J. H., Cantwell, D. P., Lesser, L. I., and Podosin, R. L. Physiological studies of the hyperkinetic child: I. *American Journal of Psychiatry,* **128,** 1972, 1418–1425.

Satterfield, J. H. and Dawson, M. E. Electrodermal correlates of hyperactivity in children. *Psychophysiology,* **8,** 1971, 191–197.

Sauerhoff, M. W. and Michaelson, I. A. Hyperactivity and brain catecholamines in lead-exposed developing rats. *Science,* **182,** 1973, 1022–1024.

Silbergeld, E. K. and Goldberg, A. M. A lead-induced behavioral disorder. *Life Sciences,* **13,** 1973, 1275–1283.

Silbergeld, E. K. and Goldberg, A. M. Lead-induced behavioral dysfunction: An animal model of hyperactivity. *Experimental Neurology,* **42,** 1974, 146–157.

Sleator, E. K., von Neumann, A., and Sprague, R. L. Hyperactive children: A continuous long-term placebo-controlled follow-up. *Journal of the American Medical Association,* **229,** 1974, 316–317.

Sprague, R. L., Barnes, K. R., and Werry, J. S. Methylphenidate and thioridazine: Learning, reaction time, activity and classroom behavior in emotionally disturbed children. *American Journal of Orthopsychiatry,* **40,** 1970, 615–628.

Sprague, R. L. and Sleator, E. K. Effects of psychopharmacologic agents on learning disorders. *Pediatric Clinics of North America,* **20,** 1973, 719–735.

Stevens, J. R., Sachdev, K., and Milstein. V. Behavior disorders of childhood and the electroencephalogram. *Archives of Neurology,* **18,** 1968, 160–177.

Stewart, M. A., Pitts, F. N. Jr., Craig, A. G., and Dieruf, W. The hyperactive child syndrome. *American Journal of Orthopsychiatry,* **36,** 1966, 861–867.

Sykes, D. H. Douglas, V. I., and Morgenstern, G. The effects of methylphenidate (Ritalin) on sustained attention in hyperactive children. *Psychopharmacologia (Berlin),* **25,** 1972, 262–274.

Sykes, D. H., Douglas, V. I., and Weiss, G. Attention in hyperactive children and the effects of methylphenidate (Ritalin). *Journal of Child Psychology and Psychiatry,* **12,** 1971, 129–139.

Weiss, G., Minde, K., Werry, J. S., Douglas, V., and Nemeth, E. Studies on the hyperactive child. VIII. Five year follow-up. *Archives of General Psychiatry,* **24,** 1971, 409–414.

Wender, P. H. *Minimal Brain Dysfunction in Children.* New York, Wiley, 1971.

Wender, P. H. The minimal brain dysfunction syndrome in children. *Journal of Nervous and Mental Disease,* **155,** 1972, 55–71.

Werry, J. S. Developmental hyperactivity. *Pediatric Clinics of North America,* **15,** 1968, 581–599.

Wikler, A., Dixon, J. F., and Parker, J. B., Jr. Brain function in problem children and controls: Psychometric, neurological, and electroencephalographic comparisons. *American Journal of Psychiatry,* **127,** 1970, 634–645.

Witter, C. Drugging and schooling. *Trans-Action,* July/August 1971, 31–34.

Zimmerman, F. T. and Burgermeister, B. B. Action of methylphenidylacetate (Ritalin) and reserpine in behavior disorders in children and adults. *American Journal of Psychiatry,* **115,** 1958, 323–328.

GLOSSARY OF "STREET" TERMS

The following glossary of "street" names for various drugs is given with some qualifications: "street" names often change over time, there are regional differences; often a name may be used for a number of different drugs; finally, because of alteration of "street" drugs, there is no guarantee that a particular drug is really what it is purported to be.

"A" Amphetamines; speed.
Acapulco gold High-grade marihuana.
Acid Lysergic acid diethylamide (LSD).
Amys Amyl nitrite ampules (potent, short-acting vasodilator).
Angel dust PCP (Phencyclidine or "Sernyl®," a veterinary anesthetic—in pill form called "Peace Pill," "Hog," or "Elephant"). Inhaled or swallowed in a powdered form; mixed with marihuana or oregano and smoked.
Barb(s) Barbiturates.
Benny Benzedrine®.
Bernice Cocaine.
Bhang Drink made in India of the flowering tops, stems, and leaves of cannabis. Produces mild hallucinogenic effects.
Big bloke Cocaine.
Big C Cocaine.
Big D LSD.
Big O Opium.
Black beauties Biphetamine® capsules (amphetamines).
Black magic LSD.
Black stuff Opium.
Blue angles, bluebirds, blue heaven, blue devils, blues Amobarbital sodium, a barbiturate.
Blue velvet 1 Mixture of Elixir Terpin Hydrate and Pyribenzamine® (antihistamine). 2 Mixture of paregoric and antihistamine.
Boo Marihuana.
Bombida Methamphetamine.
Bombita Amphetamine injection, occasionally with heroin.
Boy Heroin.
Brain pills Amphetamines.

Brick Compressed block made of marihuana.
Brown Heroin from Mexico—usually light brown in color (may be due to dilution with powdered coffee).
Browns Multicolored capsules that are long-acting amphetamine sulfate.
Brown dots LSD.
Bullets Seconal®—a barbiturate.
Bush Marihuana.
Businessman's trip Dimethyltryptamine (DMT)—relatively short-acting hallucinogen.
Buttons Dried tops of the lophophora cactus (peyote).
"C" Cocaine.
Ca-ca 1 Heroin. 2 Inferior quality of hashish, heroin, or LSD. 3 Imitation or counterfeit heroin.
California sunshine LSD.
Candy Barbiturates.
Cartwheels Amphetamine tablets scored crossways.
Carrie Cocaine.
CB also CIBA Doriden ®tablet (glutethimide)—nonbarbiturate hypnotic.
Cecil Cocaine.
Chicken powder Some amphetamine powder.
Chief LSD.
Chloral Chloral hydrate, sedative hypnotic, mild "sleeper."
Christmas trees Tuinal® barbiturates, Eskatrol® contains amphetamines and a phenothiazine or Dexamyl® amphetamine-barbiturate mixture.
Chocolate chips LSD.
Cholley Cocaine.
Cibas See CB.
Cibees See CB.
Coast-to-coast Long-acting amphetamines.
Coke Cocaine.
Co-pilots Amphetamine tablets.
Corrine Cocaine.
Crank Methamphetamine crystals.
Crinic Methamphetamine.
Cris Methamphetamine.
Cristina Methamphetamine.
Crossroads Amphetamine tablets.
Crystal Methamphetamine; cocaine.
Cube juice Morphine.
Cup cakes LSD.
"D" See CB.
"D" LSD.

"STREET" TERMS

DET Diethyltryptamine (hallucinogen).
Dexies Dexedrine® tablets or capsules (amphetamines).
DMT Dimethyltryptamine (see Businessman's Trip).
Dollies Dolophine® tablets (methadone).
DOM STP (2,5 dimethoxy-4-methylamphetamine) hallucinogen, see text.
Domes LSD tablets.
Doojee Heroin.
Dope To a heroin user, dope is heroin; to marihuana smokers, dope is anything used to get high.
Double trouble Tuinal® capsule (barbiturate).
Downers Nonnarcotic central nervous system depressants.
Dream Cocaine.
Dujie Heroin.
Dust Heroin, cocaine.
Dust of angels Phencyclidine base (see angel dust).
Dynamite 1 High quality of heroin and cocaine taken together. 2 Strong drug.
Elephant See Angel dust.
Emsel Morphine.
Eye openers Amphetamines.
Flake Cocaine.
Flats LSD tablets.
Flea powder Poor quality heroin or heroin that is greatly diluted.
Foolish powder Heroin.
Footballs Amphetamine tablets or capsules that are oval shaped.
Fu Marihuana.
GB's Seconal®, Tuinal®, or Doriden® (Downers).
Gage Marihuana.
Girl Cocaine.
Gold dust Cocaine.
Goofball Barbiturate.
Gorilla pills Doriden® (see CB).
Grape Parfait LSD.
Greenies Mixture of barbiturates and amphetamines in Dexamyl®.
Griefo Marihuana.
"H" Heroin.
Happy dust Cocaine.
Harry Heroin.
Hash Hashish.
Hawaiian sunshine LSD.
Hay Marihuana.
Hearts Amphetamine tablets, heart-shaped Benzedrine®.

Heavenly blue   Morning glory seeds.
Heaven dust   Cocaine.
Hocus   Morphine.
Hog   Vegetable material that has phencyclidine in it (see Angel dust).
Hop   Opium.
Horse   Heroin.
Hot sticks   Marihuana cigarettes.
Indian bay   Marihuana.
Indian hay   Marihuana.
Jay   Marihuana cigarette.
Jelly beans   Tuinal®, barbiturate.
Joint   Marihuana cigarette.
Jolly beans   Pep pills.
Joy powder   Cocaine.
Junk   1 Heroin. 2 Can denote any drug.
Keif   Hashish or high-quality marihuana.
L.A. turnabouts   Various colored capsules that are long-acting amphetamine sulfate.
Lid poppers   Amphetamines.
Loco weed   Marihuana or jimson weed (*Datura stramonium*).
Love drug   1 MDA (methylene dioxyamphetamine), mild hallucinogen. 2 Methaqualone (Soper®, Quāālude®, Parest®)-downer.
Ludes   Quāāludes® (methaqualone).
Magic mushroom   Mushroom that contains psylocibin.
Magic pumpkin   SPT Tablet (see DOM) that is shaped like a pumpkin seed.
Mesc   Mescaline (hallucinogenic drug from the peyote cactus).
Meth   Usually Methamphetamine or Methadrine®—occasionally methadone or methaqualone.
Mickey   Chloral hydrate (hypnotic).
Mickey Finn   Mixture of chloral hydrate plus alcohol.
Micro dots   LSD.
Mikes   Micrograms (millionths of a gram)—refers to LSD dose.
Miss Emma   Morphine.
Monster   Methamphetamine.
Nembies   Pentobarbital sodium (Nembutal®).
Nibies   Nembies.
Noise   Heroin.
Nose candy   Cocaine.
O.J.   Opium joint—a marihuana cigarette that has been dipped or smeared in opium.
Oranges   Heart-shaped amphetamine tablets containing Dexedrine®.

"STREET" TERMS

Orange sunshine   LSD.
Orange wedges   LSD.
Owsley's acid   LSD.
PCP   Phencyclidine (see Angel dust).
Pee   Heroin powder.
PG   Paregoric.
PO   Paregoric.
Panama red   Potent grade of marihuana from Panama.
Peace   LSD tablets or DOM.
Peace pill   Phencyclidine (see Angel dust).
Peanuts   Barbiturates.
Pearly gates   Morning glory seeds.
Peter   Chloral hydrate.
Pinks   Barbiturates; Seconal® capsules.
Pin yen   Opium.
Poppers   Amyl nitrite ampules (see Amys).
Product IV   Combination capsules of PCP and LSD.
Purple barrels, Purple haze, Purple ozolone   LSD.
Purple hearts   Dexamyl® (brand of dextroamphetamine sulfate and amobarbital sodium).
Purple rock   Mixture of caffeine, barbiturates, heroin, and strychnine.
Rainbows   Tuinal® capsules (barbiturates).
Red birds, Red devils, Red lillies, Reds   Secobarbital capsules.
Red rock   See purple rock.
Robe   Robitussin® AC cough syrup.
Robo   Codeine.
Roses   Benzedrine® tablets, amphetamines.
Scag   Heroin.
School boy   Codeine.
Serenity, tranquility, and peace   STP (see DOM).
Shit   1 Heroin. 2 Poor quality of heroin, hashish, or LSD. 3 Drugs.
Sleepers   Barbiturates.
Smack, Smeck, Schmeck   Heroin.
Smash   Marihuana that has been cooked with acetone. Oil that results is added to hashish.
Smears   LSD.
Smoke   1 Wood alcohol. 2 Marihuana.
Snappers   Amyl nitrite ampules (see Amys).
Snow   Cocaine crystals.
Sopers   Methaqualone (sleeping pill).
Sound   Benactyzine.
Spaghetti sauce   Robitussin® AC cough syrup.

Speed   Amphetamines, usually methamphetamine.
Speedball   Mixture of heroin and cocaine that is taken intravenously.
Splash   Amphetamine or methamphetamine powder.
Spots   Dextroamphetamine.
Squirrels   LSD.
Star dust   Cocaine.
Stoppers   Barbiturates.
Strawberry field   LSD.
Stumblers   1 Barbiturates. 2 Tranquilizers.
Sunshine   LSD.
Syrup   Codeine.
TMA   Combination of tetrahydrocannabinol, mescaline, and LSD (acid); or the compound 3,4,5-trimethoxyphenylisopropylamine (a mescaline-like drug).
Tar   Opium.
Tea   Marihuana.
Thai sticks   Buds from marihuana tied to sticks with thin threads—very potent.
TNT   Heroin.
Tooies or Tuies   Tuinal® capsules (barbiturates).
Turps   Elixir Terpin Hydrate and codeine—a cough syrup.
Upper(s), Ups   Amphetamine tablets.
Wake ups   Amphetamines, also may refer to the first shot of heroin of the day.
Wedges   1 Dexedrine® tablets (amphetamines). 2 LSD tablets.
Wen shee   Gum opium.
White lighting   LSD, also an old term for "moonshine" (bootleg) whiskey.
Windowpane   Square gelatin flake that contains LSD.
Yellow dimples   LSD.
Yellows, Yellow birds, Yellow jackets, Yellow submarines   Nembutal® capsules (Pentobarbital sodium).

This glossary was drawn from the published glossaries listed below that were provided by Susan Christenson, librarian, and *STASH* (The Student Association for the Study of Hallucinogens, Inc., Madison, Wisconsin), who also suggested some additional terms. Final editing of the glossary was done with the help of local students.

Glossary of drug-related terms. *Journal of Psychedelic Drugs,* **4,** 1971.

Heidbreder, G. A. and Woolley, B. Current street language for various drugs that are abused. *California Medicine,* **116,** 1972.

Lampe, M. Brief list of street terms in J. R. Gamage (Ed.) *Management of Adolescent Drug Misuse: Clinical, Psychological, and Legal Perspectives.* Beloit, Wisconsin, Stash Press, 1973, pp. 138–139.

Winek, C. L. *Everything You Wanted to Know About Drug Abuse . . . but were afraid to ask.* New York, Dekker, 1974, pp. 164–184.

AUTHOR INDEX

Ahlquist, R. P., 164, 174
Allan, W. F., 67
Allen, J. R., 215, 218
Allen, R. P., 246, 251
Alles, G. A., 164, 173
Altschul, S., 148
Anden, N. E., 77, 79
Armenti, N. P., 153, 154, 163
Aronow, L., 21
Asatoor, A., 106, 114

Bagdon, R. E., 115
Bain, G., 89, 90, 102, 124, 135, 201, 221
Banerjee, S. P., 102, 174
Barcai, A., 238, 240, 249
Barnes, K. R., 234, 238, 251
Barr, H. L., 207, 218
Barros, G. G., 210, 222
Barry, H., III, 152, 154, 163
Barsky, J., 116
Beck, L. H., 102, 251
Beckett, H. D., 190, 219
Beecher, H. K., 35, 36, 43, 44, 122, 135, 147, 167, 174
Begleiter, H., 152, 163
Belleville, R. E., 143, 148, 163
Bender, L., 235, 249
Bennett, C. C., 207, 219
Benton, A. L., 228, 249
Bewley, T. H., 200, 219
Bloom, F. E., 77, 79
Bloomberg, W., 164, 174
Boakes, R. J., 169, 173
Bonnie, R. J., 211, 213, 219
Bourne, P. G., 195, 219
Bouthilet, L., 43, 44
Bowen, M., 235, 249
Bradley, C., 235, 239, 249
Bradley, P. B., 92, 101, 141, 147, 168, 169, 173
Bransome, E. D., 102, 251
Brawley, P., 203, 204, 207, 219
Brazier, M. A. B., 141, 147
Brecher, E. M., 152, 163, 187, 188, 189, 211, 212, 213, 216, 219
Bremer, F., 67, 68
Brooks, C. McC., 49, 62
Buchanan, R. A., 182, 184
Burgermeister, B. B., 239, 252
Byck, R., 101, 107, 108, 114

Cade, J. F. J., 99
Cajal, R. S., 67
Campbell, A. M. G., 214, 219
Candy, J. M., 169, 173
Cannon, W. B., 47, 62
Cantwell, D. P., 230, 251
Carlton, P. L., 58, 62
Carpenter, J. A., 153, 154, 163
Casey, K. L., 125, 135
Cavanaugh, J., 173
Charpentier, 86
Chaucer, G., 23
Chayet, N. L., 190, 219
Chein, I., 193, 195, 196, 219
Chen, K. K., 164
Claussen, U., 220
Clements, S. D., 228, 249
Coatsworth, J. J., 179, 180, 184
Cochin, J., 132, 135, 201, 219
Coffey, E. M., 102
Cohen, S., 207, 209, 219
Cohen, P. J., 216, 221
Cole, J. O., 100, 101, 109, 110, 115, 224, 249
Collington, F., 235, 249
Conners, C. K., 224, 234, 236, 237, 238, 240, 241, 242, 249, 250
Cook, L., 90, 101, 113, 115
Cooper, J. R., 77, 79
Craig, A. G., 251
Crancer, H., 215, 219
Cruickshank, W. M., 223

Dahlström, A., 79
Darley, C. F., 221
Davis, J. M., 171, 173
Dawson, M. E., 234, 251

De La Cruz, F. F., 224, 250
Delay, J. C., 86, 219
De Long, F. L., 215, 219
del Pozo, E. C., 204, 219
Denhoff, E., 231, 233, 245, 250
Deniker, P., 86
De Quincey, T., 187
Dewey, W. L., 220
Dews, P. B., 108, 115, 142, 143, 147
Dieruf, W., 251
Dille, J. M., 219
DiMascio, A., 9, 10, 11, 12, 21, 88, 101, 106, 108, 111, 115
Divoky, D., 246, 250
Dixon, J. F., 229, 234, 252
Dohan, J. L., 33, 44
Dole, V. P., 201, 219
Domino, E. F., 124, 135
Dorf, J., 167, 173
Douglas, V. I., 237, 244, 251, 252
Dripps, R. D., 216, 221
Duffield, J. C., 203, 204, 207, 219

Eccles, A. K., 235, 239, 251
Efron, D. H., 209, 219
Eisenberg, L., 224, 233, 238, 240, 242, 247, 248, 249, 250
Eisenman, A. J., 148, 163
Eliasson, M., 93, 94, 101, 102
Elkes, J., 169, 173
Elliot, L. L., 144, 148
El-Yousef, M. K., 171, 173
Epstein, L. C., 237, 239, 250
Ervin, R., 178, 184
Essig, C. F., 147
Evans, M., 219

Fingl, E., 21, 184
FitzGerald, M. X., 221, 222
Fish, B., 224, 236, 250
Fisher, A. E., 69, 80
Fisher, S., 35, 36, 37, 38, 44, 236, 250
Fishman, V. S., 173
Flanary, H. G., 135, 148
Fouts, J. R., 116
Fowler, G., 224, 236, 251
Fox, B. H., 250
Frank, I. M., 221
Fraser, H. F., 136, 144, 147, 148, 163
Frazer, J. G., 39, 44
Freedman, A. M., 190, 219
Freedman, D. X., 217, 218, 220
Freeman, R. D., 236, 251
Friedler, G., 201, 220
Friedman, M. A., 220
Frisk, M., 233, 250
Fuxe, K., 79

Gaddum, J. H., 78, 79
Gaensler, E. A., 221, 222
Gallagher, B. B., 182, 184
Gallagher, C. E., 246, 250
Gastant, H., 231, 250
Gattozzi, A. A., 99, 101
Geller, J., 113, 115
Gerard, D. L., 192, 193, 194, 195, 197, 219, 220
Glaser, R., 190, 220
Goldberg, A. M., 232, 251
Goldberg, S. R., 191, 220
Goldberger, L., 218
Goldstein, A., 21
Goodnow, R. E., 144, 147
Gorodetsky, G. W., 220
Goth, A., 21, 62
Gould, I. A., 221
Grant, G. R., 224, 250
Green, E., 239, 249
Greenberg, D., 102, 174
Griffith, J. D., 170, 173
Grinker, R. R., 139, 147
Grinspoon, L., 212, 213, 220
Gritz, E. R., 15, 21
Grossman, S. P., 63, 74, 79
Groves, P. M., 68, 79
Grunthal, E., 108

Haertzen, C. A., 190, 220
Hallahan, D. P., 223
Hallgren, B., 233, 250
Hanrahan, G. E., 86, 102
Harl, J. M., 86
Harper, C. E., 221
Harris, L. S., 211, 220
Hart, E. R., 168, 174
Harvey, S. C., 140, 146, 148
Haykin, M. D., 219
Heidbreder, G. A., 258
Heise, G. A., 115
Held, J., 173
Heniger, G., 115
Henry, C. E., 236, 237, 250
Hill, H. E., 122, 123, 135, 143, 148, 190, 220
Hinton, G., 239, 250
Hofmann, A., 205, 220
Hollister, L. E., 101, 221
Holmstedt, B., 209, 219
Holt, R. R., 218
Hortling, H., 250
Huckabee, W., 33
Hunter, J., 231, 250
Hussar, A. E., 171, 174
Hutt, P. P., 190, 222

AUTHOR INDEX

Innes, I. R., 166, 172, 173
Isbell, H., 136, 144, 147, 148, 156, 163, 215, 220

Jaffe, J. H., 119, 172, 173, 186, 199, 201, 203, 217, 220
Janowsky, D. S., 171, 173
Jarvik, M. E., 15, 21, 98, 101, 107, 115, 207, 220
Jasinksi, D., 220
Jasper, H., 71, 72, 79, 176, 178, 183, 184
Jernigan, A. J., 193, 220
Johanson, C. E., 132, 135
Johnson, N., 244, 245, 251
Jones, E., 216, 220
Judson, W. E., 83, 102

Kalman, S. M., 21
Kalow, W., 18, 21
Keith, E. F., 115
Kelleher, R. T., 113, 115
Kessler, E. K., 144, 148, 167, 173
Key, B. J., 168, 173
Khantzian, E. J., 194, 195, 220
Killam, E. K., 92, 101, 124, 135, 168, 169, 173
Killam, K. F., 92, 101
Kirchheimer, W. F., 116
Kissin, B., 152, 163
Klein, G. S., 218
Klerman, G. L., 109, 115
Klett, C. J., 102
Kletzkin, M., 112, 115
Kline, N. S., 82, 83, 101, 102, 104, 115, 209, 219
Klüver, H., 204, 221
Knapp, P. H., 171, 173
Knights, R. M., 239, 250
Knobel, M., 237, 250
Koelle, G. B., 62
Koizumi, K., 49, 62
Kopell, B. S., 221
Kornetsky, C., 9, 10, 11, 12, 21, 89, 90, 91, 93, 94, 101, 102, 108, 111, 115, 122, 124, 125, 127, 135, 144, 148, 167, 171, 173, 192, 194, 195, 197, 201, 219, 220, 221
Korte, F., 220
Kramer, J. C., 171, 173

Lampe, M., 258
Langes, R. J., 218
Lapa, A. J., 210, 222
Larsson, K., 79
Lasagna, L., 32, 33, 35, 36, 43, 44, 210, 221, 239, 250
Laties, V. G., 33, 44, 111, 113, 115, 123, 136, 167, 174
Laufer, M. W., 233, 234, 245, 250
Leake, C. D., 159, 162, 163, 164, 166, 170, 174
Lee, R. S., 193, 195, 219
Lee, Y. E., 221
Lehmann, H. E., 86, 102
Lesser, L. I., 230, 251
Levi, A. J., 114
Levine, J., 43, 44
Levine, R. R., 21
Levy, B., 164, 174
Levy, B. I., 215, 219
Lindsley, D. B., 236, 237, 250
Lipper, S., 91, 102
Littlefield, D. C., 173
Livingston, A. E., 130, 135
Loewi, O., 47, 48, 62
Loomis, T. A., 111, 115
Low, L. A., 91, 102
Lucretius, 175
Lytton, G. V., 237, 250

Macht, D. I., 117, 119, 135
McGlothlin, W. H., 215, 218, 221
McKenzie, R. E., 144, 148
McLaren, A., 18
Magoun, H. W., 66, 68, 79, 141, 148
Marazzi, A. S., 168, 174
Marcus, R., 125, 127, 135
Martin, W. R., 124, 133, 135
Mattson, R. H., 183, 184
Maugh II, T. H., 214, 221
May, P. R. A., 100, 102
Mello, N. K., 155, 157, 158, 163
Mendelson, J. H., 157, 158, 163, 216, 221
Mendelson, W., 244, 245, 251
Menkes, J. H., 243, 251
Menkes, M. M., 243, 244, 251
Merritt, H. H., 180, 184
Meyer, R. E., 200, 201, 202, 216, 221
Michaelson, I. A., 232, 251
Michie, D., 18
Mikus, P., 222
Miller, A. T., Jr., 168, 174
Millichap, J. G., 178, 184, 224, 226, 236, 238, 242, 251
Milne, M. D., 114
Milner, P., 70, 79
Milstein, V., 229, 234, 251
Minde, K., 244, 251, 252
Mirsky, A. F., 67, 73, 74, 79, 89, 93–94, 102, 141, 148, 167, 171, 173, 251
Modell, W., 23, 44, 171, 174
Molitch, M., 235, 239, 251
Morgenstern, G., 237, 251
Morrissey, W., 222

AUTHOR INDEX

Moruzzi, G., 66, 68, 79, 141, 148
Mosteller, F., 35, 44, 147
Munson, A. E., 220
Musto, D. F., 187, 189, 221

Nahas, G. G., 210, 214, 221
Nathanson, M. H., 167, 174
Nelsen, J. M., 125, 126, 135, 215, 222
Nemeth, E., 244, 251
Nickerson, M., 166, 172, 173
Noback, C. R., 62
Nyswander, M. E., 201, 219

Oates, J. A., 173
Olds, J., 70, 79
Olson, L., 79
Oswald, J., 141, 148

Parker, J. B., Jr., 229, 234, 252
Penfield, W., 71, 72, 79, 176, 178, 183, 184
Penry, J. K., 179, 180, 184
Pescor, F. T., 191, 222
Pinsky, R. H., 34, 35, 44
Pitts, F. N. Jr., 251
Podosin, R. L., 230, 251
Poslun, D., 91, 102
Prien, R. F., 100, 102
Prinzmetal, M., 164, 174
Putnam, T. J., 180, 184

Randall, L. O., 113, 115
Rich, E., 214, 215, 222
Richie, J. M., 152, 163, 216, 221
Roberts, R. H., 224, 250
Robins, L. N., 192, 197, 198, 221
Robinson, E., 249
Rodriguez, A., 250
Rosenfeld, E., 193, 195, 219
Rossi, A. M., 216, 221
Rosvold, H. E., 88, 102, 237, 251
Roth, R. H., 77, 79
Roth, W. T., 215, 221
Rothschild, G. H., 234, 237, 238, 239, 249
Routtenberg, A., 5, 21
Rowe, J. S., 243, 251

Sachdev, K., 229, 234, 251
Safer, D. V., 246, 251
Sarason, I., 102, 251
Satterfield, J. H., 230, 234, 251
Sauerhoff, M. W., 232, 251
Schallek, W., 115
Schiele, B. C., 43, 44
Schildkraut, J., 108, 115
Schindel, L. E., 32, 36, 44
Schmidt, C. F., 130, 135, 164
Schmidt, R. P., 184

Schneider, N. G., 15, 21
Schuster, C. R., 132, 135, 191, 220
Scott, W., 23
Seevers, M. H., 132, 135
Seifter, J., 113, 115
Sem-Jacobsen, C. W., 70, 79, 127, 135
Sertürner, 118
Shader, R. I., 9, 10, 11, 12, 21, 88, 106, 111, 115
Shakespeare, W., 153
Shapiro, A. K., 23, 44
Shapiro, B. J., 221
Sharpe, L., 238, 249
Sharpless, S. K., 139, 140, 148
Shaw, E. N., 78, 80
Shuster, L., 132, 135
Shwartz, L., 249
Sidman, M., 63, 80
Sidman, R. L., 63, 80
Silbergeld, E. K., 232, 251
Silverman, M., 159, 162, 163
Sleator, E. K., 237, 245, 251
Smith, G. M., 167, 174
Snyder, S. H., 96, 102, 169, 170, 174, 211, 221
Solliday, N. H., 221
Solomons, G., 231, 250
Speigel, J. P., 139, 147
Sprague, R. L., 234, 237, 238, 245, 251
Spulak, F., 220
Stevens, J. R., 229, 230, 231, 234, 251
Stewart, M. A., 227, 244, 245, 251
Stowe, F. R., Jr., 168, 174
Sulkowski, A., 214, 215, 222
Sullivan, J. P., 235, 251
Swan, K., 112, 115
Swazey, J., 86, 102
Sykes, D. H., 237, 251, 252

Tagiuri, R., 147
Tashkin, D. P., 211, 214, 221
Tecce, J. J., 94, 102, 141, 148
Tenhunen, T., 250
Teitelbaum, P., 69, 80
Thompson, J. L. G., 219
Thompson, R. F., 63, 67, 69, 74, 80
Tinklenberg, J. R., 221
Torkildsen, A., 70, 79, 127, 135

Ungerstedt, U., 79
Uridil, J. E., 47, 62

Vachon, L., 211, 214, 215, 221, 222
Valenstein, E. S., 70, 80, 125, 135
Valle, J. R., 210, 222
Van Orden, L. S., 116
Vates, T. S., 144, 148

AUTHOR INDEX

Vaughan, E., 69, 80
Voltaire, 23
von Beyer, A., 138
von Felsinger, J. M., 35, 36, 44
von Neumann, A., 245, 251

Walgren, H., 152, 154, 163
Wallace, J. E., 219
Ward, P. M., 190, 222
Way, E. L., 132, 136
Weeks, J. R., 132, 136
Wegelius, B., 250
Weidley, E., 90, 101
Weil, A. T., 215, 222
Weiss, B., 113, 115, 123, 136, 167, 174
Weiss, G., 237, 244, 251, 252
Wender, P. H., 224, 227, 232, 233, 252
Werry, J. S., 224, 234, 238, 244, 252
West, L. J., 215, 218, 222
West, T. C., 111, 115
Whitaker, C. A., 221
Whitebread II, C. H., 211, 213, 219

Wikler, A., 124, 133, 135, 136, 143, 147, 148, 163, 186, 191, 222, 229, 230, 231, 234, 252
Wilkens, R. W., 83, 102
Williams, M. J., 219
Windholm, O., 250
Winek, C. L., 258
Witter, C., 246, 247, 252
Wolf, S., 33, 34, 35, 36, 42, 44
Woodbury, D. M., 21, 184
Woods, L. A., 132, 135
Wooley, D. W., 78, 80
Woolley, B., 258
Wurmser, L., 194, 195, 222

Yamamura, H. I., 102, 174
Young, J. H., 24, 44

Zbinden, G., 114, 115
Zeller, E. A., 104, 116
Zimmerman, F. T., 239, 252
Zinberg, N. E., 215, 222

SUBJECT INDEX

Acetophenazine, 88
Acetylcholine (ACh), 47, 49, 56
  in central nervous system, 74-75
  in somatic nervous system, 52
Acetylcholinesterase (AChE), 54
ACTH, adrenocorticotropic hormone, 97
Action potential, 54
Addiction see Drug addiction
Adipsia, 69
Adrenal gland, 48-49, 53
Adrenal medulla, 48, 59-60
Adrenalin®, see Epinephrine
Adrenaline, see Epinephrine
Adrenergic blocking agents, 61-62
Adrenergic drugs, 59
Adrenergic nerves, 50
Adrenergic receptors, 56
Adrenergic sweating, 49
Adrenocorticotropic hormone (ACTH), 97
Affinity, 7
Agonist, 7
Akathesia, 97
Akinesia, 97
Alcohol, 12
  absorption, metabolism, excretion, 150
  automobile accidents, 152
  on behavior, 152
  blood levels in intoxication, 151
  butyl, 162
  on cardiovascular system, 152-153
  central nervous system effects, 151-152
  chemistry, 150
  in depression, 103
  hangover, 154-155
  history, 148-149
  liver, effects in, 153
  with methaqualone, 146
  methyl, 163
  with monoamine oxidase inhibitors, 105
  narcotic comparison, 185
  physical dependence, 155-156
  proof scale, 161-162
  on sexual behavior, 153-154
  tolerance to, 155
  wood, 162
Alcoholic beverages, 158-162
  chemical constituents, 150, 162
Alcoholism, 156-158
Aliphatic phenothiazines, 86-87
Alkaloids, 57
Allergic responses, 13-14
Alpha adrenergic blocking agents, 56, 61
Alpha receptors, 56, 60
  stimulation of, 56
Amanita muscaria, 57, 208
Amitriptyline, 107
  chemistry, 105-106
Amobarbital, 139
Amphetamine, 60
Amphetamine abuse, 171-172
Amphetamine hallucinations, 171
Amphetamine psychosis, 170-171
Amphetamine use, legal issues, 172
Amphetamines, absorption, fate, excretion, 165
  abuse in MBD children, 244-245
  in animal model of MBD, 233
  on appetite, 167-168
  athletic performance, 167
  on attention in MBD, 237
  autonomic effects, 165-166
  on behavior in MBD, 236
  biochemical effects, 169
  cardiovascular effects, 170
  central nervous system effects, 166-169
  chemistry, 164-165
  on classroom behavior, 241-242
  in depression, 103
  on EEG, 169
  on EEG in MBD, 236
  in epilepsy, 179
  history, 164
  lethal dose, 170
  in MBD, 224, 226, 234, 242-243
  on performance, 166-167
  on photo-Metrazol test in MBD, 232
  on physical growth in MBD children, 246
  on reticular formation, 92

265

SUBJECT INDEX

in schizophrenics, 171
on school performance in MBD, 235
on skeletel muscles, 166
therapeutic use, 172
tolerance, physical dependence, 172
toxicity, 170
Ampliactil®, see Chlorpromazine
Amygdala, see Limbic system
emotion, 69
stimulation, electrical, 70
Amygdalectomy, 69-70
Amytal®, 139
Analgesia, amphetamine, 168
morphine, 121-123
Anaphylactic reactions, 13
Angioneurotic edema, definition, 14
Antagonism, drug, 16
Antagonist, definition, 7
Antiadrenergic drugs, 50
Antianxiety drugs, listing, dosage, 111
Anticholinergic activity, phenothiazines, 96
Anticholinergic drugs, 50
Anticholinergic side effects, 59
Anticonvulsants, see Antiepileptic drugs
Antidepressant drugs, listing, dosage, 106
Antiemetic effects, chlorpromazine, 95
Antiepiletic drugs, indications, 180
in pregnancy, 182-183
side effects, 179-183
Antihelminthic, 57
Antihistamines, 16, 147
Antipsychotic drugs, listing, dosage, 88
Antipyretic, 15
Aphagia, 69
Apothecary terminology, 19
Areca catechu (betel nut), 57
Arecoline, 57
Ascending reticular formation (ARAS), see Reticular formation
Aspirin, 15
Association cortex, 65
Asthma, 60
Atropa belladonna, nightshade, 58
Atropine, 54-55, 58-59
as a deleriant, 203
reticular formation, 92
Atropine poisoning, 59
Attention, chlorpromazine effects, 88-89
in MBD, 227, 237-238
reticular formation, 66
Autonomic nervous system, 45-62
anatomy and physiology, 48-49, 50-51
blocking agents, 55
stimulation effects, 52-53
Aventyl®, see Nortriptyline
Averaged evoked response (AER), 73-74
amphetamine, 168

Axon, 46, 54
Ayahuasca, 209
Azacyclonal, 111

Barbital, 138-139
Barbiturates, 138-145
absorption, 139-140
anticonvulsant effects, 142
autonomic effects, 142
on CAR, 91
central nervous system effects, 140-142
chemistry, 138
chlorpromazine comparison, 87
EEG effects, 141
in epilepsy, 180
history, 138
in MBD, 233
meprobamate comparison, 111
metabolism and excretion, 140
in nursing mother, 140
physical dependence, 144-145
in pregnancy, 140
reticular formation, 92, 141-142
on sleep, 141
tolerance, 144
Barbituric acid, 138
Basal ganglia, anatomy, 65
meprobamate on, 111-112
Beer, 158-159
Belladonna alkaloids, 59
Benactyzine, 111
Benzedrine®, see Amphetamine
Benzodiazepines, 111, 113-114
behavioral effects, 113
central nervous system effects, 113
clinical use, 114
in epilepsy, 183
in MBD, 225
side effects and toxicity, 113-114
suicide, 114
Benzotropine, 96
Beta adrenergic blocking agents, 56, 61
Beta receptors, 56, 60
stimulation, 56
Betel nut, Areca catechu, 57
Bethanecol, 57
Bhang, 210
Biotransformation, 6
Blood brain barrier, 5
Blood dyscrasias, definition, 12
phenothiazines, 98
Blood vessels, autonomic effects on, 53
Brain, anatomy, 63-66
human, 64
rat, 64
Brain stem, 66
Brandy, 160

SUBJECT INDEX

Bromides, 146
  in epilepsy, 179
Bruxism, amphetamine, 171
Bufotenine, 208
Butabarbital, 139
Butisol®, 139
Butyrophenones, 81, 99

Caapi, 208
Caffeine, use in epilepsy, 179
Cannabis, see Marihuana
  effects, long term, 214
  pharmacology, 213-216
  physiological effects, 213-214
Carbachol, 57
Cardiac muscle cells, 49
Carphenazine, 88
Catecholamines, 59-60
  amphetamine, 169
  in central nervous system, 76
  chlorpromazine, 96
Caudate, 65
Caudate nucleus, phenothiazines, 95
Celontin®, see Methsuximide
Cerebral hemispheres, lesions, 65
Cerebellum, 66
Cerveau isolé, 67
Chemical warfare agents, 57
Chemoreceptor trigger zone, 95
Chloral hydrate, 139, 146
Chlordiazepoxide, 111, 113
  absorption, fate, excretion, 113
  chemistry, 112
  in MBD, 225
Chlorpromazine, absorption, 97
  amygdala, 94
  antihistiminic effects, 95
  autonomic effects, 95
  basal ganglia, 95
  behavioral effects, man, 87-88
  biochemical mechanisms, 96
  body temperature, 94
  brain stimulation, inverted "U" model, 93
  cardiovascular effects, 95
  endocrine system, 96
  history, 86
  hypothalamus, 93
  imipramine comparison, 108
  inverted "U," 93
  limbic system, 94
  local anesthetic effect, 96
  in MBD, 225, 244
  metabolism, 97
  ovulation, 96
  pituitary gland, 96
  reticular formation, 92, 94
  side effects, toxicity, 97-99

  skeletel muscles, 96
  testicular weight, 96
  tolerance, 34
Chlorprothixene, 88, 99
Cholinergic blocking agents, 58-59
Cholinergic drugs, 56-57
Cholinergic fibers, 54
Cholenergic nerves, 50
Cholinergic neuron, in CNS, 75
Cholinergic receptors, 54
Cholinesterase inhibitors, 56-57
Coca-Cola, 216
Cocaine, Freud's use, 216
  pharmacology, 216-217
  snuff, 217
Codeine, 117, 119, 128, 133
  chemistry, 120
Cogentin®, see Benztropine
Cognition, effects of chlorpromazine and pentobarbital, 89
Cohoba snuff, 208
Colliculi, 66
Compazine®, 88
Conditioned avoidance response (CAR), effects of drugs, 89-91
Conditioning, placebo, 39-40
Congener, 162
Continuous Performance Test (CPT), effects of chlorpromazine, 88-90
  in MBD, 237-238
Convulsions, barbiturate withdrawal, 144-145
  methaqualone, 145
  phenothiazines, 93-94
Convulsive disorders, see Epilepsy
Corpus striatum, phenothiazines, 95
Cortex, 66
  dopamine, 96
Craniosacral system, 49
Curare, 54
Cylert®, magnesium pemoline, 225

Dagga, 210
d-amphetamine, see Amphetamine
Datura stramonium, jimson weed, 58
Decamethonium, 55
Delerium tremens, 156
Demerol®, see Meperidine
Dendrites, 46
Denervation supersensitivity, 98
Dependence, physical, 16-17
  alcohol, 155-156
  amphetamines, 172
  barbiturates, 144-145
  chloral hydrate, 146
  chlordiazepoxide, 114
  meprobamate, 112

SUBJECT INDEX

narcotic analgesics, 129-132
Dependence, psychological, 17, 187
Desipramine, 106-107
Desmethylimipramine, *see* Imipramine
Desoxybarbiturate, 180
DET (diethyltryptamine), 209
Dextro-amphetamine, *see* Amphetamine
Diacetylmorphine, *see* Heroin
Diazepam, 111
  absorption, fate, excretion, 113
  chemistry, 112
  in epilepsy, 178
  in MBD, 225
Diencephalon, 64-65
  drive state, 69
  lesions, 66
Digestive system, autonomic effects on, 52
Digit Symbol Substitution Test (DSST), 89
Dihydromorphine, *see* Hydromorphine
Dihydroxyphenylalanine, (L-dopa), 77-78
Dihydroxyphenylethylamine, *see* Dopamine
Dilaudid®, *see* Hydromorphine
Dilantin®, *see* Diphenylhydantoin
Diphenylhydantoin, 178, 180
  absorption, 181
  combination with other drugs, 181
  hallucinations, 181
  in MBD, 237
  in pregnancy, 183
  toxic effects, 181
Distribution, drug, 5-6
DMT (*n,n*-dimethyltryptamine), 209
Dolophine®, *see* Methadone
DOM (STP), 209
Dopamine, 59
  amphetamine, 169
  brain sites, 76-78
  chemical structure, 60
  chlorpromazine, 96
  extrapyramidal system, 95
Doriden®, *see* Glutethimide
Dose-effect, definition, 8-12
  placebo, 33-34
Dose-response, *see* Dose effect
Double-blind, 41
DPH, *see* Diphenylhydantoin
Drug absorption, 2-5
Drug abuse, *see* Drug addiction
  amphetamines, 171-172
  hypnotics, 147
  in MBD, 246
  methaqualone, 146
Drug addiction, as adaptive, 194-195
  in adolescents, 192-193
  attitudes toward, 186-187
  causes, 190-197
  conditioning model, 191

definitions, 185-187
epidemic areas, characteristics, 196
psychological factors, 190-195
relapse, 191
social factors, 195-199
treatment methods, 199-203
violence, 203
Drug addicts, personality, 192-193
  pre drug behavior, 193-194, 197
  psychopathology, 194-195
  Rorschach test in, 193
Drug administration, methods, 3-5
Drug dependence, *see* Drug addiction
Drug effects, age of subject, 15
  allergic responses, 13-14
  cumulative action, 17-18
Drug interaction, 15
  additive effects, 16
  antagonism-chemical, 16
  antagonism-pharmacological, 16
  antagonism-physiological, 16
  potentiation, 16
  synergism, 16
Drug preparations, 20
d-tubocurarine, 55
Dyskinesia, 97
Dystonia, 97

Effective dose 50 (ED50), 11
Effector cells, 49
Efficacy, 7
Elavil®, *see* Amitriptyline
Electroencephalogram (EEG), alpha, blocking, 74
  abnormal, 72
  alcohol, 151
  amphetamine, 168, 172
  barbiturates, 141
  benzodiazepines, 113
  chlorpromazine, CPT, 93-94
  cholinesterase inhibitors, 58
  in epilepsy, 72, 74, 175, 177-178, 184
  in MBD, 229-231, 234, 236
  meprobamate, 111
  morphine, 125-126
  pentobarbital, CPT, 93-94
  petit mal epilepsy, 72-74
  reserpine, 84
  reticular formation lesions, 67
  reticular stimulation, 66
  sleep, 71
  spike and wave, 72
  spindling, 74
  tricyclic antidepressants, 108
Electroshock therapy (EST, ECT), 110
Encéphale isolé, 68, 168
Endocrine glands, hypothalmus, 69

SUBJECT INDEX 269

Ephedrine, 60, 164
  amphetamine use, 172
  clinical use, 61
Epilepsy, EEG, 74, 175, 177-178, 184
  etiology and drug therapy, 183-184
  history, 175-176
  incidence, 176
  pharmacotherapy, 179
  seizure classification, 176-178
Epinephrine, 48, 50, 59
  in cardiac arrest, 60
  chemistry, 60
  effects of, 60-61
  gastrointestinal tract, 61
  with local anesthetics, 60
  sweat glands, 49
Equanil®, see Meprobamate
Equipotent doses, 11
Ergonovine maleate, 61
Ergot, 206
Ergot alkaloids, 61
Ergotamine tartrate, 61
Erythroxylon coca, 216
Ethanol, see Alcohol
Ethics in placebo use, 41
Ethosuximide, 178, 180
  toxic effects, 182
Ethotoin, 180-181
Ethyl alcohol, see Alcohol
Evipal®, see Hexobarbital
Excretion, drug, 5-6
Exocrine gland, 54
Extrapyramidal effects, haloperidol, 99
  phenothiazines, 97-98
Extrapyramidal system, anatomy, 65
Eye, autonomic effects on, 52

Fantastica, see Hallucinogens
Fluphenazine, 88
Fly agaric mushroom, 208
Frenquel®, see Azacyclonol
Fusel oils, 159, 162

GABA (gamma-aminobutyric acid), 78
Ganglion, 46
Ganglionic blocking actions, 58
Gemonil®, see Metharbital
Generic drugs, definition, 20
Genital system, autonomic effects, 50
Gin, 161
Glaucoma, 57
Glandular secretary cells, 49
Globus pallidus, 65
Glutethimide, 139, 146

Hague Convention, 189
Haldol®, see Haloperidol

Half-life, 8, 18
Hallucinogens, 203-209
Haloperidol, 88, 99
Hangover, alcohol, 154-155
  barbiturates, 144
Harmine, 208
Harrison Narcotic Act, 189
Hashish, 210-211
Heart, autonomic effects on, 53
Hemeralopia, in oxazolidine therapy, 182
Henbane (Hyoscyamus niger), 58
Heroin, see Narcotic drugs
  abuse, 192
  chemistry, 120
Hexamethonium, 54
Hexobarbital, 139
Hiccups, chlorpromazine, 96
Hindbrain, 66
Hippocampus, 66-70
Histamine, 16
Humulus lupulus (hops), 159
Hydantoinates, 180
Hydromorphine, 119
5-Hydroxyindoleacetic acid, 85
5-Hydroxytryptamine (5-HT), see Serotonin
Hyoscyamus niger (henbane), 57
Hyperkinetic child, see Minimal brain dysfunction (MBD)
Hyperphagia, 69
Hypersensitivity, drug, 12-13
Hypnosis, placebo, 40
Hypnotic, definition, 137
Hypnotics, listing, dosage, 139
  over-the-counter, 147
Hyposensitivity, 12-13
Hypothalamus, 66
  amphetamine, 167
  chlorpromazine, 94
  consummatory behavior, 69
  sexual behavior, 69
  intracranial stimulation, 70
  lesions, 69

Idiosyncratic responses to drugs, 13
Imipramine, 108-109
  chemistry, 105-106
  clinical use, 109
  in MBD, 226
Inderal®, see Propranolol
Indian hemp, see Marihuana
Individual differences in response to drugs, 12-13
Inotropic effect, 56
Insecticides, 57
Intracranial self-stimulation, 70
  human, 70
  morphine, 125, 127

Intrinsic activity, 7
Ipomoea violacea, 209
Iproniazid, see MAO inhibitors
Isocarboxazid, 106
Isoniazid, 103
Isopropylarterenol, 61
Isopropylnorepinephrine, 60-61
Isoproterenol, 60
  chemical use, 61

Jaundice, in phenothiazine therapy, 98
Jimson weed (Datura stramonium), 58

Kif, 210

Lacrimal gland, 52
1-amphetamine, see Amphetamine
Largactil®, see Chlorpromazine
Laudanum, 118
Law and drug use, 190, 212-213
L-dopa (dihydroxyphenylalanine), 77-78, 96
Lemniscal pathways, see Spinothalamic tract, 66-67
Lethal dose 50 (LD50), 9
Levarterenol, 60-61
1-hyoscine, 58
1-hyoscyamine, 58
Librium®, see Chlordiazepoxide
Limbic system, 66
  dopamine, 96
  meprobamate, 111
  morphine, 124
Liqueurs, 160
Lithium, lithium carbonate, 81, 88
  history, 99
  pharmacology, 100
LSD, see Lysergic acid diethylamide
Luminal®, see Phenobarbital
Lungs, autonomic effects on, 52
Lysergic acid diethylamide (LSD), 61, 204-209
  autonomic effects, 207
  behavioral effects, 207-208
  chemistry, 206
  in MBD, 245
  physiological effects, 206-207
  reticular formation, 92
  serotonin, 78
  tolerance, 207

Magnesium pemoline, 225
Ma huang, 164
Mania, lithium, 99-100
MAO, see Monoamine oxidase
Maraguana, see Marihuana
Marihuana, 210-216
  alcohol comparison, 218
  behavioral effects, 214-216
  Federal Bureau of Narcotics, 212
  history of use, 211-213
  law and, 212-213
  legalization, 218
  Mayor's Committee, 213
  in MBD, 245
  preparation, 210
  social attitudes toward, 210
Marplan®, see Isocarboxazid
Marsilid®, see Iproniazid
Marywana, see Marihuana
MBD, see Minimal brain dysfunction
Mebaral®, see Mephobarbital
Medial forebrain bundle (MFB), 70
  morphine, 125-127
Median effective dose (ED50), 11
Median lethal dose (LD50), 9
Medulla oblongata, 66
Megaphan®, see Chlorpromazine
Mellaril®, see Thioridazine
Mental hospitals, occupancy, 81-82
Mental illness, neural transmission, 75
Meperidine, 119, 128, 132
Mephenesin, 34
Mephenytoin, 180-181
Mephobarbital, use in epilepsy, 180
Meprobamate, 110-113
  absorption, fate, excretion, 112
  behavioral effects, 111
  central nervous system effects, 111-112
  chemistry, 112
  clinical use, 112-113
  EEG effects, 111
  seizures, 111
  side effects, toxicity, 112
Me-rosh, 118
Mesantoin®, see Mephenytoin
Mescaline, 204-205
Mesencephalic reticular formation, see Reticular formation
Mesencephalon, 64-66
Metabolism, 5-6
Metencephalon, 64-66
Methacholine, 57
Methadone, 119, 133
  chemistry, 120
Methadone maintenance, 201-202
Methamphetamine, see Amphetamine
Methanol, see Alcohol
Methapyrilene, 147
Methaqualone, 139, 145-146
Metharbital, use in epilepsy, 180
Methsuximide, 178, 180
Methylatropine, 58-59
Methylphenidate in animal model of MBD, 232

SUBJECT INDEX

Methylphenidate in MBD, 224, 226, 242-243
  attention, effects on, 237
  follow-up, long term, 243-246
  on motor activity, 238
  on physical development, 241
Methyprylon, 139, 146
Migraine, 61
Miltonin®, see Phensuximide
Miltown®, see Meprobamate
Minimal brain dysfunction, adolescence, 243-244
  animal model, 233
  antidepressant drugs, 226
  attention, 227, 237-238
  barbiturates, 233
  behavioral characterestics, 226-228, 236
  benzodiazepines, 225
  biochemical abnormality, 233
  central nervous system changes, 231
  chlordiazepoxide, 225
  chlorpromazine, 225, 244
  clinical history, 227
  Continuous Performance Test, 237-238
  diazepam, 225
  diphenylhydantoin, 237
  drug abuse, 246
  drug treatment in MBD, history, 235
  dyslexia, 227-228
  EEG, 229-231, 234, 236
  experimental model, 232
  follow-up, 243-246
  galvanic skin response, 234
  genetic factors, 232-233
  House Privacy Subcommittee hearings, 246
  hyperarousal, 234
  hyperkinesis, definition, 226
  hypoarousal, 234
  imipramine, 226
  impulse control, 228, 238
  intelligence, 227, 231, 234, 239
  LSD, 245
  magnesium pemoline, 225
  marihuana use, 245
  motor activity, 238
  motor skills, 239
  neurological signs, 228-229
  organic brain damage, 231-232
  organicity, predictor of drug, response, 237
  oxazepam, 225
  pentylenetetrazol, 231-232
  phenothiazines, 225
  photo-metrazol test, 231, 234
  physical development, drug therapy, 246
  political issues, 246-249
  Porteus Maze, 238-239
  pregnancy, complications, 232
  prognosis, 243-246
  school behavior, 240
  school performance, 227, 229, 239-242
  sleep disorders, 227
  social class, 240, 242
  social factors, 248
  soft neurological signs, 228-230, 237
  thioridazine, 225, 238
  WISC, 230, 238
MMPI, addicts, 190
Monoamine oxidase (MAO), 77-78, 169
Monoamine oxidase inhibitors, 104-107
  absorption, fate, excretion, 106
  central stimulation, 107
  chemistry, 104-105
  clinical use, 110
  hypotension, 107
  interaction with food, 107
  interaction with other drugs, 105
  jaundice, 107
  nonhydrazine, 107
  toxicity, side effects, 106-107
Morning glory seeds, 209
Morphine, 117, 119
  analgesia, 121-125
  analgesia and anxiety, 122, 124
  effects on CAR, 91
  central nervous system effects, 121-128
  chemistry, 120
  EEG, 125-126
  effects on pupil, 127-128
  effects on respiration, 128
  history, 118-119
  medial forebrain bundle, 125-127
  nausea, 121
  reinforcer in man, 143
  subjective effects, 121
Motor endplate, 54-55
Motor roots, 49
Muscarine, 54, 57
Muscarinic actions, 58
Muscarinic drugs, 56
Muscarinic receptors, 54-56
Muscle, cardiac, 54
  involuntary, 49
  pilomotor, 49, 53
  smooth, 49, 54
Myasthenia gravis, 57
Aydriasis, 59
Myelencephalon, 64-66
Myelin sheath, 46
Myristicin, 209
Mysoline®, see Primidone

Nalline®, see Nalorphine

Nalorphine, 119, 133-134
 chemistry, 120
Naloxone, 119, 134, 202
Naltrexone, 119
Narcan®, see Naloxone
Narcotic analgesics, 119
 absorption, distribution and excretion, 120-121
 abuse, 186-203
 autonomic effects, 129
 gastrointestinal tract, 129
 histamine release, 129
 history of use, 187-190
 overdose, signs and symptoms, 128
 tolerance and physical dependence, 129-132
Narcotic antagonist, 133-134
 in chloral hydrate overdose, 146
 treatment model, 191-192, 203
Narcotic "high," 125, 127, 198-199
Nardil®, see Phenelzine
Navane®, see Thiothixene
Nembutal®, see Pentobarbital
Neocortex, 65
Neostigmine, 57
Nerve cell, 45
Nerve cell body, 46
Nerves, adrenergic, 50
 cholinergic, 50
 cranial, 49, 66-68
 lumbar spinal, 49
 thoracic spinal, 49
 vagus, 47-48, 68
Neural transmission, chemical, 47
 electrical, 47
Neurohumors, 53, 75
Neuromuscular blocking agents, 58
Neuromuscular junction, 57
Neuromuscular system, 45
Neuron, 45
 spinal motor, 46
Neurotransmitters, termination of action, 54
Neurotransmitters in CNS, chemistry, 76
 classification, 75-78
Nialamide, 105-106
Niamid®, see Nialamide
Nicotine, 54
Nicotinic receptors, 54-56
Nightshade (Atropa belladonna), 58
Nigrostriatal dopamine pathway, 94
Noludar®, see Methyprylon
Nonmedical use of drugs, definition, see Drug abuse; Drug addiction
Nonproprietary drug, definition, 20
Nonspecific factors in drug effects, 15, 36-38
 in abuse, 218
Noradrenaline, see Norepinephrine
Norepinephrine (NE), 47, 49
 amphetamine, 169
 chemical structure, 60
 chlorpromazine, 96
 clinical use, pharmacological actions, 61
 in CNS, 74, 76-77
Norpramine®, see Desipramine
Nortriptyline, 106, 108
Nutmeg, 209

Olfactory bulb, 64, 65
Ololiuhqui, 209
Ophthalmological preparation, pilocarpine, 57
Opiates, see Narcotic analgesics
Opium, history of medical use, 117-118
 nonmedical use, 187-188
 preparation, 117
Opium smoking, Chinese, 188-189
Opium poppy, 118
Opium war, 189
Organo-phosphate anticholinesterases, 57
Orthostatic hypotension, 34, 95
Oxazepam, 111, 113
 in MBD, 225
Oxazolidinediones, 180
 toxic effects, 182

Pain and analgesia, 121-123
 methods of study, 122-123
 placebo, 35
Papaver somniferum, 118
Paradione®, see Paramethadione
Paradoxical sleep, see REM sleep
Paragoric, 118
Paraldehyde, 146
Paramethadione, 180, 182
 in pregnancy, 183
Parasympathomimetic drugs, 51
Parasympatholytic effects, 59
Parasympathetic nervous system, 47
 anatomy, 51
 stress, 48
Parest®, see Methaqualone
Parkinsonism, 65
 atropine and scopolamine, 59
 chlorpromazine, 95, 97
 dopamine in, 77-78
Parkinson's disease, 94, 96
Parnate®, see Tranylcypromine
Peganone®, see Ethotoin
Penicillin, 4
Pentazocine, 119, 134
Pentobarbital, 139
 attention, 93-94
 behavioral effects, 142-143

SUBJECT INDEX

Continuous Performance Test, 93-94
  EEG, 94
  reaction time, 143
Pentothal®, see Thiopental
Pentylenetetrazol, antagonism with antiepileptic drugs, 181
  convulsive threshold after chlorpromazine, 94
  in MBD, 231-232
Peripheral nervous system, 45
  transmitter substance, 55
Permitil®, see Fluphenazine
Perphenazine, dosage, 88
Personality, addicts, 190-191
  drug response, 13
  placebo, 35
Pertofrane®, see Desipramine
Petit mal epilepsy, EEG, 72-73
Peyote, see Mescaline
pH, 2-3
Pharmacogenetics, 18
Pharmacology, definition, 1
Phenaglycodol, 111
Phenazocine, 119
Phenelzine, 105-106
Phenergan®, see Promethazine, 95
Phenobarbital, 138-139, 233
  in anxiety, 110
  in epilepsy, 142, 178-180, 183
Phenothiazine derivatives, 81, 86-99
  behavioral effects, man, 87-88
  chemistry, 87
  conditioned avoidance response, 91
  in depression, 109
  extrapyramidal effects, 86
  history, 86
  in MBD, 225
  relative toxicity, 86-87
  side effects, toxicity, 97
Phensuximide, 180
Phenytoin, see Diphenylhydantoin, 180
Physical dependence, 16-17
  alcohol, 155-156
  amphetamines, 172
  barbiturates, 144-145
  chloral hydrate, 146
  chlordiazepoxide, 114
  meprobamate, 112
  narcotic analgesics, 129-132
Physostigmine, 57
  reticular formation, 92
Picrotoxin, antagonism with, antiepleptic drugs, 181
  convulsive threshold after chlorpromazine, 95
Pilocarpine, 57
Pineal gland, and serotonin, 78

Piperidine phenothiazines, 86-87
Pituitary gland, 69
Placebo, 22-44
  cumulative effects, 33
  definition, 22
  ethics, 41
  history, 22-24
  mechanism of action, 39-40
  in pain relief, 35
  in research, 37, 41-43
Placebo and FDA, 41
Placebo reactor, 35
Pons, 66
Postural hypotension, 34
Potency, 9
Potentiation, 16
Preganglionic fiber, 54
Primidone, 178, 180, 183
Prinadol®, see Phenazocine, 119
Probit, 9
Prochlorperazine, dosage, 88
Proketazine®, see Carphenazine
Prolixin®, see Fluphenazine
Promazine, dosage, 88
Promethazine, 95
Propanediols, 111
Propranolol, 61
  clinical use, 62
Propyl alcohol, 162
Psilocin, 208
Psilocybin, 208
Psychedelics, see Hallucinogens
Psychodysleptics, see Hallucinogens
Psychological dependence, 17, 187
Psychosis, alcohol withdrawal, 156
  amphetamine, 170-171
  barbiturate withdrawal, 144
  bromides, 145
  toxic, 203
Psychotherapy, in depression, 110
  in schizophrenia, 100
Psychotomimetics, see Hallucinogens
Putamen, 65
  phenothiazines, 95
Pyramidal system, 65, 95

Quāalude®, see Methaqualone

Raphé nucleus, serotonin, 77
Rapid Eye Movement (REM), 72, 141, 146
Rauwolfia derivatives, 81
Rauwolfia serpentina, 83
Receptor, 7
REM (rapid eye movement), 72
REM sleep, effects of barbiturates, 141
  chloral hydrate, 146
Renshaw cells, 75

SUBJECT INDEX

Research, active control, 41
  double-blind, 41-43
  placebo, 37, 41-43
  standard drug, 41
Reserpine, 83-85, 104
  absorption, 85
  autonomic effects, 83-84
  biochemical effects, 84-85
  catecholamines, 84
  central nervous system effects, 84-85
  chemistry, 83
  conditioned avoidance response, 91
  dosage, 88
  EEG, 84
  endocrine system, 85
  in epilepsy, 84-85
  history, 83
  metabolism, 85
  parkinsonism, 85
  pentylenetetrazol (Metrazol®), 84
  seizure threshold, 84
  serotonin, 84-85
  sexual drive, 85
  side effects and toxicity, 85
Ritalin®, see Methylphenidate
Reticular formation, 66-69
  amphetamine, 168-169
  attention, 66
  barbiturates, 141-142
  meprobamate, 112
  morphine, 124-125
  phenothiazines, 92, 95
  sleep, 66, 68
  stimulation, 66
  transection, 67
Rivea corymbosa, 209
Rorschach, in addicts, 193
  placebo, 36
Rosh, 118
Rum, 161
"Rum fits," 156

Sacral spinal nerves, 49
Salivary gland, autonomic effects, 53
Schizophrenia, 34
  amphetamine, 171
  drug treatment, 81
  psychotherapy versus drug therapy, 100
Scopolamine, 54-55, 58
  as a deleriant, 203
Secobarbital, 139
Seconal®, see Secobarbital
Sedation, definition, 137
Septum, 66
Serax®, see Oxazepam, 111
Serotonin, (5-hydroxytryptamine, 5-HT), 78, 104-105

lysergic acid diethylamide, 78
  phenothiazines, 96
  pineal gland, 78
Serpasil®, see Reserpine
Set and expectation, 15
Sex, alcohol, 153-154
Side effects, definition, 14
  placebo, 34
Single blind, 41
Sleep, 137
  EEG, 71
  reticular formation, 68
Solacen®, see Tybamate
Somatic nervous system, 45, 58
  blocking agents, 55
Sopor®, see Methaqualone
Sparine®, see Promazine
Speedball, 217
Spinal cord, preganglionic fibers, 49
Spinothalamic tract, (lemniscal pathways), 66-67
Status epilepticus, 142, 180, 183
Stelazine®, see Trifluoperazine
STP, (2,5-dimethoxy-4-methyl-amphetamine), 209
Street drugs, labeling, 209, 253-258; see also Glossary
Stress, autonomic nervous system, 47
Structure-activity relationship, 7
Strychnine, antagonism with antiepileptic drugs, 181
  convulsive threshold after chlorpromazine, 94
Suavitil®, see Benactyzine
Substantia nigra, 95
Succinimides, 180
Sweat glands, 49, 53
Sympathetic nervous system, 47
  anatomy, 50
  stimulation, 48
  stress, 47
Sympathin, 47
Sympathomimetic drugs, 51, 59-60, 164
Sympathomimetic effects, amphetamine, 165-166
Syanon, 200
Synapse, 46
  axo-somatic, 46
  dendro-dendritic, 46
  inhibitory, 54
Synaptic cleft, 46-47, 54
Synergism, 16

Tachyphylaxis, 7, 17
  narcotic analgesics, 131
Talwin®, see Pentazocine
Taractan®, see Chlorprothixene

SUBJECT INDEX

Tardive dyskinesia, 98
Telencephalon, 64-66
Tetrahydrocannabinol (THC), 210
Thalamus, 66
THC, (delta-9-tetrahydrocannabinol), 210
Therapeutic Index, 111
Thiopental, 4, 139
Thioridazine, in depression, 109-110
   dosage, 88
   in MBD, 225, 238
Thiothixene, 88
Thioxanthene derivatives, 81, 99
Thoracolumbar system, 49
Thorazine®, see Chlorpromazine
Time-effect curve, placebo, 33
Tindal®, see Acetophenazine
Tofranil®, see Imipramine
Tolerance, behavioral, 16-17
   definition, 16-17
   LSD, 207
   placebo, 33
   theories, narcotic analgesics, 130-131
Tranquilizers, minor, 91
Tranylcypromine, 105-107
Tricyclic antidepressants, 106-109
   absorption, distribution and fate, 108
   autonomic effects, 108
   behavioral effects, 108
   central nervous system effects, 108
   EEG, 108
   MAO interaction, 109
   side effects and toxicity, 108-109
Tridione®, use in pregnancy, see Trimethadione

Trifluoperazine, 88
Trifluperidol, 99
Triflupromazine, 88
Trilafon®, see Perphenazine
Trimethadione, 178, 180-182
3, 4, 5-trimethoxyphenethylamine, see Mescaline
Tybamate, 111

Ultran®, see Phenaglycodal

Vagus nerve, 47-48, 68
Vagusstoff, 47
Valium®, see Diazepam
Vegetative nervous system, see Autonomic nervous system
Vermifuge, 57
Veronal®, see Barbital
Vesprin®, see Triflupromazine
Viet Nam, drug use, 192, 197-198
Vigilance, effects of chlorpromazine and pentobarbital, 89
Vodka, 161

Weights and measures-table, 19
Whiskey, 160
Wines, 159-160
Withdrawal syndrome, see Physical dependence

Yage, 208

Zarontin®, see Ethosuximide